PRAISE FOR

eating for pregnancy

"As nutrition specialists we often see postpregnancy patients and wish they had received good nutrition counseling prior to and during pregnancy. This guide should be on the bookshelves of all obstetricians as they counsel their pregnant patients. It is a must-have for all pregnant patients who want to have a healthy peripartum experience."

—CAROLINE M. APOVIAN, MD, FACP, FACN

"A food-friendly guide to pregnancy and beyond. . . . The more than 150 recipes in the book are presented in categories that fit with contemporary lifestyles. . . . It's a realistic approach at a time when more and more meals take place outside the home."

—*The Washington Post*

"As an obstetrician this is a welcome resource for our patients. We often wish we had more time during prenatal visits to review healthy eating and recommendations for adequate nutrition. This book is a welcome addition!"

—DIANE SNYDER, MD, OBGYN

"*Eating for Pregnancy* has features that distinguish it from other books in the pregnancy category, including a family approach to eating and cooking during pregnancy, diabetic exchanges, an extensive chapter on vegetarian cooking, and tips for coping with morning sickness. It's a book for motherhood in the 21st century."

—*Pittsburgh Tribune-Review*

"This book is full of information that is vital to maintaining a healthy pregnancy. The recipes are creatively delicious and make eating nutritiously an exciting and achievable goal."

—DIANE FORLEY, *chef-owner of Verbena Restaurant, New York City*

"From an overview on nutrition and pregnancy through the recipes . . . this book is a must-have. The recipes reflect an appealing fresh and light approach."

—*ForeWord Magazine*

"Delicately balancing optimum and unnecessary weight gain . . . simple yet flavorful dishes . . . an overwhelming amount of information."

—*Publishers Weekly*

"Whether you want to get pregnant, are pregnant or adopting a baby, I encourage you to buy this book because it is full of simple, delicious recipes and lots of sound advice on how to eat better and enjoy a healthier lifestyle."

—CINDY PAWLCYN, *chef and restaurateur*

"Every pregnant woman knows that what she eats impacts the health of her baby. But coming up with healthy menus day in and day out can be as daunting as delivery itself. For well-meaning moms everywhere, the simple solution is *Eating for Pregnancy*. . . . If your idea of the perfect meal is equal parts easy, delicious and nutritious, this book is for you."

—*New Parents Magazine*

"Finally . . . a cookbook for mothers-to-be. . . . A new cookbook that offers nutrition guidelines for moms-to-be and includes recipes the entire family will enjoy."

—*Saginaw News*

"Everything in the book is intended to be not only easy to prepare, but also healthy and appealing to every member of the family."

—*Monadnock Ledger*

"A must for mothers-to-be."

—*Cape Gazette*

"A compact and informative nutrition guide with recipes that are easy and clear-cut. It will see you through nine months and beyond."

—MARIA THERESA GUEVARA-HENSEN, MD, OBGYN

ABOUT THE AUTHORS

CATHERINE JONES, an award-winning cookbook author and freelance food, health, and travel writer, is a graduate of Connecticut College and La Varenne Culinary School in France. She travels the world with her husband, a Foreign Service Officer, and their two children, ages nine and twelve.

ROSE ANN HUDSON, RD, LD, a perinatal nutritionist and registered dietician, served on the staff of Columbia Hospital for Women in Washington, D.C., for thirteen years. She has been on the staff of Inova Fairfax Hospital in Fairfax, Virginia, for twelve years, and has a private practice. She is the mother of two daughters, ages seventeen and twenty.

CONTRIBUTORS

ELAINE B. TRUJILLO, MS, RD, a national leader in nutrition, works at the National Cancer Institute, National Institutes of Health (NIH). She designed the original Stay Balanced Diet for the critically acclaimed book she co-authored with Catherine Jones, *Eating for Lower Cholesterol: A Balanced Approach to Heart Health with Recipes Everyone Will Love.*

SHOSHANA S. BENNETT, PHD, Founder and Director of Postpartum Assistance for Mothers, shares her knowledge on nutrition and exercise to combat postpartum depression. She is the author of *Beyond the Blues*, *Postpartum Depression for Dummies*, and *Pregnant on Prozac.*

LINDA WADE, PHD, a clinical psychologist in private practice, offers answers to frequently asked questions about weight-loss issues. Her approach is based primarily on the Internal Family Systems Model.

VICTOR PALO, a personal trainer for professional athletes, created the exercise menu for weight loss and toning specifically for women.

OTHER BOOKS BY CATHERINE JONES

Eating for Lower Cholesterol: A Balanced Approach to Heart Health with Recipes Everyone Will Love

A Year of Russian Feasts

catherine jones WITH rose ann hudson, RD, LD

eating for
pregnancy

~

**THE ESSENTIAL NUTRITION
GUIDE AND COOKBOOK
FOR TODAY'S MOTHERS-TO-BE**

2nd Edition

Completely Revised and Expanded

Da Capo

LIFE
LONG

A Member of the Perseus Books Group

Set in 10.5 point Fairfield by the Perseus Books Group

Cataloging-in-Publication data for this book is available from the Library of Congress.

First Da Capo Press edition 2009
ISBN-13: 978-0-7382-1352-1

Published by Da Capo Press
A Member of the Perseus Books Group
www.dacapopress.com

Note: The information in this book is true and complete to the best of our knowledge. This book is intended only as an informative guide for those wishing to know more about health issues. In no way is this book intended to replace, countermand, or conflict with the advice given to you by your own physician. The ultimate decision concerning care should be made between you and your doctor. We strongly recommend you follow his or her advice. Information in this book is general and is offered with no guarantees on the part of the authors or Da Capo Press. The authors and publisher disclaim all liability in connection with the use of this book. The names and identifying details of people associated with events described in this book have been changed. Any similarity to actual persons is coincidental.

Da Capo Press books are available at special discounts for bulk purchases in the U.S. by corporations, institutions, and other organizations. For more information, please contact the Special Markets Department at the Perseus Books Group, 2300 Chestnut Street, Suite 200, Philadelphia, PA, 19103, or call (800) 810-4145, ext. 5000, or e-mail special.markets@perseusbooks.com.

10 9 8 7 6 5 4 3 2

for all mothers-to-be
and their families

CONTENTS

How to Buy and Cook Fish and Shellfish ▪ FAQs about Mercury in Fish and Shellfish ▪ Why Choose Wild Salmon Over Farm-Raised? Spaghetti with Meat Sauce v Best-Ever American Meat Loaf ▪ Flank Steak with Salsa Verde ▪ Quick and Easy Chicken Curry ▪ Chicken or Veal Cutlets with Mushroom-Caper Sauce ▪ Mary Mulard's Baked Chicken ▪ Marinated Grilled Chicken or Beef Fajitas ▪ Moroccan-Style Chicken Stew ▪ Chicken with Homemade Barbecue Sauce ▪ Juicy Turkey Burgers ▪ Homemade Chicken Tenders ▪ Spice-Rubbed Pork Chops ▪ Marinated Grilled or Broiled Lamb Chops ▪ Sautéed Shrimp with Pasta ▪ Shrimp and Vegetable Stir-Fry ▪ Crab Cakes with Red Bell Pepper Sauce ▪ Sautéed Salmon on a Bed of Greens with Citrus Vinaigrette ▪ Roasted Salmon with Papaya Salsa ▪ Tilapia Mediterranean-Style ▪ Shrimp with Asparagus and Red Bell Peppers ▪ Grilled Arctic Char with Artichoke-Green Olive Tapenade ▪ Sautéed Halibut with Garlic-Herb Butter ▪ Canned Wild Salmon Patties with Dill-Yogurt Sauce ▪ Marinated Grilled Chicken with Cilantro Dipping Sauce ▪ Beef with Broccoli

Artificial Sweeteners during Pregnancy ▪ Bed Rest ▪ Leg Cramps: A Common Annoyance ▪ Exercise Tips: Fitness for Two ▪ Healthy Snacks for About 100 to 200 Calories ▪ Pelvic Floor (Kegel) Exercises ▪ Dairy Calcium Sources ▪ Vitamin A and C Fruit and Vegetable Sources ▪ Iron Sources

Peach and Blackberry Cobbler ▪ Apple-Blueberry Granola Crisp ▪ Strawberry Whole Wheat Shortcake ▪ No-Bake Fresh Strawberry-Raspberry Pie ▪ Reduced-Fat Ricotta Cheesecake ▪ Pumpkin Pie ▪ Carrot Cake with Cream Cheese Frosting ▪ Angel Food Cake with Lemon Drizzle ▪ Vanilla Flan with Fresh Berries ▪ Orange, Blueberry, and Date Salad with Frozen Yogurt ▪ Patricia Terry's Pumpkin Bread ▪ Fruit-Filled Granola ▪ Rhubarb Sauce ▪ Applesauce with Dried Apricots and Cranberries ▪ Walnut Spice Coffee Cake ▪ Blueberry Buckle

Nutrition for Breastfeeding Mothers ▪ Postpartum Depression: How Diet and Exercise Can Help ▪ Stay Balanced Diet for Mothers ▪ Get in Shape After Baby . . . or Before If You Need To

▓ DEAR READER ▓

THERE IS NOTHING like a positive pregnancy test to focus your attention on your lifestyle and eating habits. Suddenly you realize that everything you eat, drink, and do with your body can directly affect the new life you are carrying. And, if you are like most mothers-to-be, this profound realization makes you want the best for your baby, even before he or she is born. *Eating for Pregnancy* was written to help you achieve that goal, and this updated edition brings you all the very latest nutritional information with practical, easy ways to meet those needs.

In keeping with our first edition, we are committed to focusing on the realities of life. Not all pregnancies are nine months of bliss—in fact, most aren't. You will probably experience some form of mild turbulence along the way, be it morning sickness, constipation, or indigestion. Some complications, such as gestational diabetes and gestational hypertension, are more serious and can require a special diet or bed rest.

Catherine experienced gestational hypertension in both of her pregnancies, so she understands firsthand the difficulties, stress, and fears involved with a high-risk pregnancy. Rose Ann, on the other hand, had relatively easy pregnancies, but from her twenty-plus years of experience as a perinatal nutritionist, she has seen or heard just about everything imaginable. Wherever you find yourself, between the two of us, we've probably either been there or gained insight from someone who has.

If this is your first pregnancy, you will most likely have more time to take care of yourself, and you should. If you're a seasoned mom, with a toddler clinging to your leg, knocking over plants, or crying for dinner, you undoubtedly face a much greater challenge to finding time to put a healthy meal on the table. Considering our time-pressured lives, we tried to make this book as quick to read and user-friendly as possible. At-a-glance nutrient sources, pantry lists, and cooking tips are designed to make your life easier in the grocery store and in front of the stove.

Our nutrition information is thorough, and in absolutely *no way* intended to scare you. We believe that knowledge gives you the power to make the smartest choices possible, whether you are in a health food store looking for herbal teas (there are some to be avoided) or along the highway at a fast food joint (you might think twice about ordering that sky-scraper burger with salty fries). You will probably never get listeriosis or pica, but you should know what they are.

Being a trained chef, Catherine knows how to cook, but those skills became useless when she was confined to bed rest. Her experience convinced her that the recipes in this book had to be healthy, tasty, and easy to prepare. To this end, she gathered together some of her favorite recipes and made them healthier and simpler. To guarantee the results, each of the 150 recipes has been tested by someone like you, a first-time mom or a veteran mother (and some partners too), at various levels of cooking skill.

Every recipe comes with the question, What's in this for baby and me? The answers tell you exactly what nutrients you are getting. Complete Meal Ideas help you piece together menus to come up with an eating program that balances eating healthfully and gaining weight appropriately. We also offer diabetic exchanges and carbohydrate counts should you need them.

By popular demand, we have expanded our vegetarian section and incorporated information for vegans. We have created even more delicious vegetarian dishes, along with thirty-five vegan recipes, that non-vegetarians will enjoy too. Everyone—moms, dads, and children—benefits by eating more nutrient-rich vegetables, fruits, and plant protein.

A new section called "Nine Months Later" offers nutritional advice for optimal breast-feeding nutrition. And when you are ready to start taking off some of that baby weight, we give you the Stay Balanced Diet for Mothers. An illustrated exercise menu guides you through exercises you can do at home. We also offer tips from an expert on combating postpartum depression with diet and exercise.

We hope that you *always* demand the best for your family. Eating healthfully and exercising before, during, and after pregnancy is the greatest gift you can give your baby and yourself. We use the recipes in *Eating for Pregnancy* all the time—our friends and their friends tell us they do too. We hope the recipes find a permanent home in your kitchen.

Rose Ann continues to enjoy working with expectant mothers. She approaches each woman knowing what a very special time this is, and encourages her to enjoy these nine months as best she can. We are both committed to making your pregnancy as healthy and pleasant as possible.

Catherine Jones and Rose Ann Hudson

all the nutrition information you need to know

⌐⌐

I F YOU HAVE picked up this book because you are pregnant, congratulations! If you are reading it with the intention of becoming pregnant, give yourself a gold star. By planning ahead for pregnancy, you can create optimal conditions for fetal development, especially during the critical first three to eight weeks of life following conception. Improving your own health will positively influence the health of your baby, facilitate delivery, and prepare you for the hectic duties of motherhood that lie ahead.

Eating for Pregnancy was written to inform you of your specific nutritional needs before, during, and after pregnancy, and to give you delicious, easy ways to meet them— whether you are cooking at home, lunching at your desk, or on bed rest. Looking at the nutritional math of pregnancy is admittedly daunting, and meeting all of the daily dietary goals is indeed a challenge. But there is certainly more to a healthy pregnancy than consuming the perfect amounts of calcium and iron. Aim for balance. Combine a healthy eating plan with exercise and relaxation to make your prepregnancy months, and pregnancy, a healthy and enjoyable time.

SOME BASIC ADVICE FOR WOMEN TRYING TO CONCEIVE

- Get prenatal care *before you conceive*. Inform your health care provider of your desire to start a family and discuss your general health and any concerns you may have. Inform your doctor of all medications, vitamins, supplements, birth control pills, or other substances you are taking (including Accutane or Retin A).
- A prenatal vitamin or folic acid supplement will most likely be prescribed by your health care provider in preparation for conception. If not, start taking a folic acid supplement at least one month and up to three months *before* conception. Because half of all pregnancies are unplanned, a daily folic acid supplement of at least 400 micrograms is advisable for *all* women of child-bearing age, especially for women who are trying to conceive (see Folic Acid Before Conception, page 21).

- Lose weight if your doctor advises you to or if you need to. Why? Because it will help you control your weight gain during pregnancy, it will help prevent high blood pressure and gestational diabetes, and it will be easier to lose weight after delivery. If your weight qualifies you as obese, check with your doctor about any additional folic acid supplements or other supplements you should take prior to conception. The "Nine Months Later" chapter offers advice on healthy postpregnancy dieting and exercise, but both plans can be used for prepregnancy weight loss.
- Gain weight if your doctor advises you to or if you need to. Underweight women can have a harder time conceiving, and they are more at risk for premature delivery and babies with low birth weight.
- Stop smoking. While there are no conclusive studies reporting that smoking interferes with conception, quitting smoking will greatly improve your own health, and lead to a healthier pregnancy and baby.
- Stop drinking alcohol. Since you don't know when the magic moment of conception might occur, it is advisable to cease drinking while trying to get pregnant. If you are a heavy drinker, please seek treatment prior to pregnancy. Heavy drinking can lower your chances of conceiving, and cause serious damage to your health and the health of your baby.
- If you are having trouble conceiving, severely cut back or eliminate your consumption of caffeine. Studies show that pregnant women who consumed more than 200 milligrams of caffeine a day (about two cups of coffee) had twice the risk of miscarriage as the women who consumed no caffeine at all.[1]
- Make exercise a habit. Getting physically fit before pregnancy will most likely allow you to exercise throughout your pregnancy, and soon after delivery. Likewise, not being in shape can lead to difficulty when trying to begin an exercise routine during pregnancy, and it can make delivery and postpregnancy weight loss significantly more difficult.
- Diabetics should get their blood sugar under control at least three to six months *prior* to pregnancy. Inform you doctor and diabetes educator of your desire to conceive.
- If you've had bariatric surgery, your doctor will need to evaluate any nutritional disturbances that should be corrected before conception.

healthy foods for conception

1. **Whole grain cereal fortified with 100% RDA folic acid (folic acid)**

2. **Wild salmon (DHA omega-3)**

3. **Ground flaxseed (ALA omega-3)**

4. **Lentils (iron and folic acid)**

5. **Whole milk (calcium)**

6. **Yogurt (calcium)**

7. **Spinach (iron)**

8. **Black beans (protein)**

9. **Asparagus (folic acid)**

10. **Tofu (protein)**

▪ Breathe. Relax. Think positive thoughts.

We wish you success . . . and in the end, whether your pregnancy was meticulously planned, medically coaxed, or happened by surprise, one thing is certain—your life will never be the same. You will soon learn to share your body and your life with another human being who is totally dependent on you.

If you have been pregnant before, you know much about what lies ahead, but as you have probably been told, every pregnancy is different. Countless women have gone before you and countless will follow; however, *your* pregnancy is the most important thing at the moment. Following is some general advice to make the next nine months as trouble- and worry-free as possible.

SOME BASIC ADVICE FOR PREGNANT WOMEN

▪ Consult your doctor or health care provider if you think you may be pregnant or if your at-home pregnancy test result is positive.

▪ Quit smoking, stop drinking alcohol, and strictly limit or give up caffeinated beverages (including coffee, tea, and soft drinks). Inform your doctor of any prescription, over-the-counter, and/or illicit drugs you are taking.

▪ Reevaluate your eating habits. Do you skip breakfast? Eat fast food for lunch? Graze on junk food for dinner? Follow a well-balanced diet to meet your nutritional needs during pregnancy. Learn what foods are good for you and try to incorporate them into your diet.

▪ Get moving. A little exercise will help you maintain an appropriate pregnancy weight and can help prevent gestational diabetes and gestational hypertension. Exercise will increase your energy and help control insomnia, stress, anxiety, and depression. It also can alleviate gas, heartburn, and constipation (see Exercise Tips: Fitness for Two, page 379).

avoid alcohol

Avoid *all* alcohol during pregnancy, which includes over-the-counter medications that contain alcohol, such as cough and cold remedies. Alcohol in a mother's bloodstream quickly crosses the placenta to her fetus. Drinking everyday can cause miscarriage, mental and physical deficiencies, learning disabilities, and numerous other behavioral problems. Heavy consumption, four to five drinks per day, may lead to fetal alcohol exposure (FAE) and fetal alcohol syndrome (FAS), resulting in physical defects to the heart, limbs, and facial structure, in addition to other health issues.

- Eliminate as much stress as possible from your work and home environment. This will help you cope with the intense fatigue of pregnancy; it will also help keep you emotionally stable when your hormones play tricks on you. Try to let go and relax as much as possible.
- Get plenty of rest. Your body needs the extra sleep for a reason—don't fight it. Plan a fatigue schedule for added downtime, especially during the first and third trimesters. During the first trimester, the increased level of progesterone causes sleepiness, and during the third, carrying the extra body weight increases fatigue. Try to get eight hours of sleep at night, and take short naps with your legs elevated during the day.
- Avoid X-rays, hot tubs, saunas, massages (unless by a trained pre-natal therapist), and inverted yoga poses.
- Avoid all raw, rare, and undercooked meat, poultry, and seafood.
- Pregnant women should be aware of certain dangerous food-borne illnesses and take precautions to avoid them. These include listeriosis (see Listeriosis Warning, page 129), toxoplasmosis (see Toxoplasmosis Warning, page 297), *E. coli* (see *E. Coli* Warning, page 285), and *salmonellosis* (see *Salmonella* Warning, page 330, and Eggs and *Salmonella enteritidis*, page 79).
- Pregnant women should limit their consumption of certain large fish that could potentially contain high levels of methylmercury, such as swordfish and shark (see Limitations on Certain Fish Consumption, page 335).

quit smoking before you get pregnant

Smoking deprives the fetus and placenta of oxygen, causing extreme harm to the developing baby.

Three Good Reasons to Quit Smoking

1. **Increased risk for premature birth, babies with low birth weight, stillbirth, and miscarriage.**

2. **Increased risk for intellectual deficiencies, learning disabilities, and behavioral problems later in childhood.**

3. **Increased risk for breathing problems and other health problems, including SIDS (sudden infant death syndrome).**

Good Eating Habits
and Gradual Weight Gain

A healthy diet helps make a healthy baby. During pregnancy, good eating habits are more important than ever. It is not the time to skip meals, feast on junk food, or load up on empty calories for quick energy. The foods you eat have a direct effect on the development of your baby from conception to birth. Strike a balance between healthy weight gain and nutritional intake. Try to keep in mind that you are not eating for two, you are eating carefully for one.

It is critical to learn about the nutritional value of the foods you eat and to select your diet with care. Selecting a variety of nutrient-rich foods versus calorie-rich foods will help prevent excessive weight gain, which can put you at risk for high blood pressure, gestational diabetes, and permanent obesity. Conversely, a diet too restricted in calories can be inadequate in protein, fats, vitamins, and minerals. Insufficient calorie intake can result in the breakdown of stored fat (or ketones) in the mother's blood and urine, which can be harmful for the fetus.

So, what is the ideal diet? The ideal diet is one diet that fits into your lifestyle and at the same time meets all the nutritional requirements of your pregnancy. Your goal should be to follow a well-balanced meal plan that ensures optimal weight gain. A pregnant woman should increase her caloric intake by about 300 calories per day above her prepregnant state, assuming that her prior caloric intake was adequate. Certain factors may increase the nutritional requirements above the estimated demands of pregnancy—including poor nutritional status, obesity, young maternal age (teenage pregnancy), multiple pregnancy, closely spaced births, breastfeeding one or more children while pregnant, continued high level of physical activity, certain disease states (such as diabetes), and use of cigarettes, alcohol, and legal or illegal drugs. Women who fit into any of these categories or who are experiencing a high-risk pregnancy should consult a registered dietitian for customized nutritional advice.

A pregnant woman should consume between 1,800 and 3,000 calories per day, depending on her prepregnant height and weight, and whether her nutritional needs are compromised in any way. For example, assuming prepregnant weight is within the "normal range" according to the Calorie and Protein Requirements for Pregnant Women with a Normal Body Mass Index (page 433), a woman who is 5'3" would require approximately 1,900 to 2,400 calories and at least 60 grams of protein per day, while a woman who is 5'7" would require approximately 2,100 to 2,700 calories and 70 grams of protein per day.

make your 300 extra calories count

Be wise about your 300-calorie additional intake. Choose to eat a sandwich with a glass of milk instead of candy bars and high-calorie sodas and soft drinks.

Just as important as the total number of pounds gained is the rate at which the weight is gained: aim for about 2 to 5

your prepregnant weight and expected weight gain

WEIGHT GAIN	PREPREGNANT WEIGHT/CONDITION
25 to 35 lbs (11.3 to 15.9 kg)	average prepregnant weight (within ideal body weight range)
28 to 40 lbs (12.7 to 18.1 kg)	underweight prepregnant weight (10% below ideal body weight)
15 to 25 lbs (6.8 to 11.3 kg)	overweight prepregnant weight (20% above ideal body weight)
40 to 45 lbs (15.9 to 20.5 kg)	woman carrying twins

pounds for the first trimester (fourteen weeks) and 3.5 pounds per month for the remainder of the pregnancy (fourteen to forty weeks). Ideally, the total weight gain during pregnancy should be between 25 and 35 pounds.

Don't become obsessed with your weight gain—in fact, feel free to put away your scale. Your weight will be closely monitored by your doctor during each office visit. A trend of excessive or inadequate weight gain in more than one month (a gain of more than 5 pounds or less than 2 pounds) indicates that your dietary intake may need to be evaluated. If your weight is excessive and on an upward trend overall, take an inventory of your eating habits to pinpoint problem areas. Try cutting down on fried or fatty foods, fast foods, convenience foods, desserts, and soft drinks. Also, monitor your portion sizes more closely.

PRODUCTS OF CONCEPTION[2]

NUMBER OF POUNDS	SOURCE OF WEIGHT GAIN
4–6	Maternal stores (fat, protein, and other nutrients)
2–3	Increased fluid volume
3–4	Increased blood volume
1–2	Breast enlargement
2	Uterus
6–8	Baby
2	Amniotic fluid
1.5	Placenta (tissue connecting mother and baby that brings nourishment and takes away waste)

If you do not fit into the normal range of the body mass index table, if you are carrying multiples, or if you are a teenager, use the following variations for determining calorie requirements during pregnancy. You should consult your doctor or dietitian for your individual protein needs.

If underweight (90% below your IBW):
40 cals × ideal body weight in kilograms
If overweight (20% above your IBW):
25 cals × current body weight in kilograms
If obese (50% above your IBW):
12 cals × current body weight in kilograms
For twins:
Add 300 cals to your requirements
For triplets:
Add 600 cals to your requirements
For teenagers:
40 cals × ideal body weight in kilograms

If inadequate weight gain or weight loss is an issue, evaluate your exercise plan (especially if you exercise every day), because you may be burning off essential calories and not replacing them. Also, try increasing the amount of protein and calcium-rich foods in your diet. Adding nonfat dry milk powder to milk, milk shakes, smoothies, hot cereals, dips, and soups is a way of getting extra protein, calcium, and calories. One-third cup of pasteurized instant nonfat dry milk provides 80 calories and 8 grams of protein. Keep in mind that it is not unusual to have a large one-month weight gain sometime in the second trimester. This may be attributed to a 25 percent increase in blood and fluid volume for the mother.

Planning a Healthy, Well-Balanced Diet

Planning a healthy, well-balanced diet to meet your pregnancy needs does not have to be difficult or time-consuming. Following is a Food Groups Guide for Pregnancy. For a list of foods and serving sizes that fit into these food categories, see Food Groups and Serving Sizes for Pregnant Women, page 37. A Vegetarian Food Groups Guide for Pregnancy is located in chapter 4: Vegetarian and Vegan Delights, on page 180.

FOOD GROUPS GUIDE FOR PREGNANCY[3]

Dairy products = 4 or more servings per day
Meat, poultry, fish, beans, and eggs = 2 or more servings per day
Grains = 6 to 9 servings per day
Vegetables = 4 or more servings per day
Fruits = 3 or more servings per day
Fats = no minimum requirement

making sense of nutrition lingo

▶ **RDA: A recommended dietary allowance is the average daily dietary intake level that is sufficient to meet the nutrient requirement of nearly all healthy individuals (97.5%) for a given gender and stage of life. The process for setting an RDA depends on being able to set an estimated average requirement (EAR).**

▶ **EAR: An estimated average requirement is a nutrient intake value that is estimated to meet the requirement of half the healthy individuals in a given group.**

▶ **AI: Adequate intake is a goal value based on observed or experimentally determined approximations of nutrient intake by a group (or groups) of healthy people. It is used when an RDA cannot be determined.**

▶ **DV: Daily value is the amount of the daily nutrient requirement that a certain food contains. This measurement is commonly found on food, multivitamin, and mineral supplement labels.**

It is helpful to understand some of the most important nutrients and their role in your baby's development. Daily Nutrients for Pregnancy and Lactation illustrates all of the extra nutrients needed. Pregnant teens should consult a dietitian to determine the best intakes for their growing bodies and developing babies. Other conditions during pregnancy, such as multiples and diabetes, may also require special nutrient allowances.

Prenatal vitamins and supplements act as a safety net to your diet during pregnancy, and they should be taken as directed by your doctor. Keep in mind that they do not replace real food. During the first trimester, morning sickness can be exacerbated by certain prenatal vitamins. If you suspect this, try taking your vitamin with food, before bedtime, or ask your doctor to switch vitamin brands. If you stop taking your vitamin for any reason, you should continue to take a folic acid supplement throughout pregnancy.

Macronutrients

Energy

Energy comes from protein, carbohydrates, and fats. Calorie intakes during pregnancy vary from woman to woman depending on a number of factors, such as her metabolism, prepregnancy weight, stage of pregnancy, and physical activity level. It is estimated that, on average, a pregnant woman requires a total of 85,000 additional calories over the course of 40 weeks of pregnancy. This breaks down to approximately 300 extra calories per day.[4] During the first trimester, energy needs are generally low, and 300 additional daily calories are not required. Needs begin to pick up in the fourth month as the uterus, mammary glands, placenta, and fetus grow and blood volume increases. In the later

DAILY NUTRIENTS FOR PREGNANCY AND LACTATION[5]

NUTRIENT	ADULT WOMEN	PREGNANCY	LACTATION
Protein (g)	46	71	60
Carbohydrates (g)	130	175	210
Total Fiber (g)	25	28	29
Linoleic Acid (LA) (g) omega-6	12	13	13
Alpha-Linoleic Acid (ALA) (g) omega-3	12	13	13
Vitamin A (mcg)	700	770	1,300
Vitamin D (mcg)	5/200	5/200	5/200
Vitamin E (mg)	15	15	19
Vitamin K (mcg)	90	90	90
Vitamin C (mg)	75	85	120
Thiamin (mg)	1.1	1.4	1.4
Riboflavin (mg)	1.1	1.4	1.6
Vitamin B_6 (mg)	1.3	1.9	2.0
Niacin (mg)	14	18	17
Folate (mcg)	400	600	500
Vitamin B_{12} (mcg)	2.4	2.6	2.8
Pantothenic Acid (mg)	5	6	7
Biotin (mcg)	30	30	35
Choline (mg)	425	450	550
Calcium (mg)	1,000	1,000	1,000
Phosphorus (mg)	700	700	700
Magnesium (mg)	320	350	310
Iron (mg)	18	27	9
Zinc (mg)	8	11	12
Iodine (mcg)	150	220	290
Selenium (mcg)	55	60	70
Fluoride (mg)	3	3	3
Manganese (mg)	1.8	2.0	2.6
Molybdenum (mcg)	45	50	50
Chromium (mcg)	25	30	45
Copper (mcg)	900	1,000	1,300
Sodium (mg)	2,300	2,300	2,300
Potassium (mg)	4,700	4,700	5,100

stages of pregnancy, energy needs climb to support the growing fetus and the extra weight of the mother.

▶ *Protein*

During pregnancy extra protein is needed to help with fetal brain development and with muscle and tissue formation. Inadequate amounts of dietary protein can impair the development of the placenta and fetus, resulting in low birth weight and intrauterine growth retardation. For the mother, protein is essential for the increase in maternal blood volume and for the formation of amniotic fluid. During labor, delivery, and lactation, protein storage reserves are tapped, making it vital to have an excess amount. Most women will need to consume between 60 and 70 grams of protein per day (see Calorie and Protein Requirements for Pregnant Women with a Normal Body Mass Index, page 433). Some good sources of protein include: poultry, lean meats, fish, cottage cheese, pasteurized cheese, yogurt, eggs, milk, tofu, tempeh, soy products, beans, legumes, nut butters, nuts, and seeds (see Protein Sources, page 10, for a more complete list).

▶ *Carbohydrates*

Carbohydrates fuel your brain and body. Adequate intake of carbohydrates is necessary to allow protein that would otherwise be tapped for energy to be used for muscle building and tissue formation in the fetus. Always choose complex carbohydrates, such as whole grains, beans, whole wheat pasta, brown rice, fruits, and vegetables, which contain vitamins (particularly the B complex vitamins), iron, and fiber. While simple sugars, such as candy, sodas, and desserts, may give you a temporary energy boost, they are sources of empty calories and should not be substituted for nutrient-rich foods.

▶ *Fats*

Pregnancy is the wrong time to start counting fat grams. No dieting is allowed—but do not use your pregnancy as an excuse to pig out either. Fats play a central role in skin health, cell formation, and fetal brain development (60 percent of the dry weight of the brain is fat), and therefore they should not be restricted during pregnancy. All fats provide slow-burning, long-lasting energy and also help with absorption of the fat-soluble vitamins A, D, E, and K. However, not all fats are created equal, and some are better for you than others. In general, it is best to choose unsaturated fats over saturated fats, and to eliminate trans fats from your family's diet.

Questions and Answers about Omega-3 and Omega-6 Fatty Acids

▶ *What are omega-3 fatty acids?*

Within the polyunsaturated fat category, there is a key subgroup called omega-3 fatty acids, which are vital to good health throughout life, starting in the womb. There are three types of omega-3s.

UNSATURATED FATS

Unsaturated fats, also called "good" fats, are definitely the preferred fat during pregnancy and throughout life. There are two types, monounsaturated and polyunsaturated. They come primarily from plants, nuts, seeds, and cold-water fish, and they remain liquid at room temperature. Monounsaturated fats will become solid when refrigerated (olive oil is an example), but polyunsaturated fats (like fish oil) will not. Consume lots of these fats.

SATURATED FATS

Saturated fats are solid at room temperature and come mainly from animal sources. Butter, cheese, whole milk, cream, lard, meat, and poultry are common examples. Palm kernel and coconut oils are also considered saturated fats, despite their vegetable origins. Consume these fats in moderation.

TRANS FATS

Trans fats, also called partially hydrogenated oils, are synthetic saturated fats produced by passing hydrogen bubbles through heated polyunsaturated oils. Trans fats are found in hard margarines, vegetable shortening, fried and fast foods, and many other processed products on grocery shelves, including certain breakfast cereals, cookies, prepared frozen foods, and even hot cocoa mixes. While there is no scientific evidence that trans fats are particularly harmful to pregnant women, studies show that excessive consumption can decrease the body's conversion of essential omega-3 fatty acids, which are imperative for fetal brain development.[6] Everyone, not just pregnant women, should avoid these fats.

EPA and DHA naturally occur in fish and the algae they eat. They can also be synthesized in the body from ALA, the primary essential fatty acid (called "essential" because your body cannot make this fatty acid on its own).

Omega-3 Fatty Acids (n-3)

Alpha-linolenic acid (ALA)

Eicosapentaenoic acid (EPA)

Docosahexaenoic acid (DHA)

ALA can be obtained from plant sources, such as certain vegetable oils, nuts, seeds, and green leafy vegetables. Your body converts ALA to EPA and DHA, but the exact amount of conversion remains unclear, varies from person to person, and is known to be quite low. The adequate intake for ALA during pregnancy and lactation is 13 grams. We do not yet know the adequate intakes of DHA and EPA for pregnant women, but stay tuned as research results unfold in the coming years.

▶ *Why are omega-3 fatty acids important for pregnant women?*
  DHA is the most critical omega-3 for your baby's brain and eye development in the womb and during infancy. Your baby's brain will have its greatest growth spurt during the last trimester of pregnancy, and DHA is known to be a significant structural component of the brain.[7] EPA is also imperative, though it plays a cell-signaling rather than cell-structuring role in the brain.

In regard to eye development, DHA is a fundamental component of the retina (30 to 50 percent of the retina is made of DHA). Deficiency is associated with poor night vision and other visual and spatial interpretation problems.[8] Additional research results show that an increased intake of DHA through supplementation during pregnancy may help

- prevent preterm delivery,[9]
- increase head circumference and birth weight,[10]
- benefit infant problem solving at nine months and infant visual acuity at four months of age,[11] and
- prevent depression during pregnancy and postpartum.[12]

OMEGA-3 FOOD SOURCES[13]

ALA	EPA AND DHA	
Flaxseed, ground	Salmon	Trout
Vegetable oils: flaxseed	Light canned tuna	Lobster
(linseed), canola, walnut,	Sardines	Crab
soybean, pumpkin, and olive	Mackerel	Shrimp
Pumpkin seeds	Herring	Clams
Walnuts	Halibut	Scallops
Soybeans, tofu, miso	Cod	Oysters (cooked)
Wheat or barley grass	Haddock	Anchovies
Dark green, leafy vegetables	Catfish	Cod liver oil
Seaweed	Flounder	Microalgae supplements

▶ **What are sources of omega-3 fatty acids?**

Fish, fish oil, and DHA microalgae supplements are excellent sources of DHA and EPA. Some fish that are safe for pregnant women to eat are listed on page 12. Sources of ALA-enriched and some DHA-enriched products are constantly appearing on the market. They currently include eggs, fortified orange juice, peanut butter, cereal, margarines, milk, oils, pasta, and other products. (See Omega-3–Enriched Products to Add to Your Breakfast Lineup, page 40.)

▶ **If there is no Recommended Daily Intake of DHA during pregnancy, how much DHA should a pregnant woman consume?**

The best thing to do is to ask your doctor and to keep abreast of evolving information on the websites listed in the appendix. The Food and Drug Administration's (FDA's) recommendation for the *general public* is that consumers do not exceed more than a total of 3 grams (3,000 milligrams) per day of EPA and DHA omega-3s, with no more than 2 grams (2,000 milligrams) per day from a dietary supplement. People taking more than 3 grams of omega-3 fatty acids from supplements should do so only under a physician's care. Exceedingly high intakes could potentially cause excessive bleeding in women and men who are taking anticoagulants, prescription blood pressure medications, or aspirin on a daily basis, or those known to have an inherited or acquired predisposition to bleeding.[14]

▶ **Should pregnant women eat fish?**

Absolutely. Seafood is an excellent source of protein, vitamins, and minerals. Fish varieties high in DHA and EPA omega-3s, such as wild salmon, canned light tuna, trout, and catfish, which are all low in mercury, should be consumed regularly (see Safe Fish Sources with DHA and EPA Omega-3s, page 12).

▶ **Should pregnant women take DHA supplements?**

This is a question to ask your doctor. If supplements are advised, be sure to ask what amount to consume and for how long, and ideally request a brand-name recommendation. Do *not* self-prescribe omega-3s or any other supplements during pregnancy and breastfeeding.

▶ **What are omega-6 fatty acids and what do they do?**

Omega-6 fatty acids comprise another subgroup within the polyunsaturated fat category.

LA, linoleic acid, is the essential omega-6 fatty acid (again, this means that you must consume it in food because your body can't produce it). The adequate intake of LA for pregnancy and lactation is 13 grams. GLA and AA do not yet have adequate intake guidelines, but most people consume enough from eggs, meats, and dairy products.

omega-6 fatty acids (n-6)

Linoleic acid (LA)

Gamma-linoleic acid (GLA)

Arachidonic acid (AA)

AA helps form the cellular structure of the brain, and GLA (like EPA) assists with cell signaling.[15] Of the sources listed below, borage seed oil should *not* be used during pregnancy because it may be harmful to the fetus and may induce early labor.[16]

OMEGA-6 FOOD SOURCES

LA	GLA	AA
Margarines made from sunflower, corn, safflower, or soybean oils	Plant seed oils made from evening primrose, black currant, borage, and truffle oils	Egg yolks
Vegetable oils: sunflower, sesame, safflower, corn, soybean, walnut, and wheat germ oil		Meats
Walnuts and Brazil nuts; sesame, pumpkin, and sunflower seeds		Dairy products
Peanut and almond butter		
Wheat germ		
Tahini (sesame paste)		

"Omega-6 Fatty Acids," University of Maryland [Internet]. [Cited September, 2008]. Available from: http://www.umm.edu/altmed/articles/omega-6–000317.htm.

Healthy Vegetable Oils

All vegetable oils are combinations of saturated, monounsaturated, and polyunsaturated fatty acids. Each is categorized according to the predominant type of fat it contains. For instance, canola oil is considered monounsaturated because it contains 8 grams of monounsaturated fat, 4 grams of polyunsaturated fat, and .9 grams of saturated fat. Corn oil is classified as polyunsaturated because it contains 8 grams of polyunsaturated fats, 3 grams of monounsaturated fat, and 1.7 grams of saturated fat. All of these oils are good for you. As a general rule, the nut and seed oils should not be used in cooking with heat; they are ideal in salad dressings and drizzled over foods. Corn, safflower, canola, olive, and other oils can withstand heat.

VEGETABLE OIL CLASSIFICATIONS

MONOUNSATURATED OILS	POLYUNSATURATED OILS
Almond	Corn
Avocado	Flaxseed
Canola	Grape seed
Olive	Pumpkin seed
Peanut	Safflower
Sesame	Soybean
	Sunflower
	Walnut

Essential Minerals

▶ *Calcium*

Calcium is an essential mineral for bone and teeth construction for the mother and her baby. The RDA is 1,000 milligrams during pregnancy, and more for women carrying multiples and for pregnant adolescents. Bones contain 99 percent of your calcium, and the remaining 1 percent is found in your blood. If calcium intake is not adequate enough to meet a baby's needs (especially during the third trimester to accommodate rapid skeletal

calcium and osteoporosis

Pregnancy does not have to drain your bones of calcium. If your daily calcium consumption is adequate to meet your needs as well as those of your developing baby, pregnancy can actually help preserve bone mass. The high levels of estrogen during pregnancy stimulate the activation of vitamin D (which promotes calcium absorption) and increase the production of calcitonin, which inhibits bone breakdown. While menopause may seem light-years away at this point in your life, maintaining a high calcium intake is a good habit to continue.

growth), calcium reserves of the mother's bones are tapped, resulting in calcium depletion. Calcium in the bloodstream is very important, particularly during labor, when it is needed to maintain proper heartbeat, muscle contractions, nerve transmissions, and for blood clotting.

Consuming calcium through proper diet and supplements is only one phase of building and maintaining healthy bones (see Dairy Calcium Sources, page 345, and Nondairy Calcium Sources, page 185). In order for the body to absorb calcium, the calcium must be combined with vitamin D. The body can manufacture vitamin D with the help of sunlight. For those who cannot be outdoors, fortified milk, whole or skim, and vitamin D-fortified cereals are good sources of vitamin D (see Vitamin D, page 20). To prevent interference with iron absorption, calcium supplements should *not* be taken with a prenatal vitamin, and should be taken preferably between meals.

calcium supplements

Calcium supplements from natural sources such as oyster shell or bone meal may be high in lead. Synthetic supplements made from calcium carbonate have much lower levels of lead (1 milligram per tablet); about the same amount of lead found in one serving of milk. Calcium carbonate supplements—or antacids such as Caltrate 600 + D, Viactiv Soft Calcium Chews (500 + D), and TUMS (Extra Strength)—can be purchased over the counter. Consult your doctor before taking any supplements.

Lactose intolerance, or the inability to digest milk sugar contained in dairy products due to a deficiency of the enzyme lactase, is one of the major reasons women cannot meet their calcium goal. One option is yogurt made with live or active cultures whose bacteria releases lactose-digesting enzymes (see The Power of Yogurt, page 17). Or, you might consider Lactaid drops or pills, lactose-free milk products (which range from 70 percent to 100 percent lactose-free), or non-dairy, fortified beverages such as soy, almond, rice, and oat milks. Read labels carefully to select the brands that offer the most calcium, protein, and vitamins.

▶ Iron

Any woman who does not get a sufficient amount of iron during her pregnancy, or who starts her pregnancy with low iron stores, is at risk for iron deficiency anemia (see Iron Deficiency Anemia, page 25). Because it is impossible to meet your daily iron requirements through food sources alone, a prenatal vitamin that contains iron is recommended for all pregnant women.

Iron is essential for the formation of hemoglobin, which carries oxygen in the blood. An iron intake of 27 milligrams is recommended for most healthy pregnancies, while pregnant women suffering from anemia may need more. Adequate maternal iron stores are vital in protecting the mother from complications due to blood loss during pregnancy. Also, during the last trimester, a three- to four-month supply of iron is stored in the liver of the fetus for use after birth, before food stores of iron are added to an infant's diet.

the power of yogurt

Yogurt is made by heating milk and then adding culture. The fermentation process results in the breakdown of casein, or milk protein, one of the most difficult proteins to digest. Culturing, the process following fermentation, restores many of the enzymes destroyed during pasteurization, including lactase. Lactase is the enzyme that breaks down lactose (milk sugar) into glucose and galactose, and it is this breakdown that allows some people who are otherwise lactose intolerant to consume cultured yogurt without side effects (check yogurt labels for active cultures). One last bit of good news is that yogurt is so high in calcium, 6 ounces provide as much calcium as 8 ounces of reduced-fat (1% or 2%) milk.

Heme iron from animal sources is more easily absorbed by the body than non-heme iron from plant sources. One easy way to increase iron absorption is to eat high-iron foods with a source of vitamin C. While it is true that some of the highest sources of iron (such as beef and eggs) are also high in cholesterol and fat, a low-cholesterol, low-fat diet is not recommended during a normal pregnancy without complications. Cholesterol levels may rise slightly during the second half of pregnancy, but they usually resume to normal levels within the six-month postpartum period. Women with extremely elevated cholesterol levels prior to pregnancy should consult with a doctor and a registered dietitian for any special restrictions. (See Iron Sources, page 38.)

▶ *Phosphorus*

Phosphorus helps build strong bones and teeth. It is involved in the metabolism of fats, protein, and carbohydrates, and in the formation of genetic material, cell membranes, and enzymes. Pregnant women should consume 700 milligrams daily. Some good sources include meats, poultry, fish, eggs, shrimp, whole grains, beans, lentils, nuts, seeds, baked potatoes, and dairy products.

▶ *Magnesium*

Magnesium is critical for bone building, muscle function, heart health, immunity, regulation of blood sugar levels, promoting normal blood pressure, and energy metabolism synthesis. Studies show that magnesium may play a role in preventing preeclampsia, but the evidence is not conclusive.[17] The following foods can help meet the daily recommended intake of 350 milligrams: nuts, seeds, soybeans, tofu, spinach, oatmeal, potatoes with skin, wheat bran, whole grains, brown rice, almonds, lentils, avocados, bananas, orange juice, pineapple juice, molasses, and dairy products.

▶ *Zinc*

Zinc is essential for cell growth, maintaining immunity, wound healing, fat metabolism, gene expression, and sexual function. Zinc deficiency can cause poor fetal growth.

Dietary sources of zinc include seafood, meat, eggs, dairy products, zinc-fortified cereals, legumes, seeds, cashews, and whole grains. Pregnant women should consume 11 milligrams of zinc daily.

▶ *Iodine*

Iodine is critical for thyroid functioning and metabolism regulation. A daily recommended intake of 220 micrograms can be obtained from iodized salt, seaweed, cow's milk (by way of iodine-containing products used to disinfect milk-collection vessels), eggs, fish, shellfish, and pork. Iodine deficiency (unlikely in most developed nations) can result in enlargement of the thyroid gland, goiter, or hypothyroidism, which could have detrimental effects on the fetus.

▶ *Selenium*

Selenium protects cells from free-radical damage, promotes proper thyroid functioning, and boosts the immune system. Pregnant women should aim for 60 micrograms. Some good sources include Brazil nuts, peanuts, seeds, oatmeal, pork chops, fish, shrimp, poultry, eggs, tofu, mushrooms, brown rice, milk, and whole grains.

▶ *Fluoride*

Fluoride is important for tooth development and preventing tooth decay in the mother during pregnancy. Fluoride toothpaste, water (only if fluoridated), caffeine-free tea, or canned fish with bones should easily supply the 3 milligrams daily recommended intake.

▶ *Manganese*

Manganese is imperative for bone development, maintaining normal blood sugar levels, nerve cell health, thyroid functioning, and metabolism of protein, fats, and carbohydrates. The adequate intake is 2 milligrams. Some good sources include nuts, seeds, romaine lettuce, beans, spinach, soybeans, oats, lentils, brown rice, whole wheat bread, kale, baked potatoes, spinach, raspberries, bananas, pineapple, and molasses.

▶ *Molybdenum*

Molybdenum is an important trace element in the metabolism of protein and fat. Spinach, whole grains, milk, and lentils can help supply the 50 micrograms recommended daily.

▶ *Chromium*

Chromium enhances insulin and helps with carbohydrate, fat, and protein metabolism. Pork chops, chicken, broccoli, romaine lettuce, peanuts, potatoes, spinach, tomatoes, whole wheat bread, whole grains, and apples are good sources for the 30 microgram adequate intake.

Copper

Copper assists with iron utilization and other metabolic functions. Greens, mushrooms, seeds, nuts, squash, asparagus, kidney beans, soybeans, tofu, lentils, brown rice, potatoes, whole wheat bread, and pineapple juice are good sources for the daily recommended intake of 1,000 micrograms.

Sodium

Sodium is necessary for regulation of blood and bodily fluids, communication among nerves, heart activity, and certain metabolic functions. The adequate intake is 2,300 milligrams of sodium per day. Most Americans consume much more than the adequate intake; the average sodium intake for American adults is 3,400 milligrams.

Potassium

Potassium is necessary for optimal kidney, heart, digestive, and muscle function. Adequate dietary intake helps prevent osteoporosis. Low intake can lead to high blood pressure. The adequate intake of 4,700 milligrams can come from salmon, potatoes, dried apricots, bananas, orange juice, dairy products, and seeds.

Vital Vitamins

Vitamin A

Vitamin A is vital in promoting cell, bone, and tooth formation, normal vision, and healthy skin in the fetus. Pregnant women require 770 micrograms (about 2,300 IU) of vitamin A daily. Excessive intake of vitamin A (more than 3,000 IU in the form of retinol, not beta carotene) can increase the risk of birth defects, such as malformation of the head, brain, heart, or spinal cord. There is some concern about consuming too much liver, which is extremely rich in vitamin A, during pregnancy. Pregnant women should minimize their consumption of liver, if not eliminate it entirely from their diets.[18] Fruit and vegetable sources of vitamin A, such as mango, cantaloupe, tangerines, sweet potatoes, carrots, broccoli, and asparagus, are not toxic in large doses. They contain beta carotene, which the body converts to vitamin A based on need. Other good sources of vitamin A include egg yolks, pasteurized cheese, fortified dairy products, and butter (see Vitamin A Sources, page 350, for a more complete list).

Vitamin C

Vitamin C (also known as ascorbic acid) is essential for wound healing, healthy teeth and gums, maintaining resistance to infection, and iron absorption. A daily increase to 85 milligrams is recommended during pregnancy; however, don't overdo it. Excessive intake of vitamin C supplements could cause the newborn to have increased requirements for vitamin C, possibly leading to a deficiency syndrome called rebound scurvy. Pregnant women can fulfill their daily requirements of vitamin C by eating additional citrus fruits, berries, cantaloupe, tomatoes, broccoli, Brussels sprouts, and red bell peppers (see Vitamin C Sources, page 350, for a more complete list).

▶ *Vitamin D*

Vitamin D is manufactured by the body after exposure to the sun. It is necessary to promote the utilization of calcium and phosphorus by the body. Pregnant women need 5 micrograms (200 IU) of vitamin D per day. A healthy, nonpregnant woman usually gets adequate vitamin D from two twenty-minute sessions of exposure to sunlight weekly, without UVA-blocking sunscreen. Be aware that vitamin D through supplements can be toxic in doses larger than 1,000 IU. Good sources of vitamin D include egg yolks, butter, milk products (all milk pasteurized in the U.S. is fortified with vitamin D), vitamin D-fortified cereals, sardines, salmon, herring, and mackerel.

▶ *Vitamin E*

Vitamin E protects cells from damage, boosts immune function, assists with DNA repair, and supports metabolic processes. An intake of 15 milligrams (28.5 IU) can be obtained from wheat germ, vegetable oils, nuts, and seeds.

▶ *Vitamin K*

Vitamin K ensures normal blood clotting and bone mineralization. The adequate intake is 90 micrograms, which is easily met by the following sources: greens, Brussels sprouts, avocados, broccoli, romaine lettuce, cabbage, asparagus, spinach, and kelp.

▶ *The B Vitamins*

FOLIC ACID (B₉)

Folic acid (also called folacin and folate) is essential for cell division and manufacturing DNA and RNA, the molecules that transfer genetic information and translate it into tissue production. Increased amounts of folic acid are valuable in preventing neural tube defects, such as spina bifida and anencephaly. Spina bifida is caused by an incomplete closing of the bony casing around the spinal cord, which results in partial paralysis. Anencephaly is a fatal defect in which a major part of the brain never develops. Approximately 2,500 infants suffering from spina bifida are born in the U.S. each year. The

water-soluble and fat-soluble vitamins

Vitamins fall into two categories, water soluble and fat soluble.

▶ Water-soluble vitamins (all the B vitamins and C) dissolve in water and are not stored in your body. Your body uses the vitamins it needs and eliminates the rest.

▶ Fat-soluble vitamins (A, D, E, and K) are dissolved in fat and therefore can be stored in the body (specifically in the liver).

Keep in mind that any vitamin taken in extremely large doses can potentially be harmful. Vitamins A and D are toxic if taken in large doses. Check with your doctor or health provider before taking any vitamin or mineral supplements.

latest research shows that folic acid can also help prevent oral and facial birth defects, such as cleft palate.[19]

Pregnant women should consume 600 micrograms of folic acid daily. Women carrying multiples and obese pregnant women may be prescribed additional folic acid. Available evidence suggests that synthetic folic acid, found in supplements and fortified foods, is more effective at preventing neural tube defects than is folate from food; *both*, however, are recommended.[20] Some natural sources of folate include lentils, romaine lettuce, asparagus, chickpeas, beans, green leafy vegetables, citrus fruits, wheat germ, brewer's yeast, enriched breads, and fortified breakfast cereals (see Folic Acid Sources, page 141, for a more complete list).

VITAMIN B$_{12}$

Vitamin B$_{12}$ is essential in the formation of red blood cells and a healthy nervous system. It is found only in animal products, vitamin B$_{12}$–fortified cereals, and yeast. The recommended dose of 2.6 milligrams of vitamin B$_{12}$ during pregnancy is usually met through food sources; therefore, supplements are not needed, except perhaps for strict vegetarians or vegans. (For more information on vegetarian diets and vitamin B$_{12}$ supplements, see chapter 4: Vegetarian and Vegan Delights, page 180. Also see the list of Cereals that Contain 100 percent of the Daily Value of Vitamin B$_{12}$, page 43.)

VITAMIN B$_6$

Vitamin B$_6$ assists in the formation of red blood cells and the metabolism of protein and fats. In observational studies, vitamin B$_6$ has been positively associated with improved pregnancy outcomes, such as reduced incidence of preeclampsia and higher Apgar scores and neonatal behavior.[21] The extra protein allowance for pregnancy should be accompanied by an increase in vitamin B$_6$—a total intake of 1.9 milligrams per day. Good sources of vitamin B$_6$ include poultry, fish, pork, eggs, whole wheat products, and nuts (peanuts and walnuts).

THIAMINE (B$_1$)

Thiamine helps the body convert carbohydrates into energy. It is also necessary for healthy functioning of the heart and brain, and for healthy nerve cells. Pregnant women should consume 1.4

folic acid before conception

A folic acid supplement should be started at least one month before conception because spina bifida and similar birth defects occur in the first two weeks of pregnancy, often before you know you are pregnant. Since 50 percent of all pregnancies are unplanned, the U.S. Public Health Service advises that all women of child-bearing age get 400 micrograms of folic acid per day. To reach this goal, in 1996 the Food and Drug Administration authorized the addition of folic acid to enriched grain products, making the supplement mandatory in 1998. Fortification is estimated to provide an additional 100 micrograms of folic acid to the diet of women of reproductive age.

BODY BUILDING	BRAIN GROWTH AND FUNCTION	BONES AND TEETH	BLOOD SUPPLY	METABOLISM
Protein	Protein	Calcium	Iron	Carbohydrates
Iron	Fats	Phosphorus	Magnesium	Protein
Zinc	DHA and EPA omega-3s	Magnesium	Calcium	Fats
Selenium	AA omega-6	Manganese	B_{12}	All B vitamins
All B vitamins	Choline	Fluoride	B_6	Choline
Vitamin A	B_{12}	Vitamin A	Vitamin A	Pantothenic acid
Vitamin C	Copper	Vitamin D	Vitamin K	Magnesium
Vitamin E		Vitamin K		Phosphorus
				Manganese
				Selenium
				Chromium
				Potassium
				Zinc
				Molybdenum
				Sodium

milligrams of thiamine per day. Some good sources include unrefined cereal, brewer's yeast, lean pork, legumes, nuts, and seeds.

RIBOFLAVIN (B_2)

Riboflavin is important for body growth and cell reproduction. It is necessary for breaking down amino acids and releasing energy from fats, proteins, and carbohydrates. Pregnant women should consume 1.4 milligrams of riboflavin per day. Some good sources include meat, poultry, dairy products, grain products, and green vegetables such as broccoli, turnip greens, collard greens, asparagus, and spinach.

NIACIN (B_3)

Niacin assists with cell production. Pregnant women should consume 18 milligrams of niacin per day. Some good sources include poultry, meat, tuna, eggs, whole grains, nuts, legumes, and enriched breads and cereals.

BIOTIN (B_7)

Biotin aids in fat and sugar digestion and promotes a healthy nervous system. The adequate intake is 30 micrograms, and some good sources include egg yolks, green vegetables, and whole grains.

PANTOTHENIC ACID (B₅)

Pantothenic acid is a major player in the metabolism of fats, carbohydrates, and protein. It helps regulate the body's adrenal activity and is involved with the production of antibodies for wound healing. The adequate intake of 6 milligrams can come from meats, milk, eggs, salmon, and seeds.

CHOLINE

Choline is essential for fetal brain development and the formation of cell membranes throughout the body. Research studies on the safety and effectiveness of taking choline supplements during pregnancy for improving brain development are underway. Stay tuned for results as they become available. The adequate intake of 450 milligrams can be supplied by egg yolks, milk, nuts, fish, and meat.

High-Risk Pregnancies

Certain preexisting conditions or pregnancy-related complications require extra care and attention. For these high-risk pregnancies, women usually require a closely monitored, customized medical care plan, and some conditions may call for special nutrition guidelines. Following are some of the most common high-risk conditions.

▶ Obese Pregnant Women

Obesity in the U.S. and many other countries has reached epidemic proportions. From 1999 to 2002, approximately one-third of women of child-bearing age (20 to 39 years) were classified as obese, or having a body mass index greater than 29. Today, more and more women are entering pregnancy with excess weight.[22] This is of great concern because obesity in pregnancy is associated with numerous maternal and neonatal complications, some of which include difficulty conceiving, increased risk of miscarriage, fetal defects and mortality, increased risk of gestational hypertension, preeclampsia, gestational diabetes, and blood clots. The best way to prevent these potential complications is to lose as much weight as possible, through diet and exercise, *before* conception. If you've had bariatric surgery, a special assessment of your nutrient absorption should be done before conception.

Obese pregnant women need to maintain their weight, or to gain a minimal amount of weight during pregnancy, usually not more than 15 pounds. This number is likely to change in the near future—it is likely to go down—as more studies are done to figure out the optimal weight gain for overweight and obese mothers. No matter how overweight you are, dieting is *not* recommended during pregnancy because it will deprive the fetus of essential nutrients. Your doctor will want to monitor your health closely and will assign a registered dietitian who will create an individualized meal plan. Increased folic acid prior to conception may be prescribed to help prevent neural tube defects.

► High Blood Pressure During Pregnancy and Preeclampsia

Contrary to popular belief, when high blood pressure develops during pregnancy (particularly in women with no previous history of high blood pressure), following a strict low-sodium diet is usually not recommended. Instead, increasing protein and calcium seems to be most beneficial. Pregnant women with high blood pressure (also known as gestational hypertension) should ideally try to avoid high-sodium foods such as bacon, sausage, processed foods, fast foods, and canned soups (see Salt and High-Sodium Foods, page 308). For early detection of elevated blood pressure, blood pressure checks should be done on a regular basis (at least once a month) throughout pregnancy. Following are some of the most common warning symptoms of hypertension. Call your doctor right away if you notice any of them.

- Severe or constant headaches
- Swelling, especially in the face
- Blurred vision and sensitivity to light
- Pain in the upper right part of the abdomen
- Sudden weight gain of more than 1 pound per day, or 10 to 12 pounds in 5 days

Sometimes gestational hypertension can lead to a condition called preeclampsia—diagnosed as a combination of high blood pressure and protein in the urine at 20 weeks of gestation. When preeclampsia causes seizures, the condition becomes eclampsia, which can result in fetal complications, low birth weight, premature birth, stillbirth, and serious health risks for the mother.[23] At greatest risk for preeclampsia are:

- Women with chronic hypertension or high blood pressure levels before becoming pregnant
- Women who developed high blood pressure or preeclampsia during a previous pregnancy, especially if these conditions occurred early on
- Women who are obese prior to pregnancy

drugs: side effects and safety

Be sure your doctor is aware of any prescription medications or over-the-counter drugs you are taking if you are trying to get pregnant or are pregnant. All medications, including hemorrhoid treatments and cold remedies, should be cleared with your doctor or nurse if you are pregnant. Illegal drugs, such as cocaine, crack, and marijuana, may lead to premature delivery and contribute to low birth weight, fetal distress, neonatal addiction, and death. Infants born to substance abusers can suffer from withdrawal symptoms at birth, and they run the risk of sudden infant death.

- Pregnant women under the age of twenty or over the age of forty
- Pregnant women carrying multiples
- Pregnant women with diabetes, kidney disease, rheumatoid arthritis, lupus, or scleroderma

No one knows what causes preeclampsia or eclampsia or how to prevent it. New research on possible nutrition intervention indicates that diets high in fiber, potassium, calcium, magnesium, omega-3 fatty acids, antioxidants (vitamins E and C), and vitamin B_6 may help prevent them. Unfortunately, there are no conclusive guidelines to date.[24]

▶ *Iron Deficiency Anemia*

Iron deficiency anemia is most commonly caused by low iron stores prior to pregnancy, or from blood loss during pregnancy. Certain preexisting or inherited medical conditions can increase the risk of iron deficiency during pregnancy. The most common are sickle cell anemia, an inherited form of anemia occurring primarily in African-Americans and women from South and Central America, and thalassemia, an inherited form of anemia, occurring mostly in people of Mediterranean origin and some women of Asian origin.

Pregnant women suffering from iron deficiency anemia can experience fatigue, shortness of breath, paleness, dizziness, light-headedness, or heart palpitations. Anemia can lead to infection, premature labor, low birth weight, and a decreased ability to tolerate blood loss during childbirth. Increased iron supplementation and a high-iron diet (see Iron Sources, page 38) may be prescribed by a doctor. Be sure to take all iron supplements with citrus juice, not milk, as calcium can interfere with iron absorption. Leaf tea, coffee, and high-phytate foods also limit iron absorption. (For more information on iron absorption and phytate foods, see chapter 4, Vegetarian and Vegan Delights, page 180.)

▶ *Teenage Pregnancy*

Pregnant teenagers, eighteen years old or younger, have more nutritional requirements than pregnant adults. Teens have to meet their own increased nutritional needs for growth as well as the needs of the developing fetus. Generally, in addition to all of the standard nutrient intake requirements for pregnant women, a pregnant teenager requires 75 to 85 grams of protein, 1,300 milligrams of calcium, 1,250 milligrams of phosphorus, and approximately 400 to 500 additional calories (younger teens will need more calories). A pregnant adolescent should be counseled by her doctor, nurse, and registered dietitian for a meal plan that addresses all of her needs. Meal frequency should be evaluated, as teens occasionally skip meals due to school and other activities. Also, the importance of adequate weight gain should be stressed to pregnant teens who may be hesitant to gain weight for fear of becoming fat.

Teens should be strongly encouraged to give up alcohol, drugs, and smoking. Anemia, gestational hypertension, premature deliveries, depression, and babies with low birth weight can be associated with teen pregnancies. Getting prenatal care as early as possible will lead to a healthier baby and a healthier teen mother.

Pregnancy After 35

Pregnancy after 35 is not uncommon today. In fact, more and more women are following this trend. The good news is that pregnancies at this age are generally healthy, although it is good to know what possible risks are involved. Mothers who are over 35 are more likely than younger women to experience gestational diabetes, placental abnormalities, high blood pressure, preeclampsia, miscarriage, premature labor, and stillbirth. Also, babies born to older mothers are more prone to genetic disorders, premature birth, and low birth weight. All this said, older pregnant women are closely monitored by their physicians to try to prevent these problems from arising and to keep them, and their babies, as healthy as possible. Unless a condition pops up, pregnancy dietary recommendations are the same as for younger women. Exercise plans should be discussed with your health care provider, especially if exercise was not a part of your prepregnancy lifestyle.

Multiple Pregnancies

Pregnant women carrying twins, triplets, or more have a particular challenge meeting increased nutritional needs. The calorie and weight gain requirements are not double or triple that of a single pregnancy. Generally, on top of the normal pregnancy requirements, a woman carrying twins needs an additional 300 calories per day, and a woman carrying triplets needs an additional 600 calories per day. Because of this increased number of calories, a woman might prefer to eat frequent small meals during the day, which will also help control indigestion and heartburn. The total weight gain for a woman with twins is about 35 to 45 pounds, and 45 to 55 pounds for triplets. Protein, calcium, iron, magnesium, and folic acid requirements increase as well, and a doctor should be consulted for specific recommendations. A woman pregnant with multiples needs to consult a registered dietitian for a customized meal plan appropriate for her situation.

Diabetes During Pregnancy

While some women have diabetes before becoming pregnant, others develop gestational diabetes (also called GDM), usually during the third trimester of pregnancy. Gestational diabetes occurs when a pregnant woman cannot produce enough insulin, or her body tissues do not properly utilize the insulin she produces, resulting in an excess amount of glucose (blood sugar) in the blood. Gestational diabetes is usually caused by changes in a pregnant woman's metabolism and hormone production and usually goes away after the birth of the baby. However, women with gestational diabetes are at increased risk of developing diabetes in the future and of developing gestational diabetes in any later pregnancies. Women most at risk for gestational diabetes usually fit into one of the following categories:

- Women over the age of thirty
- Women obese prior to pregnancy
- Women who experience excessive weight gain during pregnancy
- Women with a family history of diabetes
- Women with a previous delivery of a 9.5-pound (or larger) baby, or a stillborn

All pregnant women should be tested for gestational diabetes using the glucose control test (GCT) between the twenty-fourth and twenty-eighth weeks of pregnancy. If diabetes is detected, your doctor, a diabetes nurse practitioner, and a registered dietitian will work closely with you to monitor your diet and exercise, your baby's weight gain, and your blood sugar level. Your doctor will also discuss possible complications during pregnancy and delivery, and potential problems with newborns. Any type of diabetes requires special nutritional attention in the form of a diabetic diet customized for pregnancy. One diabetic diet is based on the Exchange System created by the American Diabetes Association. Recipes in *Eating for Pregnancy* provide ADA exchange values and can be incorporated into a gestational diabetic diet. Another is based on counting carbohydrates.

If you have diabetes prior to pregnancy, it is critical that you plan ahead for your pregnancy. The American Diabetes Association suggests that a diabetic woman considering pregnancy should try to maintain good blood glucose control for three to six months before she plans to get pregnant. The first few weeks of pregnancy, when many women don't even know they are pregnant, is a crucial time for the development of vital organs, and tight blood glucose control is essential in order to prevent birth defects.[25]

▶ *General Recommendations for Pregnant Women with Gestational Diabetes*

- Consult a registered dietitian for an appropriate meal plan for optimal blood glucose control.
- Read food labels to know the composition of foods.
- Avoid sugar, honey, molasses, syrup, fruits canned in syrup, all sodas, sweetened beverages, candies, jams, jellies, cookies, cakes, pies, doughnuts, gum, frosted cereals, candy bars, ice cream, hot chocolate—you get the picture!
- Avoid fruit juices.
- Avoid alcohol.
- Try to eat your meals and snacks at the same time every day to avoid hypoglycemia.
- Measure your food after it is cooked, for accurate portion sizes.
- Try to include all servings in each meal.
- Do not eat anything for two hours after you finish your meals.
- Do not skip meals or snacks.
- Remember that you are on a customized diet to control your blood sugar and not to lose weight.
- See Tips for Diabetics Dining Out on page 276.

Charting a Healthy Course

From decades of experience working as a perinatal nutritionist—answering questions and giving advice to thousands of women—Rose Ann has discovered that pregnant women want not only nutritional information, they want really good, family-friendly recipes that use that information too. The recipes collected in *Eating for Pregnancy* are designed to be nutrient dense, easy to make, and pleasing to everyone—family and friends alike, including young eaters. In this section, we explain how to read the nutritional breakdowns and how to create balanced menus using home-cooked meals and store-bought foods.

UNDERSTANDING THE NUTRITIONAL BREAKDOWNS OF THE RECIPES

Deciphering nutritional information on labels and in cookbooks can be a bit difficult. In an attempt to simplify things, we ask the question, "What's in this for baby and me?" The answers that follow list nutrients that include 20 percent or more of the Daily Value per serving based on a 2,000 calorie nonpregnancy diet. You may want to go one step further to figure out exactly how these percentages compare with your pregnancy requirements. To do this you will need to review the values in the Approximate Nutritional Information at the bottom of each recipe and compare them to the Daily Nutrients for Pregnancy and Lactation chart on page 9.

The recipe headnote descriptions "excellent source of," "high in," or "rich in," preceding certain nutrients contain 20 percent or more of the Daily Values per serving and they correspond to the answers to "What's in this for baby and me?" Other nutrients listed as a "good source of" provide between 10 percent and 19 percent of the Daily Values per serving. (Both these percentage figures are based on a 2,000 calorie nonpregnancy diet.) This wording was carefully chosen to comply with the 1990 Food and Drug Administration labeling system to describe ranges of nutrient content in foods.

All the nutritional values (unless otherwise stated) were calculated using Nutritionist Pro software from First DataBank (2002 and 2004 First DataBank, Inc.). All ingredients in each recipe (except optional toppings) were included in the calculations for the Approximate Nutritional Information.

Every recipe in *Eating for Pregnancy* contains the following breakdowns: calories (cals.), protein (grams), carbohydrates (grams), fat (grams), fiber (grams), sodium (milligrams), and diabetic exchanges (based on the ADA exchange system). Vitamins and minerals are also listed if a recipe provides 20 percent or more of the Daily Value per serving. The major B vitamins—thiamine, riboflavin, and niacin—were viewed as a group. Each of their individual nutritional values had to meet the 10 percent or 20 percent of the Daily Value criteria for the food or recipe to be considered a good or an excellent source. Omega-3 and omega-6 fatty acids are not listed because they are not part of the software package.

In some recipes you will notice that the portion size listed next to the ADA exchange value was reduced to be more diabetic friendly. The word FREE mentioned in some of the ADA exchanges indicates foods with relatively few calories, less than 20 calories per serving. It is advisable for diabetics to limit FREE foods to a total of fifty to sixty calories per day, divided between meals and snacks.

Also, the ▼ symbol following some of the recipe titles at the beginning of each chapter indicates that the dish is suitable for vegan diets. There are 35 vegan recipes scattered throughout this book. Many vegetarian recipes can be made vegan by switching an ingredient or two. Tofu can be substituted for protein sources, such as chicken or beef, in many of the main-course recipes.

CREATING TASTY MENUS

Designing healthy meals is really quite simple. Think of the six major food groups—carbohydrates, proteins, dairy, grains, fruits and vegetables, and fats—and make sure you incorporate all of them daily. Each recipe (except the desserts and a few others) comes with *Complete Meal Ideas*, which is intended to give you a plan of how to combine foods to maximize your nutrient absorption.

Because some women like to have daily menus, we have included seven 2,000-calorie menus for pregnant women. If you require more than 2,000 calories, fill in with snacks (see Healthy Snacks for 100 to 200 Calories, page 346), and if you need to eliminate calories, cut back on portion sizes or do away with desserts. Chapter Four: Vegetarian and Vegan Delights (page 180) offers seven vegetarian and vegan menus. Make substitutions to suit your budget and tastes. Start with a shopping cart filled with healthy foods, and your meals will automatically get off to a healthy start. Finally, remember, meals are meant to be enjoyed.

2,000-calorie menus for seven days

Day One

Breakfast
1 cup fortified whole grain breakfast cereal
1 cup reduced-fat (2%) milk
1 slice whole wheat bread, toasted
1 tablespoon peanut butter
½ cup calcium-fortified orange juice

Lunch
1 whole wheat pita
½ cup hummus (see Healthy Hummus, page 175)
5 cherry tomatoes, 4 cucumber slices, and 1 cup mixed greens with 1 tablespoon
light salad dressing (see Four Delicious Homemade Salad Dressings, page 166)
1 peach

Snack
1 granola bar
1 cup low-fat blueberry yogurt

Dinner
4 ounces store-bought roasted chicken breast
1 medium-size baked potato
2 tablespoons reduced-fat sour cream
½ cup broccoli florets
¾ cup coleslaw (see Lemony Coleslaw, page 171)
1 cup reduced-fat 2% milk
½ cup frozen low-fat vanilla yogurt

Nutrition Information for Day One
Calories: 1,956 cals   Fat: 49 g
Carbohydrates: 294 g   Protein: 99 g
Fiber: 29 g   Iron: 35 mg
Calcium: 2,671 mg   Folic Acid: 877 mcg

Day Two

Breakfast
1 egg, scrambled
2 slices whole wheat bread
¾ cup cantaloupe
1 cup calcium-fortified orange juice

Lunch
1 sandwich made with 3 ounces leftover roasted chicken on whole wheat bread
with lettuce and tomato slices
8 baby carrots and 5 celery sticks with 2 tablespoons light ranch dressing
1 cup reduced-fat 2% milk

Snack
1 apple
1 tablespoon peanut butter

Dinner
1½ cups spaghetti with meat sauce (see Spaghetti with Meat Sauce, page 286)
1 tablespoon Parmesan cheese
2 cups romaine lettuce with 2 tablespoons light dressing
(see Four Delicious Homemade Salad Dressings, page 166)
1 cup low-fat vanilla yogurt with 3 tablespoons granola
(see Fruit-Filled Granola, page 370)

Nutrition Information for Day Two
Calories: 1,999 cals
Fat: 53 g
Carbohydrates: 274 g
Protein: 110 g
Fiber: 28 g
Iron: 16 mg
Calcium: 1,537 mg
Folic Acid: 563 mcg

Day Three

Breakfast
1 medium whole wheat bagel, toasted
2 tablespoons cream cheese
1 cup fresh papaya or mango
1 cup reduced-fat 2% milk

Lunch
1½ cups bean soup (see Black Bean Soup with Cilantro, page 100)
5 whole wheat crackers with 2 ounces cheddar cheese
1 orange
1 cup reduced-fat 2% milk

Snack
¼ cup hummus (see Healthy Hummus, page 175)
½ whole wheat pita

Dinner
4 ounces meat loaf (see Best-Ever American Meat Loaf, page 288)
1 cup brown rice
8 asparagus spears
2 cups mixed green salad with 2 tablespoons light French dressing
½ cup frozen low-fat vanilla yogurt with ½ cup fresh strawberries

Nutrition Information for Day Three
Calories: 2,074 cals
Fat: 66 g
Carbohydrates: 294 g
Protein: 99 g
Fiber: 36 g
Iron: 16 mg
Calcium: 1,672 mg
Folic Acid: 521 mcg

Day Four

Breakfast
1 pack instant oatmeal
1 cup reduced-fat 2% milk
1 banana

Lunch
1 serving grilled chicken Caesar salad (from a restaurant)
1 cup low-fat vanilla yogurt

Snack
1 plain brown rice cake
½ cup mandarin oranges, canned in natural juice

Dinner
2 slices vegetarian pizza
¾ cup sautéed zucchini
½ cup raspberry sorbet

Nutrition Information for Day Four
Calories: 1,984 cals
Fat: 77 g
Carbohydrates: 238 g
Protein: 95 g
Fiber: 19 g
Iron: 13 mg
Calcium: 1,540 mg
Folic Acid: 298 mcg

Day Five

Breakfast
1 oat bran muffin (see Bran Muffins with Dried Cranberries, Walnuts, and
Candied Ginger, page 71)
1 tablespoon peanut butter
1 fruit smoothie with yogurt (see Super Fruit Smoothies, page 76)

Lunch
1 Salad Bar Salad (2 cups romaine lettuce, 1 hard-boiled egg, ½ cup low-fat
cottage cheese, 1 tomato, 5 cucumber slices, and 2 tablespoons light salad
dressing)
1 whole wheat dinner roll
½ cup fresh pineapple slices

Snack
1 cup low-fat vanilla yogurt
¼ cup granola (see Fruit-Filled Granola, page 370)
½ cup fresh blueberries

Dinner
4 ounces grilled or broiled pork chops (see Spice-Rubbed Pork Chops,
page 311)
1 cup sweet potato or sweet potato casserole (see Southern-Style Sweet Potato
Casserole, page 239)
¾ cup green beans
1 cup reduced-fat 2% milk
½ cup unsweetened applesauce (see Applesauce with Dried Apricots and
Cranberries, page 374)

Nutrition Information for Day Five
Calories: 1,994 cals Fat: 55 g
Carbohydrates: 275 g Protein: 109 g
Fiber: 31 g Iron: 14 mg
Calcium: 1,418 mg Folic Acid: 506 mcg

Day Six

Breakfast
2 whole wheat or enriched waffles (see Whole Wheat Pecan Waffles, page 53)
2 tablespoons maple syrup
½ cup fresh blueberries
1 cup reduced-fat 2% milk

Lunch
1 grilled cheese sandwich on whole wheat bread with 2 slices of cheese
(see Grilled Cheese Sandwich, page 119)
1 cup reduced-fat 2% milk
1 oatmeal cookie with raisins
1 banana

Snack
1 fruit smoothie with yogurt (see Super Fruit Smoothies, page 76)

Dinner
4 ounces wild Atlantic salmon, grilled, sautéed, or roasted
(see Roasted Salmon with Papaya Salsa, page 327)
2 cups mixed greens with 2 tablespoons light salad dressing
1 cup whole wheat couscous
½ cup broccoli florets
¾ cup mango sorbet

Nutrition Information for Day Six
Calories: 2,010 cals
Fat: 43 g
Carbohydrates: 324 g
Protein: 87 g
Fiber: 25 g
Iron: 14 mg
Calcium: 1,518 mg
Folic Acid: 405 mcg

Day Seven

Breakfast
2 slices French toast prepared with 2% milk (see French Toast Banana
Sandwich, page 55)
1 cup calcium-fortified orange juice
1 banana

Lunch
½ cup tuna salad sandwich on whole wheat bread with romaine lettuce and
tomatoes
(see Tuna Salad Sandwich, page 123)
1 dill pickle
1 cup reduced-fat 2% milk
1 apple

Snack
⅓ cup dried apricots
1 granola bar

Dinner
4 ounces flank steak, or other lean beef steak, grilled (see Flank Steak with
Salsa Verde, page 290)
1 cup pasta salad (see Noodles with Spinach, Red Bell Peppers, and Sesame
Dressing, page 148)
½ cup asparagus
½ cup frozen low-fat vanilla yogurt

Nutrition Information for Day Seven
Calories: 1,980 cals
Fat: 55 g
Carbohydrates: 283 g
Protein: 99 g
Fiber: 28 g
Iron: 16 mg
Calcium: 1,079 mg
Folic Acid: 399 mcg

FOOD GROUPS AND SERVING SIZES
FOR PREGNANT WOMEN

▶ *Whole Grains (6 to 11 servings per day)*
   1 slice bread (preferably whole wheat or bran)
   ½ bagel or English muffin (preferably whole wheat)
   1 tortilla
   ½ cup cooked oatmeal or Cream of Wheat
   ⅓ cup cooked rice, bulgur wheat, or barley
   ½ cup bran or wheat flakes or ¾ cup unsweetened cereal
   ¼ cup wheat germ
   6 whole wheat crackers
   ½ cup cooked enriched pasta or couscous

▶ *Fruits and Vegetables*
   (Fruits: 2 to 4 servings per day, Vegetables: 3 to 5 servings per day)
   Choose at least one serving rich in vitamin A and one rich in vitamin C.
   (See Vitamin A and C Fruit and Vegetable Sources, page 350.)

▶ *Meat and Meat Substitutes (2 to 3 servings per day)*
   3 ounces lean beef, poultry, veal, or pork
   3 ounces fish (see Limitations on Certain Fish Consumption, page 335)
   6 ounces shellfish (shrimp)
   ¾ cup canned tuna
   4 ounces tofu = 1 ounce meat
   1 large Grade A egg = 1 ounce meat
   2 tablespoon peanut butter = 1 ounce meat
   1 cup cooked dried beans or peas = 1 ounce meat

▶ *Milk and Dairy (3 to 4 servings per day)*
   1 cup reduced-fat 2% milk
   ¾ cup low-fat or nonfat yogurt
   1 cup low-fat cottage cheese
   1¼ ounces low-fat pasteurized hard cheese or 2 ounces processed cheese
   ½ cup frozen yogurt or ice milk
   1 cup enriched soy beverage
   ⅓ cup pasteurized instant nonfat dry milk

▶ *Fats and Oils (use sparingly)*
   1 teaspoon margarine or butter
   1 teaspoon mayonnaise (1 tablespoon reduced-fat or light mayonnaise)
   ¼ large avocado
   1 teaspoon vegetable or plant oil
   1 tablespoon cream cheese (2 tablespoons low-fat cream cheese)
   2 tablespoons nuts
   2 tablespoons sour cream
   1 tablespoon salad dressing

iron sources

Food	Serving Size	Iron (mg)
Blackstrap molasses	2 tablespoons	7.0
All-Bran cereal	½ cup	4.5
Cooked soybeans	½ cup	4.4
Canned oysters	2 ounces	3.7
Cooked spinach	½ cup	3.2
Cooked lentils	½ cup	3.2
Baked potato with skin	1 potato	2.7
Cooked split peas	½ cup	2.5
Beef (short loin)	3 ounces	2.3
Cooked chickpeas	½ cup	2.3
Tempeh	½ cup	2.2
Green soybeans	½ cup	2.2
Cooked pinto beans	½ cup	2.2
Flour tortillas	2 tortillas	2.1
Cooked lima beans	½ cup	2.0
Molasses	2 tablespoons	1.8
Cooked black beans	½ cup	1.8
Ground beef patty	3 ounces	1.7
Tofu	4 ounces	1.7
Whole wheat bread	2 slices	1.6
Almonds, dry roasted	¼ cup	1.5
Canned kidney beans	½ cup	1.5
Quick-cooked oatmeal (prepared with water)	1 cup	1.5
Lamb loin	3 ounces	1.5
Prune juice	4 ounces	1.5
Romaine lettuce	2 cups	1.2
Sunflower seeds	¼ cup	1.2
Turkey breast	3 ounces	1.1
Dried figs	¼ cup	1.1
Dried apricots	5 halves	1.0
Wheat germ	2 tablespoons	1.0
Avocado	½ avocado	1.0

no more boring breakfasts

〜

DURING PREGNANCY you will quickly realize that you won't get very far without something in your stomach—especially if you are suffering from morning sickness. Health professionals have long considered breakfast the most important meal of the day. A nutritious breakfast provides the protein, energy, and vitamins needed to get you through the morning and the rest of the day. Admittedly, it can be hard to find the time for breakfast, especially if you have young, demanding children to dress and feed, and a deadline to get yourself out the front door. While everyone's morning routine varies, working in breakfast will become essential during the months ahead. Here are a few tips to help get your day off to a healthy start.

SOME BASIC ADVICE

- Make breakfast a habit. You'll be surprised at how quickly it becomes a good habit for the entire family.
- Wake up fifteen minutes earlier to be able to sit down for breakfast and try to eat slowly. Sitting down to breakfast and all meals will reduce indigestion during pregnancy.
- Start your day with a piece of fresh fruit or fruit juice, or a glass of water.
- Try to get something warm in your stomach. Warm cereal, eggs, decaffeinated coffee or tea, or just plain hot water will do.
- Plan a week's worth of breakfasts so you are not faced with empty cabinets in the morning.
- Use the weekends to make breakfast treats you can refrigerate or freeze to enjoy during the week.
- Women on the go or on bed rest can get a lot of mileage from muffins, particularly low-fat varieties, which can be refrigerated or frozen. Topped with nut butter, such as peanut, almond, cashew, or soy, muffins can provide a good dose of fiber and protein.
- The mini muffins are all designed to be diabetic friendly.

So, what is a healthy breakfast for pregnant women? A healthy breakfast should include protein, complex carbohydrates, milk or yogurt, fruit or fruit juice, and fat. A well-balanced breakfast, containing one-fourth of the daily calorie and protein requirements, includes about 550 calories and 20 grams of protein, depending on your height and weight. (See the Calorie and Protein Requirements During Pregnancy, page 433.)

Good protein sources for breakfast are eggs, cheese, and nut butters. Eggs can be prepared almost any way you wish as long as the white and yolk are completely cooked. Adding a bit of cheese or tofu to your omelet can give you a double-protein fix. Hard-boiled eggs are ideal. They make a portable breakfast for women on the go, an easy breakfast for women on bed rest, and a great snack any time of day. As tempting as they may be, try to avoid high-fat, salty breakfast meats such as bacon and sausage. Some health and whole foods stores carry soy breakfast strips or sausages that contain no nitrites, nitrates, or MSG, a healthier (though perhaps less satisfying) alternative to bacon.

Complex carbohydrates in the form of high-iron cereals, granola, whole grain muffins, waffles, and whole wheat toast provide essential B vitamins, fiber, and energy. Look for

omega-3-enriched products to add to your breakfast lineup

These products are enriched with ALA in the form of flaxseed. The conversion from ALA to DHA is limited, but they are still excellent choices and offer other nutritional benefits as well.

Eggland's Best, Giving Nature, Nellie's, or The Country Hen O-3-Enriched eggs (100 to 375 mg per egg; Giving Nature has 75 mg of DHA)

Kashi GOLEAN Crunch (500 mg per 1-cup serving)

Kashi TLC (Tasty Little Chewies) Honey Almond Flax (300 mg per bar)

Life Stream Flax Plus Organic Whole Grain Waffles (1,000 mg per 2 waffles)

Nature's Path Flax Plus Pumpkin Raisin Crunch (650 mg per 1-cup serving)

Nature's Path Organic Flax Plus Multibran (500 mg per 1-cup serving)

Nature's Path Organic Flax Plus Red Berry Crunch (800 mg per 1-cup serving)

Peace Cereal Ginger Hemp Granola (400 mg per 1-cup serving)

Smart Balance Omega Natural Peanut Butter (1,000 mg per 2-tablespoon serving)

Van's Wheat Free Flax Waffles (1,000 mg per 2 waffles)

Omega Plus Oil: A rich natural source of 3, 6, and 9 plus the vital antioxidants of extra-virgin cold-pressed olive, avocado, and flaxseed oils

all-natural cereal and granola bars

Cereal and granola bars can be a great way to satisfy hunger and get nutrients and protein (some contain up to 16 grams of protein per bar), especially for busy moms-to-be.

CEREAL BARS

Barbara's Puffins Cereal and Milk Bars
Cascadian Farms Organic Granola Bars
Health Valley Organic Breakfast Bars
Kashi GOLEAN High Protein and Fiber Bars

GRANOLA BARS

Nature Valley Chewy Granola
Nature's Path Organic Granola Bars
Odwalla Bars
Power Bar Pria
Pro Bars
Save the Forest Organic Cereal Bars and Trail Mix Bars
Soy Joy
Zone Perfect All Natural Nutrition Bars
Kashi TLC (Tasty Little Chewies) Honey Almond Flax

cereals fortified with 100 percent of the daily value of folic acid and iron (see Cereals that Contain 100 Percent of the Daily Value of Folic Acid, page 42). Vegetarians, particularly vegans, should choose cereals fortified with 100 percent of the daily value of vitamin B_{12} (see Cereals that Contain 100 Percent of the Daily Value of Vitamin B_{12}, page 43). Raisins and dried fruit increase your fiber intake; but if you need to watch your sugar intake, it is best to avoid cereals with dried fruit.

A source of calcium—such as milk, yogurt, or low-fat cottage cheese—is recommended at every meal, particularly breakfast. For some women, milk and other dairy products are not easily tolerated in the morning, especially during the first trimester. If this is true for you, try consuming dairy products later in the day with a snack or with another meal. Calcium-enriched products, from fruit juices to breads, are a real bonus for pregnant women. Many of the breakfast recipes give the option of a Calcium Boost by adding pasteurized instant nonfat dry milk to pancake and waffle batters, fruit smoothies, and other dishes. Experiment with your favorite recipes and store-bought products to see how powdered milk can add extra calcium to your diet.

Fruit, preferably fresh, or packed in its natural juices, has essential vitamins and calories for a quick pick-me-up in the morning. A cut-up orange or half a grapefruit is the ideal breakfast fruit because it provides vitamins and fiber. Any fresh fruit is generally a better choice than fruit juice because whole fruits contain more fiber and are metabolized more slowly. Freeze-dried fruits, such as raspberries, bananas, and mangoes (high

breakfast cereals that contain
100 percent of the daily value of folic acid

Following is a list of some cereals that are enriched with 100 percent of the Daily Value (DV) of folic acid based on a 2,000-calorie diet for nonpregnant women.

General Mills Harmony
General Mills Multi-Grain Cheerios
General Mills Multi Bran Chex
General Mills Wheat Chex
General Mills Total Corn Flakes
General Mills Whole Grain
Kellogg's All-Bran Original
Kellogg's All-Bran with Extra Fiber
Kellogg's All-Bran Bran Buds
Kellogg's Complete Wheat Bran Flakes
Kellogg's Crispix
Kellogg's Almond Crunch with Raisins
Kellogg's Low Fat Granola with Raisins
Kellogg's Low Fat Granola without Raisins
Kellogg's Müeslix
Kellogg's Just Right Fruit and Nut
Kellogg's Product 19
Kellogg's Smart Start
Kellogg's Special K

in vitamin C or A, iron, or potassium) can be added to muffin, pancake, or waffle batters; hot or cold cereals; and fruit salads.

Fat is recommended for breakfast and at every meal. However, this does not give you the liberty to drown your whole wheat bagel in cream cheese, or to make your waffles soggy with butter. It simply means that if the other components of your breakfast are completely fat-free, spread 1 teaspoon of butter or tub margarine on your toast. A small amount of fat is necessary at every meal to provide calories for energy, and as a source of the fat-soluble vitamins A, D, E, and K.

MORNING SICKNESS AND TIPS FOR COPING

Some degree of nausea and vomiting occurs in about 50 percent of all pregnancies. It usually starts around the second month of pregnancy and lasts until about the fourth. It is called morning sickness because it commonly occurs in the morning, but it can occur

cereals that contain 100 percent of the daily value of vitamin B_{12}

Following is a list of some cereals that are enriched with 100 percent of the Daily Value (DV) of vitamin B_{12} based on a 2,000-calorie diet for nonpregnant women.

Kellogg's Product 19
Kellogg's Complete All Bran Wheat Bran Flakes
Kellogg's Just Right Fruit and Nut
Kellogg's Müeslix
Kellogg's Low-Fat Granola with or without Raisins
Kellogg's All Bran Original, Bran Buds, and Extra Fiber
General Mills Total Corn Flakes
General Mills Total Whole Grain
General Mills Total Raisin Bran
General Mills Total Brown Sugar and Oats

anytime and can last all day. It is generally believed that pregnancy hormones are the culprits of morning sickness. Why some women are affected by the increased hormonal levels and others are not remains a medical mystery. There is no cure for morning sickness. Listen to your body and figure out what works best for you. Eating small, frequent, low-fat meals generally improves food tolerance.

If you are suffering from morning sickness it is vital that you keep your body hydrated and get in as much nourishment as possible to avoid weight loss and dehydration. If vomiting becomes severe or persistent, contact your physician immediately. Following are a few tips to help you get through the morning and the rest of the day.

Tips for Coping with Morning Sickness

- Before you get out of bed in the morning eat dry toast, crackers, or cookies—whatever works best. Allow about 10 minutes for the food to settle before rising.
- Move slowly upon waking—allow yourself a few extra minutes when getting out of bed to balance your body and brain.
- Keep dry crackers with you at all times to satisfy sudden hunger and to quell nausea.
- Have breakfast items on hand so you don't have to go rummaging through your cupboards or refrigerator. See page 48 for a list of breakfast items to have on hand throughout pregnancy.
- Avoid sudden movement after eating or drinking.

- Don't let your stomach go empty—eat small, frequent meals. Small meals are easier to digest than large ones.
- Try to include protein in your meals, especially dinner.
- Drink plenty of fluids, particularly if you are losing fluids through vomiting. Try to eat fruits and vegetables with a high water content, such as melons, citrus fruits, and salads.
- Don't mix liquids and solids—eat and then wait twenty minutes before drinking.
- Avoid greasy or fatty fried foods, especially fast food.
- Avoid highly seasoned foods.
- Avoid caffeinated beverages.
- Eat popsicles, fruit ice, or sherbet between meals. Chew ice or suck on an ice cube. Sip cold Gatorade, ginger ale, or lemonade.
- When you cook, open windows to eliminate cooking odors.
- Get plenty of rest. Physical and emotional fatigue can exacerbate nausea.
- Get plenty of fresh air. Go for a walk in the middle of the day. Make sure your workspace is well-ventilated and not too hot. Take deep breaths of fresh air from time to time.
- Take your prenatal vitamins at night. Consult your doctor to change brands if your vitamin makes you nauseous (some brands are more easily tolerated). Continue taking a folic acid supplement even if you stop taking a prenatal vitamin.
- Do not take any medication or supplements for nausea or vomiting unless prescribed by your doctor.

RECIPE NOTES

Almost anyone—pregnant or not—will agree that the early-morning weekday hours are a difficult time to cook and clean up. The recipes included in this chapter are intended for when you have the time and energy to make something homemade for breakfast, or when your dietary requirements call for increased protein or calcium and you need some ideas to help make that happen.

Anyone with young children knows that picky eating goes with the territory. Despite their finicky palates, it is important to continuously offer children a range of healthy foods, especially for breakfast. If you invest some time and energy into making homemade breakfast treats, you may soon hear your children (and others) asking for your special waffles, the big pizza pancake, your star-shaped French toast, or your yummy banana muffins.

no more boring breakfasts

Breakfast Pizza Pancake

Whole Wheat Pecan Waffles

French Toast Banana Sandwich

Yogurt-Vanilla Pancakes

Diabetic-Friendly Strawberry-Raspberry Syrup

Whole Wheat Popovers

Ricotta Cheese Pancakes with Quick Blueberry Sauce

Cheese Omelet with Breakfast Chili

Brunch Casserole with Spinach and Red Bell Peppers

Banana Muffins with Walnuts and Wheat Germ

Bran Muffins with Dried Cranberries, Walnuts, and Candied Ginger

Summer Fruit Salad ▼

Winter Fruit Salad

Super Fruit Smoothies

Chris Prouty's Saturday Special Blueberry Muffins

Coconut Pancakes with Yogurt, Fresh Fruit, and Honey

▼ Vegan recipe

Some notes about the recipes in this chapter:

- To avoid food-borne illnesses, be sure to thoroughly cook the yolks and whites of eggs and to follow egg safety guidelines (see Eggs and *Salmonella enteritidis*, page 79).
- Use only eggs in their shell or egg products. Avoid farm-fresh eggs.
- Choose DHA-enriched eggs if possible.
- All egg dishes (such as egg-based casseroles, quiches, flans, etc.) should be cooked to 160°F, as shown on an instant-read thermometer inserted into the center of the dish.
- The reduced-fat 2% milk called for in recipes can be replaced by whole milk or a soy beverage.
- All-purpose flour should, ideally, be enriched and unbleached.
- Unsalted butter is preferred, as the salt content varies and can interfere with taste.
- Don't be afraid to experiment and modify the recipes to suit your family's needs and tastes.

pantry items for no more boring breakfasts

Fresh Produce
Baby spinach
Bananas
Blueberries
Cantaloupe
Fresh herbs: cilantro and dill
Kiwi
Lemons
Oranges
Raspberries
Scallions
Strawberries

Dairy and Soy Products
Extra-firm tofu
Grade A large eggs
Grated sharp cheddar cheese
Low-fat or fat-free plain yogurt
Nonfat buttermilk
Part-skim ricotta cheese
Reduced-fat 2% milk
Unsalted butter
Whole milk

Dry Staples
All-Bran cereal
Baking powder
Baking soda
Calcium-enriched bread (such as
    Calcium Rich Roman Meal)
Confectioners' sugar
Desiccated coconut
Dried cranberries
Enriched all-purpose flour (preferably
    unbleached)
French or Italian baguette
Ground flaxseed
Light or dark brown sugar

Nuts: pecans, sliced almonds,
    and walnuts
Pasteurized instant nonfat dry milk
Wheat germ
Whole wheat flour

Canned, Bottled, and Jarred Staples
Black beans
Canola oil
Canola oil cooking spray
Coconut milk
Honey
Jams (any kind)
Maple syrup
Molasses
Orange marmalade
Peeled and diced tomatoes
    (14.5-ounce can)
Roasted red bell peppers

Spices and Flavorings
Candied ginger
Chili powder
Ground cinnamon
Ground cumin
Ground ginger
Pure vanilla extract

Frozen Staples
Apple juice concentrate
Blueberries
Chopped spinach (10-ounce package)
Raspberries
Strawberries
From the Salad Bar
Assorted fresh fruit

breakfast staples to have on hand

- Any whole grain cereal fortified with 100 percent folic acid and 100 percent iron that is also low in fat and sugar (less than 3 grams of sugar per ounce)

- Whole grain fresh or frozen bread, muffins, bagels, or whole wheat English muffins

- Whole grain breads fortified with calcium and folic acid

- Cereal or breakfast bars (see All-Natural Cereal and Granola Bars, page 41)

- Quick-cooking oatmeal or Cream of Wheat cereal

- Frozen whole wheat, fortified waffles

- Yogurt, preferably low-fat or nonfat

- Reduced-fat 2% milk, whole milk, or soy beverages

- Dried fruits (such as raisins, apricots, dates, or prunes) and freeze-dried fruits

- Fresh fruit, sliced fruit, or fruit cups packed in natural juices or light syrup; and no-sugar-added, calcium-fortified fruit juices

- Grade A large eggs, or a protein source such as pasteurized cheese (cottage or ricotta cheese) or nut butters

- Instant breakfast drinks

- Milk fruit shakes, smoothies, and yogurt drinks

- Wheat germ or ground flaxseed to add to cereals or yogurt

four sample breakfast menus using breakfast staples

⌒

¾ cup fortified dry cereal with 8 ounces reduced-fat 2% milk

1 medium fresh fruit or 8 ounces fruit juice

2 slices whole grain toast with 2 tablespoons peanut butter

▪

Whole wheat bagel with ¼ cup part-skim ricotta cheese

1 medium fresh fruit or 8 ounces fruit juice

8 ounces reduced-fat 2% milk or 8 ounces plain low-fat yogurt

▪

2 frozen whole wheat, enriched waffles

1 medium fresh fruit or 8 ounces fruit juice

8 ounces reduced-fat 2% milk or 8 ounces plain low-fat yogurt

▪

¾ cup oatmeal

½ whole wheat English muffin

2 tablespoons peanut butter

1 medium fresh fruit or 8 ounces fruit juice

8 ounces reduced-fat 2% milk or 8 ounces plain low-fat yogurt

PLANNING AHEAD FOR NO MORE BORING BREAKFASTS

▶ *Can Be Made the Same Day*

Breakfast Pizza Pancake

French Toast Banana Sandwich

Whole Wheat Popovers

Ricotta Cheese Pancakes with Quick Blueberry Sauce

Cheese Omelet with Breakfast Chili

Super Fruit Smoothies

Summer Fruit Salad

Winter Fruit Salad

Coconut Pancakes with Yogurt, Fresh Fruit, and Honey

▶ *Can Be Made the Night Before*

Yogurt-Vanilla Pancakes (batter)

Whole Wheat Pecan Waffles (batter)

Summer Fruit Salad

Winter Fruit Salad

Diabetic-Friendly Strawberry-Raspberry Syrup

Quick Blueberry Sauce

Banana Muffins with Walnuts and Wheat Germ

Bran Muffins with Dried Cranberries, Walnuts, and Candied Ginger

Brunch Casserole with Spinach and Red Bell Peppers (make casserole)

Chris Prouty's Saturday Special Blueberry Muffins

▶ *Can Be Refrigerated for up to 3 Days*

Banana Muffins with Walnuts and Wheat Germ

Yogurt-Vanilla Pancakes

Bran Muffins with Dried Cranberries, Walnuts, and Candied Ginger

Breakfast Chili

Diabetic-Friendly Strawberry-Raspberry Syrup

Quick Blueberry Sauce

Chris Prouty's Saturday Special Blueberry Muffins

▶ *Can Be Frozen for up to 1 Month*

Whole Wheat Pecan Waffles

Banana Muffins with Walnuts and Wheat Germ

Bran Muffins with Dried Cranberries, Walnuts, and Candied Ginger

Light and Airy Whole Wheat Popovers

Chris Prouty's Saturday Special Blueberry Muffins

breakfast pizza pancake

What's in this for baby and me? Protein and folic acid.

TOPPED WITH A thin layer of your family's favorite jam or fresh berries, this pancake, high in protein and folic acid, turns into a scrumptious breakfast pizza. Getting your little one to watch this pancake pizza bubble and rise might convince him or her to try a bite.

serves 2

½ cup reduced-fat 2% milk, warmed slightly

2 large eggs

½ cup all-purpose flour

Dash of ground cinnamon or nutmeg
   (optional)

1 tablespoon unsalted butter

OPTIONAL TOPPINGS

   3 tablespoons confectioners' sugar, or to
     taste

   Juice of ½ lemon, or to taste

   Jam

   Fresh berries, washed, and sliced if large

1. Preheat the oven to 425°F.
2. Whisk the milk and eggs in a bowl until well combined. Add the flour and cinnamon and whisk until smooth.
3. Melt the butter in a large (11- or 12-inch) ovenproof seasoned cast-iron skillet or nonstick skillet over high heat. Pour the batter into the skillet and cook over high heat for 1 minute. Transfer the skillet to the oven and bake for 15 minutes, or until puffed and golden brown.
4. Remove the pancake from the oven. Sprinkle generously with confectioners' sugar and a squeeze of lemon juice, if desired. Serve immediately. Pass extra confectioners' sugar at the table. Or, if you are making a breakfast pizza, spread a thin layer of jam over the pancake, then top with fresh berries.

▶ *Calcium Boost:* In a measuring cup, combine ¾ cup milk (instead of the ½ cup listed) with 3 level tablespoons of pasteurized instant nonfat dry milk. Mix until the milk powder has dissolved, then follow the directions in Step 2. Pancakes made with powdered milk tend to be slightly denser and to rise less, but they taste just as good.

▶ *Cooking Tip:* The order in which you mix these ingredients is very important. The wet ingredients should be mixed before adding the dry ingredients. A seasoned cast-iron skillet works best.

marmite and folic acid

The brand name Marmite comes from the French word *marmite,* or stew pot, which is the shape of the distinctive yellow-capped brown jar this 100 percent vegetarian enriched yeast extract comes in. Produced only in the United Kingdom, this salty brown spread is extremely high in folic acid and other B vitamins. Vegemite is the Australian equivalent. Generally speaking, you either love Marmite and become addicted to it or you can't stand it. If you've never tried it, the content of folic acid, B_{12}, and other B vitamins might convince you to take the plunge, especially if you are a vegetarian. It is traditionally eaten thinly spread on buttered toast (or a bagel) or on crisp bread with cottage cheese. According to the nutrition label on the jar, the percentage of daily values (based on a 2,000-calorie diet) in ½ teaspoon (4 grams) of Marmite are as follows:

25% folic acid
15% thiamine
15% riboflavin
30% niacin
10% vitamin B_{12}
2 grams protein

▶ *Diabetic Tip:* Instead of confectioners' sugar, use a low-sugar jam (such as Polaner All Fruit; 2 teaspoons are FREE), or top your pancake with 2 teaspoons (also FREE) Diabetic-Friendly Strawberry-Raspberry Syrup (page 59).

▶ *Complete Meal Ideas:* Serve this breakfast pizza pancake with:
Fresh fruit or juice of your choice
Reduced-fat 2% milk or low-fat yogurt

APPROXIMATE NUTRITIONAL INFORMATION: Serving size: ½ breakfast pizza pancake (without any topping); Calories: 273. cals; Protein: 11 g; Carbohydrates: 27 g; Fat: 13 g; Fiber: .84 g; Sodium: 95 mg; Folic Acid: .75 mcg; Diabetic Exchange: Bread/Starch 2, Fat 2, Meat (Medium Fat) 1

whole wheat pecan waffles

What's in this for baby and me? Protein and calcium.

An EXCELLENT SOURCE of protein and calcium, and a good source of iron, fiber, B vitamins, and vitamin A, these waffles are a weekend treat that can be frozen for weekday breakfast bliss. Diabetic-Friendly Strawberry-Raspberry Syrup (page 59), honey, maple syrup, molasses, and fresh berries are all fabulous toppings.

makes about eighteen 5½ x 2¼-inch waffles

¾ cup whole wheat flour

1 cup all-purpose flour

1 tablespoon baking powder

1 tablespoon sugar

½ teaspoon salt

2 large eggs plus 1 large egg white

6 tablespoons unsalted butter, melted

2 cups reduced-fat 2% milk

½ cup chopped pecans

Canola oil cooking spray, for greasing the
   waffle iron

1. Place the dry ingredients in a large bowl and whisk together.
2. In a second bowl or large measuring cup, whisk together the eggs, egg white, melted butter, and milk.
3. Add the wet ingredients to the dry ingredients and whisk together until well blended. Stir in the nuts.
4. Preheat the waffle iron. Spray the waffle grids with cooking spray. Spoon some batter onto the hot iron and spread to within ¼ inch of the edge of the grids. Close the lid and cook until the waffles are golden brown. Serve immediately.

▶ *Cooking Tip #1:* To prevent cooked waffles from getting soggy, if you are not serving them immediately, place them on a plate lined with a paper towel, or lean them up against each other in a tent-like position to allow the steam to escape. If they do get soggy or cold, toast them briefly in a toaster or place them directly on the rack of a 350°F oven for a few minutes.

▶ *Cooking Tip #2:* A Belgian waffle iron can be used to make these waffles. The yield will be about fourteen 4½ x 4-inch waffles.

▶ *Calcium Boost:* In a measuring cup, combine ⅓ cup pasteurized instant nonfat dry milk with the milk. Mix until the milk powder has dissolved, then follow the directions in Step 2. Waffles made with instant nonfat dry milk tend to be a little heavier.

▶ **Variation:** If you do not have whole wheat flour, you can use 1¾ cups all-purpose flour.

▶ **Storage Tip:** To freeze, cool the waffles, place them in a zip-lock bag, and freeze. To reheat, place the frozen waffles directly on the oven rack or on a piece of foil in a 350°F oven until heated through, about 7 minutes, or reheat them in a toaster. The waffles will keep for about one month in the freezer.

▶ **Diabetic Tip:** Reduce the unsalted butter to 4 tablespoons and omit the pecans. Use a low-sugar jam (such as Polaner All Fruit; 2 teaspoons are FREE), or top your pancake with 2 teaspoons (also FREE) Quick Diabetic-Friendly Strawberry-Raspberry Syrup (page 59).

▶ **Complete Meal Ideas:** Serve these waffles with:
    Fresh fruit or juice of your choice that contains vitamin C
    Reduced-fat 2% milk or low-fat yogurt

waffles unlimited

Frozen "designer" waffles—including multi-grain waffles; organic brands made with flax, hemp, and soy; and fiber-enhanced waffles—seem to be the latest breakfast rage. Bring along a dictionary to decipher the fancy grains. Packaged waffle mixes come in countless new varieties as well. Powdered mixes can easily be enriched with pasteurized instant non-fat dry milk. You will need to experiment to find the right amount to add. When purchasing frozen waffles or packaged waffle mixes, look for those fortified with calcium and folic acid. Add fresh, dried, or frozen berries to waffle or pancake batters for a burst of flavor and vitamin C.

APPROXIMATE NUTRITIONAL INFORMATION: Serving size: 3 whole wheat pecan waffles; Calories: 372 cals; Protein: 11g; Carbohydrates: 34 g; Fat: 22 g; Fiber: 3.3 g; Sodium: 467 mg; Calcium: 246 mg; Diabetic Exchange: Bread/Starch 2, Fat 4.5, Meat (Medium Fat) 1

french toast banana sandwich

What's in this for baby and me? Protein, calcium, and folic acid.

THIS SNAPPY FRENCH toast sandwich is an excellent source of protein, calcium, and folic acid, and a good source of vitamin C, B vitamins, iron, and fiber. It is delicious topped with syrup, honey, cinnamon and sugar, or sliced fresh fruit. This recipe specifies Calcium Rich Roman Meal bread because two slices have as much calcium as one glass of milk!

makes 4 to 5 slices of toast

2 large eggs

½ cup reduced-fat 2% milk

½ tablespoon unsalted butter or canola oil

   cooking spray, for cooking the French toast

4 to 5 slices of calcium-enriched bread (such as Calcium Rich Roman Meal)

2 bananas, sliced

Maple syrup, jam, or your favorite topping

1. In a bowl, mix the eggs and milk.
2. Melt the butter in a large nonstick skillet over medium-high heat. Place a slice of bread in the egg mixture and turn to coat both sides, then add the slice to the skillet and cook for 2 minutes on each side or until thoroughly cooked and golden brown on both sides. Repeat with the remaining bread.
3. As you cook the toast, add some of the sliced bananas to the skillet and cook them, about 2 minutes on each side.
4. Place a slice of the French toast on each plate, top with some of the banana slices, cover with another piece of toast, and serve with your favorite topping.

▶ *Storage Tip:* Cover any leftovers with plastic wrap and refrigerate. To reheat, place the French toast on a plate and microwave for a few seconds.

▶ *Diabetic Tip:* Omit the banana and top the French toast with low-sugar jam (such as Polaner All Fruit; 2 teaspoons are FREE) or 2 teaspoons (also FREE) Quick Diabetic-Friendly Strawberry-Raspberry Syrup (page 59).

▶ *Complete Meal Ideas:* Serve these French toast sandwiches with:
   Fresh fruit (if not using bananas) or juice of your choice that contains vitamin C
   Reduced-fat 2% milk or low-fat yogurt

APPROXIMATE NUTRITIONAL INFORMATION: Serving size: 2 slices of French toast made from calcium-enriched bread and 1 banana; Calories: 332 cals; Protein: 11 g; Carbohydrates: 53 g; Fat: 10 g; Fiber: 3 g; Sodium: 376 mg; Iron: 2 mg; Calcium: 246 mg; Folic Acid: 87 mcg; Diabetic Exchange: Bread/Starch 3, Fat 2, Fruit .5

healthy bagel toppings

Hard cheese (such as cheddar, Swiss, and Monterey Jack)

Ricotta cheese (whole milk or part-skim)

Neufchâtel cheese

Peanut butter or other nut butters

Hard-boiled or fully cooked eggs

Salmon spread

Egg salad (recipe, page 118)

Tuna salad (recipe, page 123)

Chicken salad (recipe, page 120)

Hummus or bean dips (recipes, pages 175 and 179)

Marmite (see page 52)

Tofu spreads

yogurt-vanilla pancakes

What's in this for baby and me? Protein, calcium, and folic acid.

THESE CRÊPE-LIKE pancakes are an excellent source of protein, calcium, and folic acid, and a good source of iron and B vitamins. Let your kids fill their pancakes and roll them up—a fun way to eat and develop fine motor skills at the same time.

makes about 12 six-inch pancakes

One 8-ounce container fat-free plain yogurt	**1 teaspoon pure vanilla extract**
1 cup reduced-fat 2% milk	**1 tablespoon sugar**
2 large eggs	**⅛ teaspoon salt**
2 tablespoons canola oil, plus 1 teaspoon canola oil or canola oil cooking spray for greasing the skillet	**¼ teaspoon baking soda**
	1 cup all-purpose flour

1. Combine the yogurt, milk, eggs, oil, and vanilla extract in a large bowl and whisk together. Add the remaining ingredients and whisk until smooth.
2. Heat the 1 teaspoon canola oil in a large nonstick skillet over medium to medium-high heat until hot, about 3 minutes. Add a little less than ⅓ cup batter to the skillet and immediately swirl the batter to form it into a thin pancake about 6 inches in diameter. Cook the pancake until the surface bubbles and then sets and the underside is golden brown, about 1 minute. Flip the pancake with a wide spatula and cook for 1 more minute. Serve warm.

▶ *Storage Tip:* Cover leftover pancakes with plastic wrap and refrigerate. Reheat in a microwave oven for a few seconds before serving.

▶ *Calcium Boost:* In a measuring cup, combine ⅓ cup pasteurized instant nonfat dry milk with the milk. Mix until the milk powder has dissolved, then follow the directions in Step 2. Pancakes made with powdered milk tend to be slightly denser.

▶ *Diabetic Tip:* Use a low-sugar jam (such as Polaner All Fruit; 2 teaspoons are FREE), or top your pancake with 2 teaspoons (also FREE) Quick Diabetic-Friendly Strawberry-Raspberry Syrup (page 59).

▶ *Complete Meal Ideas:* Serve these pancakes with:
Fresh fruit or juice of your choice that contains vitamin C
Reduced-fat 2% milk or low-fat yogurt

APPROXIMATE NUTRITIONAL INFORMATION: Serving size: 4 plain yogurt-vanilla pancakes; Calories: 387 cals; Protein: 16 g; Carbohydrates: 47 g; Fat: 15 g; Fiber: 1 g; Sodium: 368 mg; Calcium: 285 mg; Folic Acid: 94 mcg; Diabetic Exchange: Bread/Starch 3, Fat 3, Meat (Medium Fat) .5

preventing mild hypoglycemia

Hypoglycemia in people who do not have diabetes is far less common than once believed. However, it can occur under certain conditions, such as early pregnancy, prolonged fasting, and long periods of strenuous exercise. A person with hypoglycemia may feel weak, drowsy, shaky, confused, hungry, and dizzy. Paleness, headache, irritability, sweating, rapid heart beat, and a cold, clammy feeling are also signs of low blood sugar.

Hypoglycemia can be a complication of diabetes. Pregnant diabetics or women diagnosed with gestational diabetes should discuss this condition with their doctor and dietitian to develop a coping plan should it occur. Generally, including a source of protein in your breakfast, eating small frequent meals that also include a source of protein, avoiding long periods without eating, and avoiding concentrated sweets, such as sugar, candy, honey, jam, jelly, syrup, and soft drinks, may help prevent mild hypoglycemia.

diabetic-friendly
strawberry-raspberry syrup

What's in this for baby and me? Vitamin C.

THIS EASY-TO-MAKE syrup is delicious served with any type of store-bought or home-made pancakes, waffles, French toast, or oatmeal. High in vitamin C, it is also a wonderful accompaniment to yogurt, frozen yogurt, or ice cream, and it is great on top of the Reduced-Fat Ricotta Cheesecake (page 353). You can use 1 pound of strawberries (about 4 cups) instead of mixing strawberries and raspberries. You might consider adding a little more sugar to please young eaters.

makes about 2½ cups

½ cup frozen apple juice concentrate

½ cup sugar

2 cups fresh strawberries, washed, hulled, and
   quartered (see Cooking Tip below for
   frozen berries)

2 cups fresh raspberries, rinsed quickly

½ teaspoon pure vanilla extract (optional)

1. Combine the apple juice concentrate and sugar in a large nonstick skillet, stir, and bring to a boil. Reduce the heat and simmer for 5 minutes.
2. Add the berries, stir, and return to a boil. Reduce the heat and simmer, uncovered, for 10 minutes, or until the consistency of a thin syrup. Remove from heat, stir in the vanilla extract, and serve warm or at room temperature. Cover and refrigerate any leftovers.

▶ *Cooking Tip:* Four cups frozen unsweetened berries can be substituted for the fresh berries. Defrost (at room temperature or in a microwave) and drain them, then proceed with the recipe. (Frozen berries may take slightly longer to reach the thin syrup consistency.) Also, you can increase the amount of sugar and eliminate the apple juice concentrate; however, added sugar is not diabetic-friendly.

APPROXIMATE NUTRITIONAL INFORMATION: Serving size: 2 tablespoons strawberry-raspberry syrup; Calories: 81 cals; Carbohydrates: 20 g; Fat: .3 g; Fiber: 2.3 g; Sodium: 4 mg; Vitamin C: 23 mg; Diabetic Exchange: Fruit 1.5, a reduced serving size of 2 teaspoons are FREE

make coffee work for you

The amount of caffeine considered safe during pregnancy continues to be a controversial issue. Abstaining from caffeine altogether is the best approach, but some women just need their coffee. At least try limiting yourself to only one cup of any caffeinated beverage per day. To meet your daily calcium requirements and satisfy your coffee craving at the same time, try increasing the amount of milk (soy beverages included) you add to your coffee. In other words, turn your coffee into a calcium-rich café au lait. The following list of caffeine levels in beverages and food comes from the U.S. Food and Drug Administration and the National Soft Drink Association:[1]

ITEM	MILLIGRAMS OF CAFFEINE	
	AVERAGE MG	RANGE OF MG
Coffee (5-oz cup)		
Brewed, drip method	115	60–180
Brewed, percolator	80	40–170
Instant	65	30–120
Decaffeinated, brewed	3	2–5
Decaffeinated, instant	2	1–5
Espresso (single)	100*	
Cappuccino (single)	100*	
Tea (5-oz cup)		
Brewed, major U.S. brands	40	20–90
Brewed, imported brands	60	25–110
Instant	30	25–50
Iced (12-oz glass)	70	67–76
Some soft drinks (6-oz serving)	18	15–30
Cocoa beverage (5-oz cup)	4	2–20
Chocolate milk beverage (8-oz cup)	5	2–7
Milk chocolate (1 oz)	6	1–15
Dark chocolate, semi-sweet (1 oz)	20	5–35
Baker's chocolate (1 oz)	26	26
Chocolate-flavored syrup (1 oz)	4	4

* The values for espresso and cappuccino are taken from the Women's Nutrition Patient Education Resource Manual.

whole wheat popovers

What's in this for baby and me? Protein.

THESE POPOVERS ARE well worth their forty-minute baking time. High in protein, and a good source of calcium, iron, folic acid, B vitamins, and fiber, they are best eaten straight from the oven with your favorite jam or marmalade.

makes 6 large popovers

½ cup whole wheat flour

½ cup all-purpose flour

1 cup reduced-fat 2% milk

2 large eggs plus 1 large egg white

2 teaspoons canola oil

½ teaspoon salt

Canola oil cooking spray for greasing the
　popover pan

1. Preheat the oven to 450°F. Have ready a six-cup nonstick popover pan.
2. In a large mixing bowl, mix the whole wheat and all-purpose flours. Add the remaining batter ingredients and beat with an electric mixer on high speed for 30 seconds. Scrape down the sides of the bowl and beat 15 seconds more. (Note: Don't be concerned if you see tiny lumps of flour. Mash any bigger lumps against the side of the bowl with the back of a spatula.)
3. Preheat the popover pan in the oven for 2 minutes, then remove it and spray with cooking oil. Divide the batter evenly among the popover cups.
4. Bake for 20 minutes, then reduce the heat to 350°F and bake for 20 more minutes, or until golden brown and puffed. Remove the popovers from the oven and serve immediately.

▶ *Cooking Tip:* To freeze, cool completely, then place the popovers in a zip-lock bag and freeze. To reheat, place the popovers on a piece of foil in a preheated 350°F oven for about 10 minutes. Do not microwave.

▶ *Calcium Boost:* In a measuring cup, combine the milk with ⅓ cup pasteurized instant nonfat dry milk. Mix until the milk powder has dissolved, then follow the directions in Step 2. Note: Calcium-fortified popovers tend to be considerably heavier than those made according to the basic recipe.

▶ *Variation:* A total of 1 cup all-purpose flour can be used instead of whole wheat flour. Popovers made only with all-purpose flour tend to rise more and are lighter.

► *Complete Meal Ideas:* Serve these popovers with:
Fresh fruit or juice of your choice that contains vitamin C
Reduced fat 2% milk or low-fat yogurt

APPROXIMATE NUTRITIONAL INFORMATION: Serving size: 2 whole wheat popovers; Calories: 265 cals; Protein: 13 g; Carbohydrates: 35 g; Fat: 8 g; Fiber: 3 g; Sodium: 488 g; Diabetic Exchange: Bread/Starch 2.5, Fat 1.5, Meat (Medium Fat) 1

the incredible edible egg

Eggs are an excellent source of protein and vitamin B_{12}, especially for pregnant vegetarians. Designer eggs, free of antibiotics and hormones, often enriched with omega-3s, are all the rage. Buy them if you can afford to. Following is the nutritional breakdown of one large hard-boiled egg compared to the recommended daily allowances for pregnant women.

ONE LARGE EGG	RDA FOR PREGNANT WOMEN
6.2 g protein	71 g protein
25 mg calcium	1000 mg calcium
.55 mcg vitamin B_{12}	2.6 mg vitamin B_{12}
.25 mg riboflavin	1.4 mg riboflavin

ricotta cheese pancakes with
quick blueberry sauce

What's in this for baby and me? Protein, calcium, and vitamin C.

No one can turn down a bite of these protein- and calcium-packed ricotta cheese pancakes topped with vitamin C blueberry sauce. The key to making these delicate pancakes is to use as little flour as possible. They might be harder to flip, but the slightly creamy consistency of the finished pancakes is worth the effort. The sauce is also an excellent topping for ice cream or yogurt.

makes nine 2½-inch pancakes

1 cup part-skim ricotta cheese

1 large egg

2 tablespoons sugar

1 teaspoon pure vanilla extract

6 tablespoons all-purpose flour

1 tablespoon orange marmalade or apricot jam

½ tablespoon unsalted butter or canola oil cooking spray, for cooking the pancakes

Quick Blueberry Sauce (recipe follows)

1. Mix the ricotta cheese, egg, sugar, and vanilla extract in a bowl until smooth. Add the flour and orange marmalade and mix until well blended.
2. Melt the butter in a large nonstick skillet over medium-high heat. Add 1 heaping soupspoonful of the pancake batter for each pancake and flatten slightly with the back of the spoon; do not crowd the pancakes in the pan. Cook for 1½ to 2 minutes, or until the bottoms are golden brown. With a wide spatula, very carefully flip each pancake (using a blunt knife to push the pancake onto the spatula) and continue cooking until golden brown on the second side, about 1½ to 2 minutes longer.
3. Top the pancakes with the blueberry sauce and serve immediately.

quick blueberry sauce

yield: about 1 cup

1 pint (about 2 cups) fresh blueberries, washed, or 8 ounces frozen unsweetened blueberries (half a 16-ounce bag)
⅓ cup sugar, or to taste

Combine the blueberries and sugar in a saucepan and bring to a boil, stirring occasionally, over high heat. Continue to cook until the syrup has thickened slightly, about 5 minutes. Serve warm. Cover and refrigerate any leftovers.

▶ **Variation:** An equal amount of pasteurized farmer's cheese can be substituted for the ricotta cheese, although the calcium value will decrease.

▶ **Complete Meal Ideas:** Serve these pancakes with:
   Fresh fruit or juice of your choice
   Reduced-fat 2% milk or low-fat yogurt

APPROXIMATE NUTRITIONAL INFORMATION: Serving size: 3 cheese pancakes; Calories: 260 cals; Protein: 13 g; Carbohydrates: 29 g; Fat: 10 g; Fiber: .7 g; Sodium: 128 mg; Calcium: 237 mg; Diabetic Exchange: Bread/Starch 2, Fat 2

APPROXIMATE NUTRITIONAL INFORMATION: Serving size: 5 tablespoons blueberry sauce; Calories: 135 cals; Protein: .6 g; Carbohydrates: 35 g; Fat: .4 g; Fiber: 3 g; Sodium: 6 mg; Vitamin C: 12 mg; Diabetic Exchange: Fruit 2.5

cheese omelet with breakfast chili

What's in this for baby and me? Protein and vitamin C.

Eggs are an excellent source of protein, especially for vegetarians or women who have an aversion to meat during pregnancy. This omelet is also a good source of calcium, folic acid, and vitamin A. By altering the amounts of yolks and whites in your omelet, you can increase or decrease your iron and cholesterol intake. If your dietary needs call for lots of iron, use the 2 whole eggs in your omelet, because the iron is in the yolk. If you need to watch your cholesterol, use 1 whole egg and 1 egg white.

An excellent source of vitamin C and a good source of protein, calcium, iron, folic acid, and fiber, the breakfast chili is a nutritional powerhouse. Leftovers are delicious for lunch or dinner over rice, topped with grated cheese, or as a snack with baked tortilla chips and melted cheese.

Cheese Omelet

serves 1

2 large eggs
½ teaspoon unsalted butter

2 tablespoons grated cheddar cheese (or any cheese of your choice)
Breakfast Chili (recipe follows)

1. Whisk the eggs and pepper in a bowl; set aside. Melt the butter in a small nonstick skillet over medium-high heat. Add the eggs and allow to cook for about 20 seconds, then, while tilting the skillet, use a spatula to push the cooked egg toward the center of the pan, allowing the raw egg to hit the skillet. Distribute the cheese on top of the eggs, reduce heat to low, and cook for 1 to 2 minutes or until the eggs are cooked through.
2. Flip the omelet in half, cook 10 seconds longer or until there is no visible liquid egg, then transfer to a serving plate. Place some of the breakfast chili on the side and serve immediately.

Breakfast Chili

makes about 4 cups

2 teaspoons canola oil or olive oil
1½ teaspoons chili powder
½ teaspoon ground cumin
One 14.5-ounce can diced tomatoes (do not drain)

1 cup canned black beans, rinsed and drained
4 ounces extra firm tofu, cut into ½-inch cubes and blotted dry with paper towels
¼ cup chopped fresh cilantro

Heat the oil in a large nonstick skillet over medium-high heat. Add the chili powder and cumin and cook for 30 seconds, then add the tomatoes, beans, and tofu, reduce heat to low, and cook for 5 minutes. Mix in the cilantro, and set aside.

▶ *Cooking Tip:* Any leftover black beans or tofu can be tossed into a salad.

▶ *Health Tip 1:* Be sure to cook your eggs thoroughly (both whites and yolks) during pregnancy (see Eggs and *Salmonella enteritidis*, page 79).

▶ *Health Tip 2:* If your doctor has restricted your fat intake, use canola oil cooking spray instead of unsalted butter and use a reduced-fat cheese or omit the cheese.

▶ *Complete Meal Ideas:* Serve this omelet with:
  Fresh fruit or juice of your choice that contains vitamin C
  Reduced-fat 2% milk or low-fat yogurt
  2 slices toast (preferably whole wheat)

APPROXIMATE NUTRITIONAL INFORMATION: Serving size: 1 cheese omelet made with 2 large eggs; Calories: 224 cals; Protein: 16 g; Carbohydrates: 1 g; Fat: 17 g; Fiber: 0 g; Sodium: 214 mg; Diabetic Exchange: Meat/Protein 2, Fat 1

APPROXIMATE NUTRITIONAL INFORMATION: Serving size: ¾ cup breakfast chili; Calories: 128 cals; Protein: 8 g; Carbohydrates: 15 g; Fat: 4 g; Fiber: 5 g; Sodium: 341 mg; Calcium: 95 mg; Vitamin C: 16 mg; Folic Acid: 65 mcg; Diabetic Exchange: Bread/Starch 1, Meat (Medium Fat) 1

swallow your iron supplement with orange juice

Iron and vitamin C are a natural pair. You can increase the amount of iron your body absorbs by consuming a source of vitamin C with iron-rich foods or with your iron supplement. Try not to take your iron supplement with calcium-fortified juices, as calcium can interfere with iron absorption.

brunch casserole
with spinach and red bell peppers

What's in this for baby and me? Protein, calcium, vitamins A and C, and folic acid.

THE CHEESE, EGGS, and milk are all excellent sources of protein and calcium, and the spinach and red peppers are high in vitamins A and C and folic acid. This casserole also gets a good rating for iron, B vitamins, and fiber. One of its best features is that it can be assembled the night before baking.

Vary the ingredients to suit your family's tastes. To avoid a soggy mess, be sure that any fresh vegetables that have a high water content, such as mushrooms, bell peppers, or squash, are sautéed before adding. Almost any type of bread can be used; however, stale slices of French or Italian bread work best. Also, any type of good melting cheese, such as Havarti, Gruyère, Monterey Jack, Fontina, or Colby, can be substituted for the sharp cheddar. For a decadent splurge, half-and-half can be substituted for the whole milk.

serves 6

- 1 tablespoon unsalted butter, softened
- 1 supermarket French or Italian baguette, cut into enough ½-inch slices to make two layers in an 8 x 8 x 2-inch baking dish, spread out on a baking sheet or tray, and left out to dry
- One 10-ounce package chopped frozen spinach, thawed and squeezed dry
- 6 ounces (about 1¾ cups) grated sharp cheddar cheese
- ½ cup jarred roasted red peppers, drained and chopped
- 2 scallions, trimmed and thinly sliced
- 2 tablespoons chopped fresh dill
- 6 large eggs
- 1¾ cups whole milk
- 1½ teaspoons salt
- Freshly ground pepper, to taste

1. Grease an 8 x 8 x 2-inch Pyrex baking dish with most of the butter. Spread any leftover butter on as many bread slices as possible; set aside.
2. Arrange half of the bread slices in a single layer in the baking dish. Scatter half of the spinach, cheese, red peppers, and scallions and dill over the slices. Arrange a second layer of bread on top of the first and cover with the remaining spinach, red peppers, scallions, and dill. Sprinkle half of the remaining cheese on top. Cover the remaining cheese and set aside.
3. Whisk the eggs, milk, salt, and pepper in a bowl. Pour evenly over the casserole and cover with plastic wrap, pressing it directly against the surface. Press gently to make sure that the bread absorbs the liquid. Then place a weight (such as a bag

of rice or a couple of cans) on top of the plastic wrap to keep the bread submerged. Refrigerate for at least 1 hour, or overnight.

4. Remove the casserole from the refrigerator and preheat the oven to 350°F.

5. Just before baking, remove the plastic wrap from the casserole and sprinkle the remaining cheese over the top. Bake for 40 minutes, or until puffed and the middle has set. (Note: The internal temperature of this casserole should reach 165°F on an instant-read thermometer inserted into the center of the dish.) Remove the casserole from the oven and let cool for 10 minutes before serving.

► *Calcium Boost:* In a measuring cup, combine ⅓ cup pasteurized instant nonfat dry milk with the whole milk. Mix until the milk powder has dissolved, then follow the directions in Step 2.

► *Health Tip:* If your doctor has restricted your fat intake use tub margarine instead of unsalted butter, reduced-fat cheddar cheese, and reduced-fat 2% milk. If you need to watch your sodium intake, reduce the salt to ½ teaspoon.

► *Complete Meal Ideas:* Serve this casserole with:
  Fresh fruit or juice of your choice that contains vitamin C
  Reduced-fat 2% milk or low-fat yogurt
  2 slices toast (preferably whole wheat)

APPROXIMATE NUTRITIONAL INFORMATION: Serving size: One-sixth of this brunch casserole; Calories: 453 cals; Protein: 21 g; Carbohydrates: 34 g; Fat: 26 g; Fiber: 3 g; Sodium: 1195 mg; Calcium: 414 mg; Vitamin A: 4,919 IU; Vitamin C: 27 mg; Folic Acid: 136 mcg; Diabetic Exchange: Bread/Starch 2, Fat 2, Meat (Medium Fat) 2

banana muffins with walnuts and wheat germ

~

What's in this for baby and me? Protein, folic acid, and fiber.

Nothing beats a great banana muffin—any time of day. These muffins are an excellent source of protein, folic acid, and fiber, and a good source of iron, vitamin C, and B vitamins.

makes 12 regular muffins or about 40 mini muffins

Canola oil cooking spray for greasing the
   muffin pan (or use muffin cup liners)

¾ cup whole wheat flour

¾ cup all-purpose flour

⅓ cup toasted wheat germ

2 teaspoons baking soda

¼ teaspoon salt

½ cup chopped walnuts or pecans

½ cup packed light brown sugar

⅓ cup canola oil

1 large egg

¼ cup reduced-fat 2% milk

1½ cups coarsely mashed ripe bananas (3 to 4
   large bananas) (see Cooking Tip)

1. Preheat the oven to 350°F. Spray the muffin cups with cooking spray or line them with muffin liners.
2. In a large bowl, whisk together the flours, wheat germ, baking soda, salt, and walnuts until well combined.
3. In a small bowl, combine the brown sugar, canola oil, egg, and milk and whisk until well blended. Add the bananas and mix well, then add to the flour mixture and mix until well blended.
4. Divide the batter evenly among the muffin cups. Bake until a tester inserted into the center comes out clean: 25 to 30 minutes for regular muffins, 10 to 12 minutes for mini muffins. Transfer the muffins to a rack and cool slightly before eating.

▶ *Cooking Tip:* Ripe bananas can be frozen whole and unpeeled (the skin will turn completely brown when frozen) or peeled and mashed. Defrost the pulp or whole bananas at room temperature or in a microwave oven. To facilitate peeling defrosted whole bananas, start at the bottom of the banana rather than at the top stem. Mash the bananas with the back of a fork or a potato masher.

▶ *Variation:* Substitute ¾ cup all-purpose flour for the whole wheat flour.

▶ *Diabetic Tip:* Omit the nuts and use mini muffin pans for baking. Eat only 1 regular muffin or 2 mini muffins.

herbal teas to avoid

Herbal teas should be used sparingly during pregnancy, since the composition and safety of most are unknown. Some herbal teas are probably safe, but several, including lobelia, sassafras, coltsfoot, comfrey, pennyroyal, black cohosh, and blue cohosh, have potentially harmful side effects.[2] All diet, cleansing, laxative, and detoxification teas should be avoided.

▶ *Complete Meal Idea:* Serve these muffins with:
Fresh fruit or juice of your choice that contains vitamin C
Reduced-fat 2% milk or low-fat yogurt (or combine the fruit and
    yogurt in a smoothie—see Super Fruit Smoothies, page 76)
Peanut butter

APPROXIMATE NUTRITIONAL INFORMATION: Serving size: 2 regular-size banana muffins; Calories: 432 cals; Protein: 10 g; Carbohydrates: 58 g; Fat: 20 g; Fiber: 5 g; Sodium: 539 mg; Folic Acid: 79 mcg; Diabetic Exchange (values per 1 muffin): Bread/Starch 2, Fat 2

bran muffins with dried cranberries, walnuts, and candied ginger

What's in this for baby and me? Folic acid and fiber.

QUICK, SIMPLE, AND super tasty, these bran muffins are high in folic acid and fiber, and they are a good source of protein, vitamin C, and B vitamins. The cranberries, ginger, and walnuts are all optional. Feel free to substitute your favorite ingredients—such as raisins, diced dried apricots or pears, and dried cherries.

makes 15 regular muffins or about 52 mini muffins

Cooking spray for greasing the muffin pan (or use muffin cup liners)

3½ cups All Bran cereal

1 cup boiling water

¼ cup canola oil

¾ cup sugar

1 cup nonfat buttermilk

1 large egg

1¼ cups all-purpose flour

1¼ teaspoons baking soda

¼ teaspoon salt

½ teaspoon ground ginger

½ cup dried cranberries or chopped dried apricots

½ cup chopped walnuts

⅓ cup chopped candied ginger

1. Preheat the oven to 400°F. Spray the muffin cups with cooking spray or line with muffin liners.
2. Place the cereal in a small bowl and pour the boiling water over it—do not stir. Set aside.
3. Combine the canola oil and sugar in a large bowl and whisk together. Add the buttermilk and egg and whisk again. Add the flour, baking soda, salt, and ground ginger, if using, and whisk just until well combined. Add the All Bran mixture and mix with a spoon, then add the remaining cranberries, walnuts, and/or candied ginger, if using, and mix just until combined. (The batter will be quite thick.) Let the batter sit at room temperature for 10 minutes.
4. Gently stir the batter, then divide evenly among the muffin cups. Bake until a tester inserted in the center of a muffin comes out clean: about 20 minutes for regular muffins, about 12 minutes for mini muffins. Transfer the muffins to a rack and cool slightly before eating.

▶ *Diabetic Tip:* Omit the dried cranberries, walnuts, and candied ginger. Use mini muffin pans for baking.

▶ **Complete Meal Idea:** Serve these muffins with:
    Fresh fruit or juice of your choice
    Reduced-fat 2% milk or low-fat yogurt (combine the fruit and yogurt
        into a smoothie—see Super Fruit Smoothies, page 76)
    Peanut butter

APPROXIMATE NUTRITIONAL INFORMATION: Serving size: 1 regular bran muffin; Calories: 194 cals; Protein: 5 g; Carbohydrates: 33 g; Fat: 7 g; Fiber: 5 g; Sodium: 203 mg; Folic Acid: 208 mcg; Diabetic Exchange: Bread/Starch 2, Fat 1.5

choosing the right breakfast cereal

▶ **Look for cereals fortified with 100 percent folic acid and 100 percent iron. (See Cereals That Contain 100 Percent of the Daily Value of Folic Acid, page 42.)**

▶ **Look for cereals containing the following first on their ingredient lists: *whole wheat*, *whole grain*, *whole oat flour*, or *rolled oats*. This ensures that the product has not been subject to fiber-robbing refining processes.**

▶ **Look for cereals containing at least 2 grams of fiber per serving. Whole grain products contain fiber, but refined grain products do not.**

▶ **Look for cereals low in sugar. A maximum of 5 grams of sugar (about 1 teaspoon) per serving is advised. Cereals containing dried fruit, such as raisins, are likely to have a higher sugar content, but the nutritional benefits are generally worth the extra sugar.**

▶ **Look for cereals with no more than 2 grams of fat per serving.**

▶ **Vegans and non–meat eaters should look for cereals fortified with 100 percent B_{12}. (See Cereals that Contain 100 Percent of the Daily Value of Vitamin B_{12}, page 43.)**

TOP THREE HIGH-FIBER CEREALS

1. **General Mills Fiber One Cereal (14 g fiber per ½ cup serving)**

2. **Kellogg's All-Bran Cereal (10 g fiber per ½ cup serving)**

3. **Kashi GOLEAN Crunch (8 g fiber per serving)**

winter fruit salad

⌒

What's in this for baby and me? Vitamin C and fiber.

UNLESS YOU LIVE in a tropical climate, or can afford to pay top dollar, summer's sweet fresh fruit becomes a distant memory by late October. Apples, grapes, pears, oranges, and bananas make a wonderful off-season fruit salad. This salad is an excellent source of vitamin C and fiber (especially if the apples and pears are left unpeeled), and the optional yogurt provides calcium. A container of fruit salad kept in a cooler is a fantastic snack and an excellent source of hydration for women on bed rest.

makes about 4 cups

FRUIT SALAD
2 oranges, peeled and sliced into segments (See Cooking Tip below)
1 apple, washed and diced
1 pear, washed and diced
1 cup red or white seedless grapes, washed
1 ripe banana, sliced
1 kiwi, peeled and sliced

OPTIONAL TOPPINGS
Low-fat plain or fruit yogurt
Honey or molasses
Wheat germ, granola, or ground flaxseed (see Fruit-Filled Granola, page 370)

1. Combine all of the fruit salad ingredients in a large bowl and mix gently. Cover and refrigerate if not serving immediately.
2. To serve, place some fruit salad in a bowl and add one or more toppings, if desired.

▶ *Cooking Tip:* To prepare orange segments: Using a sharp knife, slice off the top and bottom of the orange to expose the flesh. Stand the orange on the counter. Then, working from top to the bottom, and using your first slice as your guide to the thickness of the orange peel, slice the peel off the orange in wide strips. Working over a bowl to catch the juices, hold the orange in one hand and slice out the orange segments from beneath the membranes, holding your knife as close to the membranes as possible; let the segments drop into the bowl. Then squeeze as much juice as possible from the membranes into the bowl.

▶ *Time-Saving Tip:* Make fruit salad from a salad bar. Or use canned mandarin orange segments instead of fresh orange slices.

APPROXIMATE NUTRITIONAL INFORMATION: Serving size: 1 cup winter fruit salad; Calories: 144 cals; Protein: 2 g; Carbohydrates: 36 g; Fat: .9 g; Fiber: 5 g; Sodium: 1 mg; Vitamin C: 64 mg; Diabetic Exchange: Fruit 2.5

summer fruit salad

What's in this for baby and me? Vitamins C and A and fiber.

During summer this fruit salad, high in vitamins C and A, and fiber (with a good dose of folic acid), is perfect for breakfast or brunch, a snack, or dessert. Use any fresh fruits in any proportions you wish. For a tropical twist, with an even more serious supply of vitamins A and C, try combining mangoes, papaya, kiwi, and pineapple with fresh passion fruit juice instead of orange juice.

Serve fruit salad soon after it's made—the berries tend to get a bit soggy if allowed to sit for too long. If there is any leftover salad, throw it in the blender, add some yogurt and pasteurized instant nonfat-dry milk, and whip it into a fruit smoothie (see Super Fruit Smoothies, page 76). Talking about the shapes and colors of the various fruits in this salad might be a way to get your little one to try a bite.

makes about 4 cups

1 cup fresh raspberries, rinsed quickly

1½ cups fresh strawberries, washed, hulled, and quartered

1 cup fresh blueberries, washed

1½ cups cantaloupe balls or cubes (from about half a melon)

1 kiwi, peeled and sliced

1 banana, sliced

¼ cup orange juice

Combine all of the ingredients in a large bowl and mix gently. Cover and refrigerate if not serving immediately.

▶ *Timesaving Tip:* Make fruit salad from a salad bar.

APPROXIMATE NUTRITIONAL INFORMATION: Serving size: 1 cup summer fruit salad; Calories: 118 cals; Protein: 2 g; Carbohydrates: 29 g; Fat: .9 g; Fiber: 6 g; Sodium: 10 mg; Vitamin C: 97 mg; Vitamin A: 2,113 IU; Diabetic Exchange: Fruit 2

get juiced up

Today, juices come in seemingly endless varieties, with a spectrum of benefits from which to choose. Some are fortified with calcium and antioxidants, others have low acid and extra pulp, while still others are juice combinations that offer a blast of vitamins and calories. To control your calorie intake, it is advisable to limit your juice consumption to 8 ounces per day. Following is a list of fruit juices (8-ounce servings) and their primary vitamin and calorie values based on the recommended daily allowances (RDA) for a 2,000-calorie diet.

JUICE	VITAMIN	CALORIES
Orange	C = 207%	111 cals
Grapefruit	C = 156%	96 cals
Carrot	A = 539%, C = 35%	98 cals
Mango	C = 130%	130 cals
Tangerine	C = 128%	106 cals
Pineapple	C = 45%	140 cals
Cranberry	C = 149%	144 cals
Tomato	C = 74%, A = 27%	41 cals
V-8 juice	C = 100%, A = 40%	50 cals

super fruit smoothies

~

What's in this for baby and me? Protein, calcium, and vitamins.

Smoothies are in! These protein-, calcium-, and vitamin-packed fruit smoothies are great any time of day.

The following recipe for the Fresh or Frozen Banana Smoothie can be modified to suit your taste. The variations that follow offer some ideas, but feel free to change anything except the amounts of yogurt and dry milk. Using these amounts of yogurt and dry milk is equivalent to drinking about 2 cups of milk. Different yogurts can be used, soy instead of regular, and flavored instead of plain. On the fruit scene, frozen bananas (or other frozen fruit) are ideal because they cool the smoothie without using any ice. All of the variations call for half a large fresh or frozen banana combined with approximately ½ cup of another fresh, frozen, or canned fruit.

Each smoothie make about 2 cups

fresh or frozen basic banana smoothie

¾ cup low-fat plain yogurt

⅓ cup pasteurized instant nonfat dry milk

1 large ripe banana, frozen if desired

1 teaspoon apple juice concentrate or sugar, or to taste

A drop of pure vanilla extract (optional)

1–2 ice cubes

Place all of the ingredients in a blender and process until smooth. Serve immediately.

▶ *Cooking Tip:* Use a paring knife to peel the frozen banana. If the peel is too hard, hold it under running hot water for about 30 seconds.

▶ *Timesaving Tip:* Mix 8 ounces fat-free frozen smoothie mix with ¾ cup low-fat plain yogurt, ⅓ cup pasteurized instant nonfat dry milk, and ice. Add more smoothie mix to taste.

▶ *Calorie Boost:* For a richer, more caloric smoothie, substitute ¾ cup frozen yogurt, ice cream, or soy ice cream for the low-fat plain yogurt; or add Carnation Instant Breakfast powder according to the package directions.

▶ *Diabetic Tip:* Halve the recipe to yield 1 cup smoothie and omit the apple juice concentrate or sugar.

designer smoothies

Smoothies are getting fancier (and pricier) by the day. Power-packed with nutrition and flavor, they offer a huge nutritional bang for your calorie buck. Because they are extremely fortified and filling, you may want to consume one 16-ounce bottle over the course of two days. Bolthouse Farms, Naked, and Stonyfield Farm Organic smoothies are enriched with vitamins, minerals, fiber, protein, and calcium.

APPROXIMATE NUTRITIONAL INFORMATION: Serving size: 1 banana smoothie (about 2 cups); Calories: 385 cals; Protein: 25 g; Carbohydrates: 65 g; Fat: 4 g; Fiber: 3 g; Sodium: 344 mg; Diabetic Exchange (values per 1 cup smoothie): Skim Milk 2, Fruit .5

FUN VARIATIONS

fresh or frozen strawberry-banana smoothie

¾ cup low-fat plain yogurt

⅓ cup pasteurized instant nonfat dry milk

6 large strawberries (about ½ cup), washed and hulled

½ large ripe banana, frozen if desired

1 teaspoon apple juice concentrate or sugar, or to taste

1 drop of pure vanilla extract (optional)

1–2 ice cubes

APPROXIMATE NUTRITIONAL INFORMATION: Serving size: 1 strawberry-banana smoothie (about 2 cups); Calories: 352 cals; Protein: 25 g; Carbohydrates: 57 g; Fat: 4 g; Fiber: 3 g; Sodium: 344 mg; Calcium: 853 mg; Vitamin C: 50 mg; Diabetic Exchange (values per 1 cup smoothie): Skim Milk 2, Fruit .5

fresh or frozen raspberry-banana smoothie

¾ cup low-fat plain yogurt

⅓ cup pasteurized instant nonfat dry milk

½ cup fresh raspberries, rinsed quickly

½ large ripe banana, frozen if desired

1 teaspoon apple juice concentrate or sugar, or to taste

1 drop of pure vanilla extract (optional)

1–2 ice cubes

APPROXIMATE NUTRITIONAL INFORMATION: Serving size: 1 raspberry-banana smoothie (about 2 cups); Calories: 360 cals; Protein: 25 g; Carbohydrates: 59 g; Fat: 4 g; Fiber: 6 g; Sodium: 343 mg; Calcium: 856 mg; Vitamin C: 25 mg; Diabetic Exchange: (values per 1 cup smoothie) Skim Milk 2, Fruit .5

fresh, frozen, or canned peach-banana smoothie

¾ cup low-fat plain yogurt

⅓ cup pasteurized instant nonfat dry milk

½ small ripe peach, washed and quartered, or

    ½ cup frozen (unthawed) or canned peaches

½ large ripe banana, frozen if desired

1 teaspoon apple juice concentrate or sugar,

    or to taste

1 drop of pure vanilla extract (optional)

1–2 ice cubes

APPROXIMATE NUTRITIONAL INFORMATION: Serving size: 1 peach-banana smoothie (about 2 cups); Calories: 351 cals; Protein: 25 g; Carbohydrates: 56 g; Fat: 3 g; Fiber: 2 g; Sodium: 343 mg; Calcium: 845 mg; Vitamin C: 13 mg; Diabetic Exchange (values per 1 cup smoothie): Skim Milk 2, Fruit .5

fresh or canned pineapple-banana smoothie

¾ cup low-fat plain yogurt

⅓ cup pasteurized instant nonfat dry milk

½ cup diced fresh pineapple or ½ cup canned

    pineapple in its own juice

½ large ripe banana, frozen if desired

1 teaspoon apple juice concentrate or sugar,

    or to taste

1 drop of pure vanilla extract (optional)

1–2 ice cubes

APPROXIMATE NUTRITIONAL INFORMATION: Serving size: 1 pineapple-banana smoothie (about 2 cups); Calories: 400 cals; Protein: 25 g; Carbohydrates: 69 g; Fat: 3 g; Fiber: 2 g; Sodium: 353 mg; Calcium: 843 mg; Vitamin C: 22 mg; Diabetic Exchange (values per 1 cup smoothie): Skim Milk 2, Fruit .5

eggs and salmonella enteritidis

~

While salmonella can be contracted a number of different ways, contaminated raw eggs are of particular concern for pregnant women. (See page 330 for more information on other causes of salmonellosis.) Unbroken fresh eggs in their shells that appear perfectly normal may contain bacteria called *Salmonella enteritidis* (SE), which can cause food-borne illness. SE silently infects the ovaries of healthy-appearing hens and contaminates the eggs before the shells are formed. SE bacteria are usually in the yolk, but it's possible that the bacteria are in the whites as well.[3]

People with health problems, the very young, seniors, and pregnant women (the risk is to the unborn child) are particularly vulnerable to SE infections. The symptoms include fever, abdominal cramps, and diarrhea.[4] Proper refrigeration, cooking, and handling of raw eggs should prevent most contamination problems. People can and should enjoy eggs and egg dishes, provided they follow these safe handling guidelines[5]:

▶ Don't eat raw eggs—including raw eggs contained in milk shakes, Caesar salad dressing, Hollandaise sauce, homemade mayonnaise, ice cream, or eggnog. Also, avoid tasting any batters (such as cake and cookie batters) that contain raw egg.

▶ Choose Grade A or AA eggs with clean, uncracked shells. Don't wash eggs.

▶ Buy only refrigerated eggs and keep them refrigerated in their original egg carton in the coldest part of the refrigerator, and not in the door.

▶ Don't keep eggs out of the refrigerator for more than two hours. Bacteria grow rapidly at room temperature.

▶ Use raw eggs within three to five weeks of purchase. Use any leftover yolks or whites within four days. Hard-cooked eggs can be kept in the refrigerator for one week.

▶ Handle eggs safely. Wash hands, utensils, equipment, and work areas with warm soapy water before and after contact with raw eggs and dishes containing raw eggs.

▶ Keep raw eggs separate from other foods that will be cooked.

▶ Cook eggs thoroughly until the yolk and whites are firm. Scrambled eggs should not be runny and there should be no visible liquid egg. Casseroles and other egg-based dishes should be cooked to 160°F on an instant-read thermometer.

▶ Eat eggs promptly after cooking. Refrigerate any leftovers, and consume within three to four days.

Commercially manufactured ice cream and eggnog made with pasteurized eggs have not been linked to SE infections. Dry meringue shells and cookies are safe to eat. It is advisable to avoid meringue-topped pies, chiffon and fruit pies made with raw whipped egg whites, and any custard-based desserts in which the eggs might not have reached a safe internal temperature of 160°F.

chris prouty's saturday special blueberry muffins

What's in this for baby and me? A delicious treat on a weekend morning.

THESE MOUTHWATERING MUFFINS provide a good source of B vitamins, folic acid, and fiber. The streusel topping is optional, but adds a wonderful texture and cinnamony sweetness—a perfect wake-up call on a Saturday morning.

Makes 12 regular muffins or about 40 mini muffins

STREUSEL TOPPING
⅓ cup brown sugar
⅓ cup all-purpose flour
3 tablespoons unsalted butter
1 teaspoon ground cinnamon

MUFFINS
Canola oil cooking spray for greasing the
    muffin pan (or use muffin cup liners)
2 cups fresh blueberries, washed and drained
1½ cups all-purpose flour, plus 1 tablespoon
    for the blueberries
½ cup sugar
½ teaspoon salt
2 teaspoons baking powder
⅓ cup ground flaxseed (optional)
⅓ cup canola oil
1 large egg
About ¾ cup whole milk (see Step 5)
1 teaspoon lemon zest

1. To make the streusel topping, in a small bowl, combine all ingredients and quickly mix with your fingers to the consistency of coarse cornmeal. Refrigerate until ready to use.
2. Preheat the oven to 400°F. Spray the muffin cups with cooking spray or line them with muffin liners.
3. To make the muffins, mix the blueberries with 1 tablespoon of the flour and set aside.
4. In a large bowl, whisk together the remaining flour, sugar, salt, baking powder, and flaxseed until well combined.
5. Place the canola oil in a 2-cup measuring cup, add the egg, and then add enough milk for the contents level to reach the 1¼-cup mark on the measuring cup (this will be about ¾ cup milk). Whisk this mixture, then add it to the dry ingredients and mix until combined. Fold in the lemon zest and the reserved blueberries.

6. Divide the batter evenly among the muffin cups. Top each muffin with a bit of the reserved streusel topping. Bake 20 to 25 minutes for regular muffins, 12 to 15 minutes for mini muffins, or until a tester inserted in the center comes out clean. Transfer the muffins to a rack and cool slightly before eating.

▶ *Diabetic Tip:* Omit the streusel topping and use mini-muffin pans for baking. Eat only one mini muffin.

▶ *Complete Meal Ideas:* Serve these muffins with:
   One packet instant oatmeal
   Reduced-fat 2% milk or low-fat yogurt
   Fresh fruit

APPROXIMATE NUTRITIONAL INFORMATION: Serving size: 1 regular-size blueberry muffin; Calories: 248 cals; Protein: 4 g; Carbohydrates: 32 g; Fat: 12 g; Fiber: 3 g; Sodium: 114 mg; Diabetic Exchange: Bread/Starch: 2, Fat 2

coconut pancakes with yogurt, fresh fruit, and honey

What's in this for baby and me? Folic acid.

Mᴀᴅᴇ ᴡɪᴛʜ ᴄᴏᴄᴏɴᴜᴛ milk, these pancakes are an excellent source of folic acid, and a fine source of protein, vitamin C, B vitamins, iron, and fiber. The toppings of fresh fruit and yogurt transform these pancakes into a hearty meal. Make small silver-dollar-size pancakes for a satisfying snack anytime.

Makes about 12 four-inch pancakes

1 cup all-purpose flour

3 tablespoons sugar

½ teaspoon baking soda

½ cup desiccated coconut (dry shredded coconut)

1 cup coconut milk

⅓ cup pasteurized instant nonfat dry milk

1 large egg

Canola oil cooking spray for greasing the skillet

TOPPINGS

1½ cups plain low-fat yogurt

1½ cups fresh berries (any kind)

Honey, to taste

1. In a medium bowl, whisk the flour, sugar, baking soda, and desiccated coconut until well combined. Set aside.
2. In a separate bowl, whisk together the coconut milk, dry milk, egg, and a ½ cup of water. Add to the dry mixture and mix until well blended.
3. Heat a large nonstick skillet over medium heat. Spray with canola oil cooking spray, then add ¼-cup portions of batter for each pancake onto the skillet (you will probably fit 3 or 4), and spread into 4-inch rounds. Cook for 2 minutes or until the surface bubbles and then slightly sets and the underside is golden brown. Flip the pancakes and continue cooking about 2 minutes longer. Serve warm with the toppings on the side. Refrigerate leftovers.

▶ *Diabetic Tip:* Use a low-sugar jam, such as Polaner All Fruit (2 teaspoons are FREE; 2 teaspoons (also FREE) Quick Diabetic-Friendly Strawberry-Raspberry Syrup (page 59), or lightly dust the pancakes with powdered sugar.

▶ *Complete Meal Ideas:* Serve these pancakes and toppings with:
   A glass of calcium-fortified orange juice

APPROXIMATE NUTRITIONAL INFORMATION: Serving size: 3 coconut pancakes with one-quarter of the toppings; Calories: 396 cals; Protein: 10 g; Carbohydrates: 50 g; Fat: 19 g; Fiber: 3 g; Sodium: 252 mg; Folic Acid: 82 mcg; Diabetic Exchange: Bread/Starch 2, Fat 3, Milk 1

soups and sandwiches
to savor

◯N A COLD day, there is nothing homier than walking into a kitchen where soup is simmering on the stove, perfuming the air with each waft of steam. And on a hot day, a bowl of chilled soup is a refreshing treat. Vitamins, minerals, calcium, protein, and fiber—soups have them all, and, being pregnant, you need them all. In particular, women on bed rest can get good mileage out of soups in a thermos, and women on the go can get a longer-lasting fix from soup than from a cup of coffee.

Homemade soups are undoubtedly the best. They are generally healthier than their store-bought cousins, which are usually high in sodium and often contain MSG. Making soups from scratch is surprisingly easy. No special skills are required, and there is no single perfect outcome. Adapt recipes to your liking—soups can be creamy, chunky, packed with spice, or plain and simple.

Sandwiches are just as forgiving and versatile as soups. There is no right answer—cater to your own tastes and nutritional needs. And when you need a simple, healthy fallback, there's always good old peanut butter and jelly.

RECIPE NOTES

Soup Notes

- To save time, pick up vegetables from a salad bar, buy pre-cut bagged vegetables, or use frozen ones.
- Pureeing soups, as called for in some of the recipes, is optional.
- Almost any soup can be adapted to a vegetarian diet by using vegetable stock and omitting meat products. Vegans can also omit dairy products.
- To increase the calcium content of creamy vegetable soups, mix $\frac{1}{3}$ cup of instant nonfat dry milk to the milk, buttermilk, or half-and-half going into the soup.
- For convenience, soups can be frozen in meal-size portions in plastic containers or freezer bags. Be sure to label and date all frozen foods.

- Vegetable soups should be frozen after they are pureed and before adding dairy products such as buttermilk or half-and-half.
- Tub margarine or vegetable oils can be substituted for unsalted butter.
- Starting and stopping the cooking process usually does not affect the outcome, especially of longer-cooking soups.
- Choose fat-free, low-sodium canned stocks whenever possible.
- Bouillon cubes (meat, poultry, vegetable, or vegan) dissolved in water can be substituted for the amount of stock or water called for in the recipes. They are cheaper than canned stock and take up less storage space in kitchen cupboards. Choose MSG-free brands.
- All herbs and spices are optional. Young children may object to green things in their soup, or they may prefer a blander flavor.
- Thin soups to the desired consistency gradually, adding about 2 tablespoons of liquid at a time. It is always easier to thin a soup than to thicken one. To thicken a soup, add a quick-dissolving thickener according to the package directions.
- A flame tamer buffers the heat for longer-cooking soups.
- As a general rule, soups cooked in a slow cooker require less water than those cooked on the stove as there is almost no evaporation. Vegetables take a surprisingly long time to cook in a slow cooker, so they should be thinly sliced and placed on the bottom of the pot. Meat should follow the vegetables. Because it is impossible to predict their liquid absorption, avoid adding uncooked pasta, rice, or any other raw grain to soups cooked in a slow cooker unless you follow specific directions in a recipe. Also, while sautéing onions, garlic, and other vegetables and seasonings before adding them to the cooker may seem like more work, it greatly improves the flavor of the finished soup.

Sandwich Notes

Sliced turkey, ham, roast beef (well-done), chicken, or your favorite deli meats or tofu provide protein. Purchase home-style or all-natural meats, because they contain little or no preservatives. To prevent listeriosis, be sure to thoroughly heat all lunch meats before eating them (see Listeriosis Warning, page 129). Try to avoid the following sandwich meats because of their high fat, nitrite, or nitrate content: salami, bacon, Spam, corned beef, and bologna. Pasteurized cheese is a tasty addition to any sandwich. Choose low-fat varieties (less than 2 grams of fat per ounce) if you need to restrict your fat intake.

Salad Suggestions

Egg, chicken, salmon, tuna, crab, shrimp, or lobster salads (homemade or store-bought) make delicious sandwiches and add some protein to your diet.

soups and sandwiches to savor

SOUPS

Creamy Asparagus-Artichoke Soup

Cheesy Cauliflower-Potato Soup

Great Green Broccoli-Spinach Soup

Butternut Squash–Carrot Soup with Ginger

Greek-Style Chicken, Lemon, and Egg Soup

Black Bean Soup with Cilantro ▼

Lentil Soup with Brown Rice and Spinach ▼

Turkish-Style Red Lentil Soup ▼

Mediterranean Pasta, Bean, and Vegetable Soup ▼

Green Split Pea Soup ▼

Beef, Barley, and Vegetable Soup

Gazpacho ▼

Basic Chicken Stock

Basic Vegetable Stock ▼

SANDWICHES

Pr-egg-o Salad Sandwich

Chicken Salad with Dried Apricots and Almonds

Grilled Cheese Sandwich

Tuna Salad Sandwich

Wraps and Rolls

Keep-It-Simple Lobster Salad Sandwich

▼ Vegan recipe

high-calcium dairy products without the fat

If you have been advised to watch your fat intake, these dairy products are a great way to get your calcium with less than 5 grams of fat. Keep this list handy post-delivery when you are trying to shed baby fat but want to keep your calcium high.

High-Calcium Dairy Products with Less Than 5 Grams of Fat per Serving

FOOD	SERVING SIZE	CALCIUM (MG)
Nonfat plain yogurt	1 cup	488
Low-fat plain yogurt	1 cup	448
Reduced-fat Alpine Lace Swiss cheese*	1 slice	350
Nonfat milk	8 ounces	301
Reduced-fat 1% milk	8 ounces	300
Nonfat dry milk	⅓ cup	283
Part-skim mozzarella cheese	1 ounce	222
Cracker Barrel 2% milk cheddar cheese**	1 ounce	200
Fat-free ricotta cheese	¼ cup	200
Weight Watchers Fat-free Swiss cheese	2 slices	150
Fat-free American cheese	1 slice	150
Reduced-fat buttermilk	½ cup	142
Fat-free frozen yogurt (not chocolate)	½ cup	138
Parmesan cheese	2 tablespoons	138
Reduced-fat crumbled feta cheese	¼ cup	80
Low-fat 2% cottage cheese	½ cup	78
Fat-free cottage cheese	½ cup	60
The Laughing Cow Light Swiss cheese	¾ ounce wedge	60
Fat-free sour cream	2 tablespoons	40

*Reduced-fat Alpine Lace Swiss cheese (1 slice) contains 7 grams of fat.

**Cracker Barrel 2% Milk cheddar cheese contains 6 grams of fat.

Spread Suggestions

As an alternative to high-quality light mayonnaise, try pasteurized cheese spreads such as Boursin or other flavored cheese spreads, pasteurized goat cheese (chevre), Neufchâtel, or flavored cream cheeses, plain ricotta cheese or Roasted Red Pepper and Cheese Dip (page 174), guacamole (store-bought or Homemade Guacamole, page 173), hummus (store-bought or Healthy Hummus, page 175), pesto (store-bought or Basil Pesto, page 147), or any other prepared spread, to give your sandwich a flavor boost.

Vegetable Suggestions

Salad—romaine, loose-leaf, Boston, Bibb, mesclun, and watercress—tomatoes, cucumbers, green peppers, and shredded carrots are all great sources of fiber and vitamins. Leftover grilled, roasted, or stir-fried vegetables are a fabulous addition to any sandwich, particularly wraps. (Keep in mind that romaine lettuce has the highest folic acid content of all the greens listed above.)

Bread Suggestions

Choose whole grain, bran, or calcium-enriched bread whenever possible. Flat breads or tortillas are perfect for wrap sandwiches. Try to stay away from white bread that has little nutritional value unless it is fortified with calcium, iron, or other nutrients.

choosing the healthiest breads

Look for whole wheat or whole grain breads that are high in fiber and low in added fat. Avoid those with trans fats. The top two high-fiber breads on the shelves today are Fiber One Multigrain (7 grams per slice) and Pepperidge Farm Whole Grain Double Fiber (6 grams per slice). Keep in mind that just because breads are brown does not mean that they contain whole grains.

GOOD BREAD CHOICES

Alvarado Street Bakery breads

Fiber One Multigrain breads

Mestemacher All Natural Famous German breads

Milton's Whole Grain breads

Pepperidge Farm Natural Whole Grain Double Fiber breads

Roman Meal Sandwich Bread Calcium Rich breads

Shiloh Farms breads

The Baker breads

Vermont Bread Company breads

pantry items for
soups and sandwiches to savor

SOUP PANTRY

Fresh Produce

Asparagus

Baby spinach (5- and 6-ounce packages)

Broccoli and broccoli florets

Butternut squash

Carrots (peeled baby carrots or regular carrots)

Cauliflower

Celery

Cucumbers

Fresh herbs: cilantro, dill, and parsley

Garlic

Ginger

Lemons

Mushrooms (preferably cremini)

Onions: regular and Vidalia or other sweet onions

Potatoes (any kind)

Scallions

Swiss chard

Tomatoes

Zucchini

Dairy and Soy Products

Cheese: grated Fontina, Monterey Jack, Parmesan, and/or sharp cheddar

Extra-firm tofu

Grade A large eggs

Half-and-half (preferably ultra-pasteurized)

Low-fat or fat-free plain yogurt

Nonfat buttermilk

Unsalted butter

Whole milk

Canned, Bottled, and Jarred Staples

Artichoke hearts packed in water or brine (13.75-ounce can)

Balsamic vinegar or any other vinegar

Black beans (19-ounce can)

Canola oil

Fat-free low-sodium stock (any kind)

Great Northern white beans (15.5-ounce can)

Olive oil

Peeled and diced tomatoes (14.5-ounce can)

Roasted red peppers

V-8 juice (low-sodium preferred) or tomato juice

Dry Staples

Brown rice and any other rice except instant

Croutons

Dried apricots

Green lentils

Green split peas

Pasteurized instant nonfat dry milk

Pearl barley

Red lentils

Small pasta (such as ditalini or alphabet pasta)

Herbs and Spices

Bay leaves

Bouillon cubes (any flavor)

Chili powder

Dried marjoram

Dried mint

Dried oregano

Dried tarragon

Dried thyme
Garlic powder (not garlic salt)
Ground cumin
Ground ginger
Paprika or red pepper
Pesto (store-bought or homemade)

Frozen Staples
Artichoke hearts
Spinach (6-, 8-, or 10-ounce package)

Meats and Poultry
Beef shank, bone-in
Chicken tenders
Whole chicken
Lobster

From the Salad Bar
Broccoli florets
Cauliflower florets
Diced onions
Sliced mushrooms

SANDWICH PANTRY

Fresh Produce
Avocados
Bananas
Celery
Cucumbers
Fresh herbs: cilantro, dill, and parsley
Lemons
Lettuce
Red bell peppers
Scallions
Tomatoes

Dairy
2% Milk Singles (cheese slices)
Cheese for sandwiches
Grade A large eggs
Grated Parmesan cheese

Canned, Bottled, and Jarred Staples
Caesar salad dressing (preferably reduced-fat)
Canola oil
Light tuna in spring water
Hoisin sauce
Light mayonnaise
Mustard (any kind)
Peanut butter (preferably reduced-fat)
Roasted red peppers
Salsa
Thai-style peanut sauce

Dry Staples
Dried apricots
Sliced almonds
Burrito-size tortillas (10-inch)
Calcium-enriched bread (such as Calcium Enriched Roman Meal)
Whole wheat, enriched bread
Hot dog rolls with a top slit

Miscellaneous Staples
Chicken tenders or leftover cooked chicken
Hummus (store-bought or homemade)
Tabbouleh (store-bought or homemade)
Lunch meats

From the Salad Bar
Sliced cucumbers
Sliced red bell peppers
Sliced tomatoes
Washed lettuce

creamy asparagus-artichoke soup

What's in this for baby and me? Vitamin C and folic acid.

IF YOUR CHILDREN are fond of green vegetables, they could acquire a taste for this soup, which is high in vitamin C and folic acid, and a good source of protein, vitamin A, and fiber.

serves 6 (makes about 7 cups)

3 tablespoons unsalted butter

1 medium onion, chopped

1 medium potato, peeled and diced

4 cups fat-free low-sodium stock

½ teaspoon salt, or to taste

1 pound green asparagus, washed, tough ends trimmed, and stalks cut into 1-inch pieces

One 13.75-ounce can artichoke hearts, drained

1½ teaspoons dried tarragon (optional)

½ cup half-and-half or whole milk (optional)

Freshly ground pepper, to taste

Squeeze of fresh lemon juice (optional)

1. Melt the butter in a 6-quart saucepan over medium-high heat. Add the onion and sauté for 3 minutes. Add the potato, stock, and salt and bring to a boil. Add the asparagus, artichoke hearts, and tarragon, if using, and return to a boil, then reduce the heat and simmer, uncovered, for 10 to 15 minutes, or until the potatoes are tender. Remove from the heat.

2. Allow the soup to cool slightly, then puree it. Return the pureed soup to the rinsed-out saucepan, add the half-and-half, if using, and bring just to a boil over medium-high heat. Adjust the seasoning, add the lemon juice, if desired, and serve immediately, or let cool to room temperature, refrigerate, and serve chilled.

▶ *Timesaving Tip:* Use 1 pound frozen asparagus instead of the fresh. Rinse the frozen asparagus under hot water to dissolve any ice, then proceed with the recipe.

▶ *Storage Tip:* This soup keeps refrigerated for about 5 days. It can be frozen, before the half-and-half or whole milk is added, for up to 1 month.

▶ *Health Tip:* If your doctor has restricted your fat intake, substitute margarine for the butter and additional fat-free stock or water for the half-and-half.

▶ **Complete Meal Ideas:** Serve this soup with:

    3 ounces protein (you might want to try the Tomato and
        Mozzarella Salad with Fresh Basil, page 157)
    Whole wheat bread
    Reduced-fat 2% milk or low-fat yogurt
    Fresh fruit

APPROXIMATE NUTRITIONAL INFORMATION: Serving size: 1 cup asparagus-artichoke soup; Calories: 152 cals; Protein: 6 g; Carbohydrates: 15 g; Fat: 9 g; Fiber: 4 g; Sodium: 284 mg; Vitamin C: 19 mg; Folic Acid: 86 mcg; Diabetic Exchange: Bread/Starch 1, Fat 2

cheesy cauliflower-potato soup

What's in this for baby and me? Protein, calcium, and vitamin C.

THIS SOUP IS rich in protein, calcium, and vitamin C, and a good source of vitamin A, folic acid, and fiber. For a chunkier soup, puree all but 2 cups of the soup. Garnish with chopped fresh cilantro or parsley.

serves 6 (makes about 7 cups)

3 tablespoons unsalted butter

1 medium onion, chopped

4 cups cauliflower florets (about 1 pound),
   washed and cut into small florets

1 medium-large potato, peeled and diced

½ teaspoon salt, or to taste

4 cups fat-free low-sodium stock

1½ cups whole milk

1 cup grated sharp cheddar cheese, Fontina,
   or Monterey Jack

Freshly ground pepper, to taste

¼ cup chopped fresh parsley or cilantro

1. Melt the butter in a 6-quart saucepan over medium-high heat. Add the onion and sauté for 3 minutes. Add the cauliflower florets, potato, salt, and stock and bring to a boil, then reduce the heat and simmer for 15 to 20 minutes, or until the potatoes and cauliflower are tender. Remove from the heat.

2. Allow the soup to cool slightly, then puree it. Return the pureed soup to the rinsed-out saucepan. Add the milk and bring just to a boil over medium-high heat. Add the cheese, reduce the heat to low, and stir until the cheese is melted—do not let the soup boil after adding the cheese.

3. Adjust the seasoning, garnish with the parsley, and serve.

▶ **Storage Tip:** This soup keeps refrigerated for about 5 days. Do not freeze.

▶ **Complete Meal Ideas:** Serve this soup with:
   Green salad (you might want to try the Spinach Salad with
      Mandarin Oranges and Toasted Almonds, page 163, or a tossed
      salad with French-Style Tarragon Vinaigrette, page 166)
   Whole wheat bread
   Reduced-fat 2% milk or low-fat yogurt
   Fresh fruit

APPROXIMATE NUTRITIONAL INFORMATION: Serving size: 1 cup cheesy cauliflower-potato soup; Calories: 221 cals; Protein: 10 g; Carbohydrates: 15 g; Fat: 14 g; Fiber: 3 g; Sodium: 395 mg; Vitamin C: 42 mg; Calcium: 219 mg; Diabetic Exchange: Bread/Starch 1, Fat 3, Whole Milk 1.5

food aversions and cravings

What? All of a sudden you've lost your taste for vegetables? Fruits? Fish? Chicken? But you used to love a good steak with a baked potato smothered in sour cream! Fear not. Food aversions are just as common as food cravings during pregnancy. And, like cravings, they can last for an hour, a day, weeks, or even months. Also, don't be surprised if your food aversion on Monday becomes your craving on Friday, or the other way around.

The taste for certain foods varies from person to person and can change without warning at any time during pregnancy. This is usually not a problem, but some food aversions may require effort to replace lost nutrients. For example, if you have an aversion to fruit, increase your intake of vegetables—and vice versa. If chicken or beef turn you off, increase your intake of peanut butter, eggs, cheese, dried beans and peas, or tofu. If a food aversion lasts longer than one month, or the appropriate substitutions are not meeting your daily nutrient requirements, discuss the situation with your doctor or a dietitian.

great green broccoli-spinach soup

What's in this for baby and me? Calcium, vitamins A and C, and fiber.

DELICIOUSLY GREEN, THIS broccoli-spinach soup is high in calcium, vitamins A and C, and fiber, and a good source of protein, iron, and folic acid. Garnish with grated cheese or croutons.

serves 6 (makes about 7 cups)

3 tablespoons unsalted butter

1 medium onion, chopped

1 pound (about 8 cups) broccoli florets, washed and trimmed

1 medium potato, peeled and diced

4 cups fat-free low-sodium stock

1 teaspoon salt, or to taste

One 6-ounce package baby spinach, washed,

or 6–8 ounces frozen chopped spinach, thawed, drained, and squeezed

1 cup nonfat buttermilk

⅓ cup pasteurized instant nonfat dry milk (optional)

Freshly ground pepper, to taste

Shredded sharp cheddar cheese or your favorite cheese, for garnish

1. Melt the butter in a 6-quart saucepan over medium-high heat. Add the onion and sauté for 3 minutes. Add the broccoli, potato, stock, and salt and bring to a boil, then reduce the heat and simmer, covered, for about 15 minutes, or until the potatoes are tender. During the last 5 minutes, stir the spinach into the soup. Remove from the heat.

2. Allow the soup to cool slightly, then puree it in batches in a blender or food processor. Return the pureed soup to the rinsed-out saucepan.

3. In a large measuring cup or small bowl, combine the buttermilk and dry milk and whisk until smooth. Add to the pureed soup and bring the soup just to a boil over medium-high heat. Adjust the seasoning, garnish with the cheese, and serve immediately.

▶ *Storage Tip:* This soup keeps refrigerated for about 5 days. It can be frozen, before the half-and-half is added, for up to one month.

► *Complete Meal Ideas:* Serve this soup with:

   3 ounces protein (you might want to try the Grilled Cheese Sandwich, page 119)
   Whole wheat bread
   Reduced-fat 2% milk or low-fat yogurt
   Fresh fruit that contains vitamin C

APPROXIMATE NUTRITIONAL INFORMATION: Serving size: 1 cup broccoli-spinach soup; Calories: 160 cals; Protein: 9 g; Carbohydrates: 17 g; Fat: 7 g; Fiber: 6 g; Sodium: 563 mg; Calcium: 206 mg; Vitamin A: 2,930 IU; Vitamin C: 87 mg; Diabetic Exchange: Bread/Starch .5, Fat 1, Low-Fat Milk 1

butternut squash–carrot soup with ginger

⌒

What's in this for baby and me? Vitamins A and C.

Butternut squash and carrots are excellent sources of vitamins A and C. To save time, use peeled and cut-up fresh butternut squash. If it is unavailable in your area, see the Cooking Tip below for instructions on using a whole squash. For a zippier soup, feel free to replace the fresh and ground ginger with 1½ teaspoons mild curry powder.

serves 6 to 8 (makes about 8½ cups)

2 tablespoons unsalted butter

1 medium onion, chopped

2 tablespoons minced fresh ginger

1¼ pounds peeled and cut-up butternut
    squash

3 carrots, peeled and chopped, or 1½ cups
    sliced peeled baby carrots

⅓ cup dried apricots (optional)

5 cups fat-free low-sodium stock

½ teaspoon salt, or to taste

1 teaspoon ground ginger

½ cup half-and-half

¼ cup chopped fresh cilantro, for garnish

1. Melt the butter in a 6-quart saucepan over medium heat. Add the onions and fresh ginger and sauté for 3 minutes. Add the squash, carrots, apricots, if using, stock, salt, and ground ginger, if using. Bring to a boil, then reduce the heat and simmer for 10 to 15 minutes, or until the squash and carrots are tender.
2. Remove the soup from the heat and allow to cool slightly, then puree in batches. Return the pureed soup to the rinsed-out saucepan, add the half-and-half, and reheat over medium-high heat just until the soup reaches a boil. Garnish with the cilantro, if desired, and serve immediately.

▶ *Cooking Tip:* To use a whole butternut squash for this soup, preheat the oven to 375°F. Line a baking dish large enough to accommodate the squash with foil and grease the foil with 2 tablespoons canola oil. Using a sharp knife, cut a 1½-pound butternut squash lengthwise in half. Scoop out the seeds and then place the two halves cut-side down in the baking dish. Bake for 45 minutes, or until the pulp is tender. Allow the squash to cool slightly, then scoop out the flesh; you should have at least 2½ cups; set aside.

▶ *Storage Tip:* This soup keeps refrigerated for about 5 days. It can be frozen, before the half-and-half is added, for up to one month.

► **Complete Meal Ideas:** Serve this soup with:

> 3 ounces protein (you might want to try the Pr-egg-o Salad Sandwich, page 118; the iron in this sandwich will be enhanced by the vitamin C in the soup)
> Whole wheat bread
> Reduced-fat 2% milk or low-fat yogurt
> Fresh fruit

APPROXIMATE NUTRITIONAL INFORMATION: Serving size: 1 cup butternut squash–carrot soup; Calories: 135 cals; Protein: 3 g; Carbohydrates: 19 g; Fat: 6 g; Fiber: 2 g; Sodium: 230 mg; Vitamin A: 14,224 IU; Vitamin C: 21 mg; Diabetic Exchange: Bread/Starch 1, Fat 1

greek-style chicken, lemon, and egg soup

~

What's in this for baby and me? Protein and vitamin A.

THIS SOUP IS an amazing source of protein and vitamin A, and a good source of vitamin C, iron, and fiber. It is a cinch to make, especially if you have leftover chicken or turkey and canned stock.

serves 6 (makes about 8 cups)

7 cups fat-free low-sodium stock

4 carrots, peeled and thinly sliced, or 2 cups
    sliced peeled baby carrots

1 celery stalk, washed and thinly sliced

½ cup uncooked rice (any kind except instant)

½ pound chicken tenders, sliced into thirds, or
    1½ cups diced cooked chicken

3 large eggs

¼ cup freshly squeezed lemon juice (from
    about 1½ lemons), or to taste

½ teaspoon salt, or to taste

Freshly ground pepper, to taste

¼ cup chopped fresh parsley or dill, for
    garnish (optional)

1. Place the chicken stock in a 6-quart saucepan and bring to a boil. Add the carrots, celery, rice, and chicken tenders or cooked chicken and bring to a boil. Reduce heat and simmer, uncovered, for 25 minutes, or until the rice is tender. Reduce the heat to low and prepare the egg-lemon mixture.
2. In a medium bowl, beat the eggs with the lemon juice until light and frothy. Gradually whisk in 3 ladlefuls of the soup broth, then add the egg mixture to the soup, stirring constantly. Stir and cook for 5 minutes longer to cook the egg completely.
3. Adjust the seasoning, including the lemon, garnish with the parsley, if desired, and serve immediately.

▶ **Storage Tip:** This soup keeps refrigerated for about 3 days. Do not freeze.

pica: an unusual craving

It has been suggested that pica, the craving for inappropriate substances with little or no nutritional value, may be associated with iron deficiency anemia. The most common non-food substances that pregnant women crave are dirt, clay, laundry starch, and ice. Other less common cravings include chalk, air fresheners, charcoal, and mothballs. Whether pica is the cause or effect of anemia remains unknown, but the condition usually clears when the anemia is treated. Consult your doctor or health-care provider if you experience the desire to consume non-food substances.[1]

▶ *Complete Meal Ideas:* Serve this soup with:
>   3 ounces protein (such as hard cheese) if you are not using chicken
>   Whole wheat bread
>   Green salad (you might want to try a tossed salad with the
>   French-Style Tarragon Vinaigrette, page 166)
>   Reduced-fat 2% milk or low-fat yogurt
>   Fresh fruit that contains vitamin C

APPROXIMATE NUTRITIONAL INFORMATION: Serving size: 1 cup Greek-style chicken soup; Calories: 189 cals; Protein: 19 g; Carbohydrates: 18 g; Fat: 4 g; Fiber: 2 g; Sodium: 344 mg; Vitamin A: 11,598 IU; Diabetic Exchange: Bread/Starch 1, Fat 1, Meat (Lean) 2

black bean soup with cilantro

What's in this for baby and me? Protein, vitamins A and C, folic acid, and fiber.

THIS SOUP IS a fabulous source of protein, vitamins A and C, folic acid, and fiber, and a good source of iron. Canned beans are a real time-saver. The spices and garnishes are optional (especially for young eaters), but they add color and a burst of flavor. Slow Cooker Instructions follow.

serves 8 (makes about 8 cups)

2 tablespoons canola oil

1 large onion, chopped

4 carrots, peeled and sliced, or 2 cups sliced peeled baby carrots

¼ cup diced jarred roasted red peppers

3 garlic cloves, crushed

2 teaspoons ground cumin

2 teaspoons dried oregano (ground or whole) or dried basil

½ teaspoon chili powder

Two 19-ounce cans black beans, drained

5 cups fat-free low-sodium stock or water, or more as needed

1 cup V-8 juice

Salt and freshly ground pepper, to taste

Chopped fresh cilantro, for garnish (optional)

Grated cheddar cheese, for garnish (optional)

1. Heat the canola oil in a 6-quart saucepan over medium-high heat until hot. Add the onion and sauté for 3 minutes. Add the carrots, and the optional red peppers, garlic, cumin, oregano, and chili powder and sauté for 3 minutes. Add the beans, stock, and V-8 juice and bring to a boil, then reduce the heat and simmer, uncovered, for 20 minutes, or until the carrots are tender.
2. Allow the soup to cool slightly, then puree 3 cups of it. Return the pureed soup to the saucepan and stir. Add stock or water to thin the soup if desired.
3. Adjust the seasoning, add the cilantro, and serve immediately.

▶ *Cooking Tip:* Stock or water can be substituted for the V-8 juice.

▶ *Storage Tip:* This soup keeps refrigerated for about 1 week, and it can be frozen for up to 1 month.

▶ *Slow Cooker Instructions:* Use 3½ cups stock instead of 5 cups. Because this recipe calls for canned black beans, the cooking time is short, even in a slow cooker. When the carrots are soft, the soup is essentially ready, usually after 4 hours on high heat.
1. Using a large nonstick skillet instead of a saucepan, sauté the onion as directed in Step 1, then add the carrots, and the optional peppers, garlic, cumin, oregano, and chili powder, and sauté for 3 minutes.

fiber sources

FOOD	SERVING SIZE	FIBER (G)
General Mills Fiber One cereal	½ cup	14
Kellogg's All Bran cereal	½ cup	10
Raspberries	1 cup	8
Cooked lentils	½ cup	8
Cooked black beans	½ cup	7
Cooked chickpeas	½ cup	5
Potato with skin	1 potato	5
Canned kidney beans	½ cup	5
Cooked green peas	⅓ cup	4
Kellogg's Raisin Bran cereal	½ cup	4
Quick-cooked oatmeal (prepared with water)	1 cup	4
Blueberries	1 cup	4
Apple with skin	1 medium	4
Whole wheat bread	2 slices	3
Strawberries	1 cup	3
Orange	1 medium	3
Wheat germ	¼ cup	3
Dried dates	5 dates	3
Broccoli	½ cup	2
Whole wheat crackers	5 items	2
Brussels sprouts	½ cup	2

▶ *Slow Cooker Instructions:* (cont.)

2. Transfer the contents of the skillet to the slow cooker, then add the black beans, stock, and V-8 juice. Cover and cook on high for 6 hours. Finish the soup as directed in Steps 2 and 3.

▶ *Complete Meal Ideas:* Serve this soup with:
Corn bread or whole wheat bread (you might also want to try the Cheese and Spinach Quesadillas, page 224)
Green salad
Reduced-fat 2% milk or low-fat yogurt
Fresh fruit that contains vitamin C

APPROXIMATE NUTRITIONAL INFORMATION: Serving size: 1 cup black bean soup; Calories: 211 cals; Protein: 11 g; Carbohydrates: 30 g; Fat: 6 g; Fiber: 10 g; Sodium: 160 mg; Vitamin A: 8,892 IU; Vitamin C: 18 mg; Folic Acid: 163 mcg; Diabetic Exchange: Bread/Starch 1.5, Fat 2

lentil soup with brown rice and spinach

What's in this for baby and me? Protein, iron, vitamin A, folic acid, and fiber.

THE COMBINATION OF lentils, brown rice, and spinach provides an impressive dose of protein, iron, vitamin A, folic acid, and fiber. For a lighter soup, omit the rice and increase the lentils to 1⅓ cups. Kids might prefer the soup without the spinach. The balsamic vinegar, added to the soup at the last minute, gives it a wonderful tang, and the olive oil adds richness. Slow Cooker Instructions follow.

serves 8 (makes about 10 cups)

2 tablespoons olive oil

1 medium onion, finely chopped

2 garlic cloves, crushed

4 carrots, peeled and finely diced, or 2 cups
  sliced peeled baby carrots

½ cup uncooked brown rice (or any rice except
  instant)

1 tablespoon dried thyme

2 bay leaves (optional)

10 cups fat-free low-sodium stock or water, or
  more as needed

1 cup green lentils, picked over and rinsed

One 5-ounce bag baby spinach, washed, or 5
  ounces (half a 10-ounce package) frozen
  spinach, thawed and drained

Salt and freshly ground pepper, to taste

Balsamic or red wine vinegar, to taste, for
  garnish (optional)

Olive oil, to taste, for garnish (optional)

1. Heat the olive oil in a 6-quart saucepan over medium heat. Add the onion and sauté for 3 minutes. Add the garlic, carrots, brown rice, thyme, and optional bay leaves and sauté for 3 minutes. Add the stock and lentils, stir, and bring to a boil. Skim off the foam with a spoon, then reduce the heat and simmer for about 35 minutes, or until the lentils are cooked. After 25 minutes of cooking, remove the bay leaves from the soup (if using), stir in the spinach.
2. If the finished soup is too thick, add more stock or water ¼ cup at a time.
3. Add a couple of drops of vinegar and olive oil, adjust the seasoning, and serve immediately.

▶ *Timesaving Tip:* Add diced vegetables to a packaged lentil soup mix and season with dried herbs and oil and vinegar if desired.

▶ *Storage Tip:* This soup keeps refrigerated for about 5 days, and can be frozen for up to 1 month.

▶ **Health Tip:** If your doctor has restricted your fat intake, omit the olive oil garnish to the finished soup.

▶ **Slow Cooker Instructions:** Use 9 cups of stock instead of 10. (If you are not omitting the brown rice and increasing the amount of lentils to 1⅓ cups, use 8 cups of stock.)
   1. Using a large nonstick skillet instead of a saucepan, sauté the onion as directed in Step 1, then add the garlic, carrots, thyme, and optional bay leaves and sauté for 3 minutes more.
   2. Transfer the contents of the skillet to the slow cooker, then add the lentils and stock. Cover and cook on high for 6 hours, or until the carrots and lentils are soft. Add the brown rice and spinach and cook 30 minutes longer. (Note: Do not leave the slow cooker unattended while cooking the brown rice.) Thin the soup with stock or water if desired, and finish the soup as directed in Step 3.

▶ **Complete Meal Ideas:** Serve this lentil soup with:
   Whole wheat bread
   Reduced-fat 2% milk or low-fat yogurt
   Fresh fruit that contains vitamin C (you might want to try the Orange, Blueberry, and Date Salad with Frozen Yogurt, page 369)

APPROXIMATE NUTRITIONAL INFORMATION: Serving size: 1 cup lentil soup with brown rice and spinach; Calories: 176 cals; Protein: 11 g; Carbohydrates: 25 g; Fat: 4 g; Fiber: 10 g; Sodium: 246 mg; Iron: 4 mg; Vitamin A: 1,841 IU; Folic Acid: 110 mcg; Diabetic Exchange: Bread/Starch 1.5, Fat, 1

turkish-style red lentil soup

What's in this for baby and me? Protein, iron, vitamin A, folic acid, and fiber.

EARTHY LENTILS ARE an excellent source of protein, iron, vitamin A, folic acid, and fiber, and a good source of vitamin C. The sautéed mint and paprika garnish is optional, but it adds a distinctive flavor. If you are short on time, simply add the mint and paprika directly to the soup during the last 20 minutes of cooking time. Slow Cooker Instructions follow.

serves 6 to 8 (makes about 7 cups)

2 tablespoons unsalted butter

1 medium onion, chopped

2 garlic cloves, crushed

3 carrots, peeled and sliced, or 1½ cups sliced peeled baby carrots

1½ cups red lentils, picked over and rinsed

7 cups fat-free low-sodium stock or water, or more as needed

Salt and freshly ground pepper, to taste

GARNISH (optional)

1½ tablespoons unsalted butter

1 teaspoon dried mint

Dash of paprika or red pepper

1. Melt the butter in a 6-quart saucepan over medium-high heat. Add the onion and sauté for 3 minutes. Add the garlic, carrots, lentils, and stock and bring to a boil. Reduce the heat and simmer, uncovered, for 30 minutes, or until the carrots are soft and the lentils are mushy.
2. Thin the finished soup with additional stock or water if desired. Adjust the seasoning and keep warm while you prepare the garnish.
3. To prepare the garnish, melt the butter in a small saucepan over medium-high heat. Add the mint and paprika and cook for 10 to 20 seconds, or just until fragrant. Add the garnish to individual soup bowls (or add it to the soup in the saucepan). (Note: You can also add the mint and paprika directly to the soup during the last 20 minutes of cooking.)

▶ *Cooking Tip:* The bright orange lentils will lose some of their color during cooking, and the finished soup will be a golden yellow color.

▶ *Storage Tip:* This soup keeps refrigerated for about 1 week, and it can be frozen for up to 1 month.

▶ *Variation:* Add your favorite diced vegetables or dried herbs and spices to this soup when you add the carrots in Step 1. Substitute a dash of mild curry powder for the chili powder.

▶ *Slow Cooker Instructions:* Use 6½ cups stock instead of 7.
1. Melt the butter in a large nonstick skillet over medium-high heat. Add the onions and sauté for 3 minutes, then add the garlic and carrots and sauté for 2 minutes.
2. Transfer the contents of the skillet to the slow cooker. Add the lentils and stock, cover, and cook on high for 4 hours, or until the carrots are tender. Follow Step 3 to finish the soup, or omit the butter and add the mint and paprika directly to the soup during the last 20 minutes of cooking.

▶ *Complete Meal Ideas:* Serve this soup with:
Whole wheat bread
Vegetable that contains vitamin C (you might want to try the
   Tomato and Mozzarella Salad with Fresh Basil, page 157)
Reduced-fat 2% milk or low-fat yogurt
Fresh fruit that contains vitamin C

APPROXIMATE NUTRITIONAL INFORMATION: Serving size: 1 cup red lentil soup; Calories: 236 cals; Protein: 15 g; Carbohydrates: 34 g; Fat: 5 g; Fiber: 6 g; Sodium: 280 mg; Vitamin A: 8,756 IU; Iron: 4 mg; Folic Acid: 106 mcg; Diabetic Exchange: Bread/Starch 2, Fat .5, Meat (Lean) 1

mediterranean pasta, bean, and vegetable soup

What's in this for baby and me? Iron, vitamins A and C, and fiber.

THIS NOURISHING SOUP is sure to become a family favorite—kids love it with alphabet pasta (add about 1½ cups) or any other small pasta. It is loaded with iron, vitamins A and C, and fiber, and a good dose of protein, folic acid, and B vitamins. For a real treat, or an elegant first course, garnish this soup with pesto (homemade, page 147, or store-bought) and grated Parmesan cheese. A pureed or strained version (without the pesto and cheese) makes a super meal for young eaters. Slow Cooker Instructions follow.

serves 6 (makes about 8 cups)

3 tablespoons olive oil or canola oil

1 medium onion, finely diced

2 garlic cloves, crushed

5 carrots, peeled, cut lengthwise in half, and sliced, or 2 cups sliced peeled baby carrots

2 teaspoons dried thyme, oregano, basil, or herbes de Provence

1 teaspoon salt, or to taste

5 cups fat-free low-sodium stock (6 cups if omitting the V-8 juice, or more if needed)

1½ cups V-8 or tomato juice (see Vegetable Variation below)

One 14.5-ounce can diced tomatoes (do not drain) or 2 cups diced fresh tomatoes

One 15.5-ounce can Great Northern white beans (or any other small canned beans), rinsed and drained

1 medium zucchini, washed, quartered lengthwise, and sliced

¾ cup ditalini pasta, or other small pasta

1 small bunch (about 10 ounces) Swiss chard, spinach, beet greens, or arugula, washed, stems removed, and thinly sliced (see Timesaving Tip below about using frozen greens)

Freshly ground pepper, to taste

Pesto, for the table (optional)

Grated Parmesan cheese or your favorite cheese, for the table (optional)

1. Heat the olive oil in a 6-quart saucepan over medium-high heat. Add the onion and sauté for 2 minutes. Add the garlic, carrots, and thyme and sauté for 3 minutes. Add the salt, stock, and V-8 juice, and bring to a boil. Reduce the heat and simmer, uncovered, for 10 minutes.

2. Add the tomatoes, beans, zucchini, and pasta, reduce the heat, and simmer for 15 to 20 minutes, or until the pasta is cooked. Add the greens during the last 10 minutes of cooking.

3. Adjust the seasoning, and thin the soup with stock or water if desired. Serve immediately and pass the pesto and cheese at the table, if desired.

▶ *Timesaving Tip:* Use one 10-ounce package frozen spinach or other greens in place of fresh. Microwave or defrost and drain well, then add to the soup during the last 5 minutes of cooking.

▶ *Vegetable Variation:* Add any favorite vegetables that require a longer cooking time (such as potatoes, winter squash, or leeks) with the carrots in Step 1; add any quick-cooking vegetables (such as broccoli or cauliflower florets, summer squash, corn, peas, and green beans or wax beans) with the zucchini in Step 2. Add any greens (fresh or frozen) during the last 5 minutes of cooking time. For a less "tomato-y" soup, omit the V-8 juice and use 7 cups stock.

▶ *Protein Variation:* Add sautéed tofu (see Instructions for Sautéing Tofu, page 228), diced cooked chicken or turkey, or any other cooked meat during the last 10 minutes of Step 2.

▶ *Storage Tip:* This soup keeps refrigerated for about 1 week, and it can be frozen for up to 1 month.

▶ *Slow Cooker Instructions:* Reduce the stock by ½ cup. Use only ½ cup pasta.
1. Using a nonstick skillet instead of a saucepan, sauté onion as directed in Step 1, then add the garlic, if using, carrots, and thyme and sauté for 3 more minutes.
2. Transfer the contents of the skillet to the slow cooker, and add the salt, stock, V-8 juice, and diced tomatoes. Cover and cook on high for 6 hours. During the last 30 minutes of cooking, add the beans, pasta, and Swiss chard. (Note: Do not leave the slow cooker unattended while cooking the pasta.) Finish the soup as directed in Step 3.

▶ *Complete Meal Ideas:* Serve this soup with:
   3 ounces protein (you might want to try the Grilled Cheese Sandwich,
      page 119, or the Hummus-Tabbouleh Roll, page 127)
   Whole wheat bread
   Reduced-fat 2% milk or low-fat yogurt
   Fresh fruit that contains vitamin C

APPROXIMATE NUTRITIONAL INFORMATION: Serving size: 1 cup pasta, bean, and vegetable soup; Calories: 210 cals; Protein: 9 g; Carbohydrates: 31 g; Fat: 6 g; Fiber: 8 g; Sodium: 667 mg; Vitamin A: 10,877 IU; Vitamin C: 32 mg; Iron: 5 mg; Diabetic Exchange: Bread/Starch 2, Fat 1

green split pea soup

What's in this for baby and me? Protein, vitamin A, folic acid, and fiber.

SPLIT PEA SOUP is an excellent source of protein, vitamin A, folic acid, and fiber, and a good source of iron. If you insist that green split pea soup needs a ham bone for flavor, this lighter recipe might convince you otherwise. Croutons make a nice garnish (see Homemade Croutons, page 165). Slow Cooker Instructions follow.

serves 6 (makes about 7 cups)

3 tablespoons olive oil	**1 teaspoon dried marjoram (optional)**
1 medium onion, finely chopped	**2 bay leaves (optional)**
2 garlic cloves, crushed	**8 cups fat free low-sodium stock or water, or**
4 carrots, peeled and sliced, or 2 cups sliced	**more as needed**
peeled baby carrots	**1½ cups (10 ounces) green split peas (see**
2 celery stalks, washed and sliced (optional)	**Cooking Tip below)**
1 teaspoon dried thyme (optional)	**Salt and freshly ground pepper, to taste**

1. Heat the olive oil in a 6-quart saucepan over medium heat. Add the onion and sauté for 3 minutes. Add the garlic, carrots, and optional celery, thyme, marjoram, and bay leaves and sauté for 3 minutes longer.
2. Add the stock and peas, stir, and bring to a boil. Skim off the foam with a spoon, then reduce the heat and simmer for about 2 hours, or until the peas are tender.
3. If the soup is too thick, add more stock or water, 2 tablespoons at a time. Adjust the seasoning, remove the bay leaves and serve immediately.

▶ *Cooking Tip:* Pick over and rinse the peas, then soak them for 8 to 12 hours in 5 cups water. Or, for faster results, place the peas in a 3-quart saucepan, add water to cover by at least 2 inches, and bring to a boil. Cook for 2 minutes, then remove from the heat and let stand, covered, at room temperature, for at least 1 hour or up to 6 hours. Drain, rinse again, and proceed with the recipe.

▶ *Timesaving Tip:* Use packaged instant split pea soup. Add your favorite cooked, diced vegetables or seasonings suggested here.

▶ *Storage Tip:* This soup keeps refrigerated for about 5 days, and it can be frozen for up to 1 month.

▶ *Slow Cooker Instructions:* It is essential to soak the peas before adding them to the slow cooker. The amount of time it takes for the peas to cook will vary; it may take up to 10 hours. Use 6 cups stock instead of 8.

1. Follow the instructions in the Cooking Tip above to soften the peas before cooking.
2. Using a large nonstick skillet instead of a saucepan, follow the instructions in Step 1.
3. Transfer the contents of the skillet to the slow cooker. Add the drained soaked peas and the stock, cover, and cook on high for 8 hours, or possibly up to 10 hours, until the peas are soft. Finish the soup as directed in Step 3.

▶ *Complete Meal Ideas:* Serve this soup with:

Whole wheat bread (you might want to try the Veggie Cheese Wrap, page 125)
Reduced-fat 2% milk or low-fat yogurt
Fresh fruit that contains vitamin C

APPROXIMATE NUTRITIONAL INFORMATION: Serving size: 1 cup green split pea soup; Calories: 203 cals; Protein: 11 g; Carbohydrates: 26 g; Fat: 7 g; Fiber: 10 g; Sodium: 306 mg; Vitamin A: 11,721 IU; Folic Acid: 100 mcg; Diabetic Exchange: Bread/Starch 1.5, Meat (Medium Fat) 1

beef, barley, and vegetable soup

What's in this for baby and me? Protein and vitamins A and C.

THE SOUP IS an excellent source of protein and vitamins A and C, as well as a good source of iron, B vitamins, and fiber. Any vegetables, from potatoes and turnips to broccoli and spinach, can be added in place of the beef to make this a hearty vegetarian soup. This soup is even better the second day. Slow Cooker Instructions follow.

serves 6 to 8 (makes about 8 cups)

2 tablespoons canola oil or olive oil

1 medium onion, finely diced

4 carrots, peeled and sliced, or 2 cups sliced
   peeled baby carrots

½ cup uncooked pearl barley, rinsed under hot
   water

1 pound beef shank, bone-in

One 14.5-ounce can peeled and diced
   tomatoes (do not drain) or 1½ cups peeled

and diced fresh tomatoes

8 cups fat-free low-sodium stock, or more as
   needed

1 zucchini, washed, halved lengthwise, and
   sliced

Salt and freshly ground pepper, to taste

¼ cup chopped fresh parsley, for garnish
   (optional)

1. Heat the canola oil in a 6-quart saucepan over medium-high heat. Add the onion and sauté for 3 minutes. Add the carrots and barley and sauté for 3 minutes. Add the beef, tomatoes, and stock and bring to a boil. Reduce the heat and simmer, uncovered, for 20 minutes.

2. Add the zucchini and simmer for about 25 minutes longer, or until the barley and meat are tender.

3. Remove the shank from the soup, and when it is cool enough to handle, remove the meat from the bone. Cut the meat into small pieces and return it to the soup.

4. Add more canned stock or water to thin the soup, if desired, and adjust the seasoning and heat through before serving. Garnish with the parsley, if desired, and serve immediately.

▶ *Storage Tip:* This soup keeps refrigerated for about 3 days, and it can be frozen for up to 1 month.

▶ *Slow Cooker Instructions:* Use 6 cups stock instead of 8. Drain the diced tomatoes.

1. Using a large nonstick skillet instead of a saucepan, sauté the onion as directed in Step 1. Add the carrots and barley and sauté for 3 minutes.

2. Transfer the contents of the skillet to the slow cooker, then add the beef shank, drained diced tomatoes, stock, and zucchini. Cover and cook on high for 6 hours.
3. Finish the soup as directed in steps 3 and 4.

▶ *Complete Meal Ideas:* Serve this soup with:
> 3 ounces protein (such as hard cheese) if you are not using the beef shank (you might want to try the Roasted Red Pepper and Cheese Dip, page 174, with bread)
> Whole wheat bread
> Reduced-fat 2% milk or low-fat yogurt
> Fresh fruit that contains vitamin C

APPROXIMATE NUTRITIONAL INFORMATION: Serving size: 1½ cups beef, barley, and vegetable soup: Calories: 240 cals; Protein: 18 g; Carbohydrates: 17 g; Fat: 11 g; Fiber: 4 g; Sodium: 312 mg; Vitamin A: 9,994 IU; Vitamin C: 18 mg; Diabetic Exchange: Bread/starch 1, Fat .5, Meat (Medium Fat) 2

crackers with a healthy crunch

Many store-bought crackers contain partially hydrogenated oil, or trans fats; try to avoid them. Whole wheat should ideally be the first ingredient listed on the label. Each of the following trans fat–free brands has at least 2 grams of fiber per serving. They are delicious topped with cheese, cottage cheese, peanut butter, hummus, artichoke dips, or any other healthy spreads or dips.

Excellent Choice Whole Wheat Crackers

365 Baked Woven Wheats
Ak-Mak 100% Whole Wheat Stone Ground Sesame Crackers
Barbara's Bakery Wheatines
Dr. Kracker High Fiber Crackers
Finn Crisp
Frookie 50% Less Fat Snack Crackers
Frookie All Natural Snack Crackers
Hain Pure Foods All Natural Baked Crackers Wheatettes
Health Valley Low-Fat Crackers, No Salt Added
Health Valley Oat Bran Graham Crackers
Hol-Grain Crackers
Kavli Crispbread
Nabisco Triscuit Baked Whole Grain Wheat Crackers Low Sodium
Ryvita Whole Grain Crisp Bread
Wasa

gazpacho

What's in this for baby and me? Vitamins A and C.

G AZPACHO IS A source of vitamins A and C, and a good source of folic acid and fiber. A quick and easy soup that involves no cooking, it is the ideal first course for a summer meal, or a refreshing snack any time of day. Puree to a chunky or smooth consistency, then add diced cucumber, tomatoes, radishes, or avocado for additional texture if desired.

serves 2 (makes about 2 cups)

1 slice white or whole wheat bread, diced

1 pound (about 3) vine-ripened tomatoes, quartered

¾ cup peeled and sliced seedless cucumber

¼ cup jarred roasted red peppers

A dash of garlic powder (optional)

¼ cup water, fat-free low-sodium stock, or V-8

juice

Leaves from 4 sprigs of fresh cilantro (optional)

Salt and freshly ground pepper, to taste

A few drops of olive oil

A few drops of balsamic vinegar

1. Combine all of the ingredients except the olive oil and balsamic vinegar in a blender or food processor and pulse until desired consistency.
2. Transfer to a bowl, cover, and refrigerate until well chilled, at least 1 hour. Stir in the olive oil and balsamic vinegar, adjust the seasoning, and serve.

▶ *Storage Tip:* This soup keeps refrigerated for up to 3 days. Do not freeze.

▶ *Health Tip:* If your doctor has restricted your fat intake, omit the olive oil.

▶ *Complete Meal Ideas:* Serve this gazpacho with:
   3 ounces protein (you might want to try the Tuna Salad, page 123)
   Whole wheat bread
   Reduced-fat 2% milk or low-fat yogurt
   Fresh fruit

APPROXIMATE NUTRITIONAL INFORMATION: Serving size: 1 cup gazpacho; Calories: 103 cals; Protein: 3 g; Carbohydrates: 17 g; Fat: 4 g; Fiber: 3 g; Sodium: 100 mg; Vitamin A: 2,133 IU; Vitamin C: 74 mg; Diabetic Exchange: Bread/Starch 1, Fat 1

drink plenty of water

Fluid intake is vital throughout pregnancy. A pregnant woman needs to drink 1 quart (4 cups) to 1½ quarts (6 cups) of water every day in addition to milk. Fruit juices are high in calories (for a list of the calorie content of juices, see Get Juiced Up, page 75), so one or two servings per day is fine, but do not drink fruit juice in place of water. If you have any concerns about bottled water, see Best Bottled Waters, page 114.

Why Is Water So Important?

To aid with digestion

To ensure proper hydration

To avoid constipation

To reduce the risk of urinary tract infections

To eliminate toxins and keep your system clean

To regulate your body temperature

To reduce swelling

To prevent dry skin

best bottled waters

There are two things to consider when purchasing bottled water: the water and the bottle. First, the water is not necessarily any purer or cleaner than the tap water in your area. In fact, much bottled water is simply tap water that has been processed and labeled as purified. Look for the source of the water on the label; if the source is not stated, call the company and ask where the water comes from. Tap water is not necessarily bad, but you shouldn't pay a high price for it.

The second conundrum is the bottle. Those numbers at the bottom of the bottle do mean something, and not all of the numbers are good. Most clear plastic water bottles are labeled #1, which is a safe plastic that should be used only once and then recycled. The safest plastics are #1 PET or PETE (polyethylene), #2 HDPE (high-density polyethylene), #4 LDPE (low-density polyethylene), and #5 PP (polypropylene). Some numbers to avoid whenever possible include #3 PVC (polyvinyl chloride or vinyl), #6 PS (polystyrene, such as Styrofoam), and #7 (polycarbonate or Lexan).

Good Bottle Numbers: 1, 2, 4, and 5

Bad Bottle Numbers: 3, 6, and 7

Why should certain plastics be avoided? Because studies show that chemicals from those plastics can leach into foods or beverages, and some chemicals, like BPA (bisphenol-A, or #7), have been associated with disruption of the estrogen hormone (though this has not been proven).[3] The FDA has not issued any warnings as of this writing, so use your best judgment. In 2006, the European Union banned all products with BPA that were made for children under the age of three, including bottles and sippy cups. The U.S. may follow at some point. For the latest information, go to the Environmental Working Group web site at www.ewg.org.

To be on the safe side, follow these three guidelines when using any plastic products: (1) Do not heat foods in plastic containers; use glass or a regular plate in the microwave oven. (2) Do not to use plastic wrap to cover foods that will be reheated in a microwave oven (use a paper towel instead). (3) Thoroughly wash any plastic bottles that you plan to reuse by hand. Do not run them through the dishwasher, where they are exposed to very high heat. Needless to say, glass baby bottles are making a comeback.

basic chicken stock

What's in this for baby and me? A homemade, all-natural stock.

USE THIS RECIPE as a blueprint—add or omit any vegetables, herbs, or spices to suit your taste. The cooked chicken from this recipe can be used for Greek-Style Chicken, Lemon, and Egg Soup (page 98), Chicken Salad with Diced Apricots and Almonds (page 120). Slow Cooker Instructions follow.

makes 7 to 8 cups

One 3¼- to 3½-pound chicken or 3¼ pound
   chicken parts, rinsed and any large chunks
   of fat removed
1 medium onion, quartered
1 large carrot, scrubbed and quartered
1 celery stalk, washed and quartered

5 fresh parsley sprigs
2 bay leaves
2 teaspoons salt, or to taste
10 to 12 cups water, or enough to completely
   cover all ingredients
Freshly ground pepper, to taste

1. In a large stockpot, combine all of the ingredients and bring to a boil. Reduce the heat and simmer, uncovered, for 1½ hours. If the water level drops below the height of the stock ingredients before the stock has simmered for 1 hour, add ½ cup of water at a time, or just enough to keep the ingredients covered.
2. Transfer the chicken to a plate; set aside. Strain the stock into a heatproof bowl. Allow the stock to cool to room temperature, then refrigerate until chilled.
3. When the chicken is cool enough to handle, remove the meat from the bones. (This is more easily done while the chicken is still warm.) Cover and refrigerate for another use.
4. Once the stock has chilled, remove it from the refrigerator and, using a large spoon, scrape off as much fat from the surface as possible. Refrigerate until needed.

▶ **Storage Tip:** This stock keeps for about 3 days refrigerated, and it can be frozen for up to 3 months. If you do not plan to use the frozen stock all at once, freeze it in smaller containers so you can defrost only what you need.

▶ *Slow Cooker Instructions:* Use a 3- to 3¼-pound whole chicken and 8 cups of water instead of 10 to 12 cups.

1. Coarsely chop the onion, carrot, and celery stalk. Arrange the onions, carrots, and celery in the bottom of a slow cooker. Add the chicken or 3¼ pounds chicken parts and the remaining ingredients. Cover and cook on high for 8 hours, or until the chicken is tender and falling off the bone.
2. Finish the stock as directed in Steps 2 through 4.

APPROXIMATE NUTRITIONAL INFORMATION: Serving size: 1 cup basic chicken stock; Calories: 30 cals; Protein: 4 g; Carbohydrates: 3 g; Fat: 0 g; Fiber: 0 g; Sodium: 885 mg; Diabetic Exchange: 1 cup FREE

basic vegetable stock

What's in this for baby and me? A homemade, all-natural stock.

KEEP THIS STOCK in your freezer for all of your soup needs.

makes about 6 cups

3 tablespoons olive oil or canola oil

1 medium onion, quartered

2 carrots, scrubbed and coarsely chopped

2 large garlic cloves, crushed

6–8 ounces mushrooms (preferably cremini), washed and cut into thick slices

1 cup boiling water

12 cups water

2 bay leaves (optional)

½ teaspoon each dried oregano and dried thyme (or 1 teaspoon of either herb)

One 14.5-ounce can peeled and diced tomatoes (do not drain) or 1½ cups peeled and diced fresh tomatoes, with their juice (optional)

1 teaspoon salt, or to taste

1. Preheat the oven to 425°F.
2. Place the olive oil in a large baking dish, add the onion, carrots, garlic, and mushrooms, and stir to lightly coat the vegetables with the oil. Roast for 30 to 40 minutes, or until the vegetables are nicely browned.
3. Transfer the roasted vegetables to a 6-quart saucepan. Add the boiling water to the baking dish and scrape up as much of the roasted bits in the bottom of the pan as possible, then add the liquid to the saucepan.
4. Add the remaining ingredients and bring to a boil, then reduce the heat and simmer gently for 1 hour, or until the stock is slightly reduced and the flavors have had a chance to develop.
5. Strain the stock into a heatproof bowl; use the back of a ladle or spoon to press against the solids to extract as much liquid as possible. Allow the stock to cool to room temperature, and refrigerate until ready to use.

▶ *Storage Tip:* This stock keeps for about 3 days refrigerated, and it can be frozen for up to 3 months. If you do not plan to use the frozen stock all at once, freeze it in smaller containers so you can defrost only what you need.

APPROXIMATE NUTRITIONAL INFORMATION: Serving size: 1 cup basic vegetable stock; Calories: 99 cals; Protein: 2 g; Carbohydrates: 8 g; Fat: 7 g; Fiber: 2 g; Sodium: 617 mg; Vitamin A: 5,799 IU; Vitamin C: 14 mg; Diabetic Exchange: Fat 1, Vegetable 1

Note: The nutrition information reflects the consumption of the vegetables in this stock.

pr-egg-o salad sandwich

What's in this for baby and me? Protein, iron, folic acid, and fiber.

A SIMPLE EGG salad sandwich is a wonderfully easy way to get protein, iron, folic acid, and fiber into your diet, especially if you're a vegetarian. This sandwich is also a good source of B vitamins and calcium. Doctor it up with your favorite seasonings, herbs, and chopped vegetables, or keep it simple.

makes 1 sandwich (makes about ½ cup salad)

2 hard-boiled large eggs, chopped
2 tablespoons diced celery (optional)
1 tablespoon light mayonnaise, or to taste
Salt and freshly ground pepper, to taste

2 slices hearty whole wheat bread or calcium-enriched bread (such as Calcium Enriched Roman Meal)

1. Gently mix the eggs, celery, if using, mayonnaise, and salt and pepper in a small bowl.
2. Spread the egg salad on one of the slices of bread, top with the remaining bread, and cut in half. (Refrigerate any leftovers.)

▶ *Variation:* For an herbal touch, add 1 tablespoon sliced scallions or chives and 1 tablespoon chopped fresh parsley, dill, tarragon, or chervil to the egg salad. Or, for a more full-flavored taste, add a dash of paprika, curry powder, mustard, or Tabasco, or a few capers or olives. For a colorful salad, add diced fresh red bell peppers or jarred red peppers.

▶ *Complete Meal Ideas:* Serve this sandwich with:
   A raw or cooked vegetable, vegetable soup, or green salad (you might
      want to try the Creamy Asparagus-Artichoke Soup, page 90,
      or the Great Green Broccoli-Spinach Soup, page 94)
   Reduced-fat 2% milk or low-fat yogurt
   Fresh fruit that contains vitamin C

APPROXIMATE NUTRITIONAL INFORMATION: Serving size: 1 egg salad sandwich (½ cup) on 2 slices whole wheat bread; Calories: 446 cals; Protein: 20 g; Carbohydrates: 47 g; Fat: 21 g; Fiber: 6 g; Sodium: 822 mg; Iron: 4 mg; Folic Acid: 80 mcg; Diabetic Exchange: Bread/Starch 3, Fat 2, Meat (Medium Fat) 2

grilled cheese sandwich

What's in this for baby and me? Protein, calcium, and fiber.

No NEED TO reinvent the wheel—but spreading the mayonnaise on the outside of the bread prevents sticking while using a minimal amount of fat. The cheese and calcium-enriched bread are great sources of protein, calcium, and fiber. To entice young children to try a bite, cut the sandwich into their favorite shapes with cookie cutters.

makes 1 sandwich

1 teaspoon light mayonnaise

2 slices of hearty whole grain bread or
  enriched bread (such as Calcium Enriched
  Roman Meal)

2 ounces sliced favorite high-calcium cheese
  (such as 2 to 3 slices 2% Milk Singles
  reduced-fat pasteurized process cheese
  with added calcium)

Mustard, to taste (optional)

1. Place a small nonstick skillet over medium-high heat. Thinly spread half of the mayonnaise on one side of a bread slice, then place the slice mayonnaise-side down in the skillet. Arrange the cheese slices on top of the bread. Spread mustard, if using, on one side of the second bread slice and the rest of the mayonnaise on the other side, and place the bread mayonnaise-side up on top of the cheese.
2. Cook the first side until nicely browned and the cheese is beginning to melt (check by lifting up the sandwich). Flip the sandwich and cook the other side until nicely browned and the cheese is entirely melted. Cut in half and serve.

▶ *Complete Meal Ideas:* Serve this sandwich with:
  A raw or cooked vegetable, a vegetable soup, or a green salad
    (you might want to try the Mediterranean Pasta, Bean, and
    Vegetable Soup, page 106, or the Gazpacho, page 112)
  Reduced-fat 2% milk or low-fat yogurt
  Fresh fruit

APPROXIMATE NUTRITIONAL INFORMATION: Serving size: 1 grilled cheese sandwich on whole grain bread; Calories: 354 cals; Protein: 17 g; Carbohydrates: 48 g; Fat: 13 g; Fiber: 6 g; Sodium: 1,220 mg; Calcium: 346 mg; Diabetic Exchange: Bread/Starch 3, Fat 2, Meat (Medium Fat) 1

chicken salad
with dried apricots
and almonds

What's in this for baby and me? Protein and vitamin C.

Hɪɢʜ ɪɴ ᴘʀᴏᴛᴇɪɴ and vitamin C and a good source of vitamin A and fiber, this chicken salad is terrific on toasted whole grain bread or on a bed of mixed greens. This salad is not designed for children, but a serving of plain cooked chicken and diced apricots can be set aside to make a perfect meal for a young eater.

makes 4 to 6 sandwiches (makes about 3 cups salad)

2 teaspoons canola oil (if using the chicken tenders)

1 pound chicken tenders or boneless, skinless chicken breasts, cut into 1-inch cubes, or about 2½ cups finely diced cooked chicken or turkey

Salt and freshly ground pepper, to taste

⅓ cup chopped dried apricots

2 tablespoons chopped fresh herbs, such as cilantro or dill

½ red bell pepper, finely diced, or ¼ cup chopped jarred roasted red peppers

½ cup sliced almonds, toasted

½ cup light mayonnaise, or to taste

1. If using chicken tenders, heat the canola oil in a large nonstick skillet over medium-high heat. Add the chicken, season with salt and pepper, and sauté for 7 minutes, or until completely cooked; transfer to a bowl to cool. Dice the cooked chicken, or tear the meat into bits with your fingers, and return to the bowl.
2. Combine the diced chicken and the remaining ingredients in a bowl and mix well. Adjust the seasoning. Refrigerate if not serving immediately. (Any leftovers should be covered and refrigerated.)

▶ *Timesaving Tip:* Buy a rotisserie chicken and cut or tear the meat into small pieces.

▶ *Variation:* Feel free to add your favorite spices, herbs, and other ingredients to the salad. Some nice additions are diced celery, toasted pine nuts, and curry powder.

► *Complete Meal Ideas:* Serve this salad with:

> Green salad (you might want to try a tossed salad with the Sun-
> Dried Tomato and Basil Dressing, page 167, or romaine
> lettuce with the Caesar Salad Dressing, page 168)
> Whole wheat roll or bread
> Reduced-fat 2% milk or low-fat yogurt
> Fresh fruit

APPROXIMATE NUTRITIONAL INFORMATION: Serving size: ¾ cup chicken salad (not including bread): Calories: 307 cals; Protein: 25 g; Carbohydrates: 13 g; Fat: 17 g; Fiber: 3 g; Sodium: 199 mg; Vitamin C: 15 mg; Diabetic Exchange: Bread/Starch 1, Fat 1, Meat (Medium Fat) 3

safe sandwiches

There are a few important points to keep in mind to ensure that your bagged lunch remains as healthy and safe as possible. Harmful bacteria multiply rapidly in the danger zone, temperatures between 40° and 140°F. Any perishable items in your lunch box, including cold cuts, hard-boiled eggs, salads made with mayonnaise, and packaged combos containing luncheon meats and cheese, should be kept cold with an ice pack and refrigerated upon arrival if possible. Food should never be left out at room temperature for more than two hours, one hour if the temperature is over 90°F. Following are a few tips to keep your lunch free of food-borne pathogens.[2]

► Insulated soft-sided lunch boxes or bags are best for keeping foods cold. Use an ice pack or frozen-juice box with any perishable foods.

► Prepare cooked food (such as tuna or egg salad, or mayonnaise-based potato or pasta salads) ahead of time to allow them to be thoroughly chilled before packing. Keep them refrigerated until ready to go.

► Use an insulated container to keep hot foods hot. Fill the container with boiling water, let stand a few minutes, drain, then add the hot food.

► When using a microwave to reheat leftovers, cover food to promote even heating and heat to 165°F. Cook frozen convenience meals according to package directions.

► Discard all used food packaging.

the perfect brown-bag lunch

Quick and easy peanut butter (or other nut butter) sandwiches made with whole wheat bread remain one of America's healthiest and most beloved sandwiches.

THE PERFECT BROWN BAG LUNCH

Peanut butter or other protein-rich sandwich

Vegetable sticks or V-8 juice

A couple of healthy oatmeal cookies

A piece of fresh fruit

8 ounces of low-fat yogurt or a glass of reduced-fat 2% milk

APPROXIMATE NUTRITIONAL INFORMATION: 1 peanut butter and jelly sandwich on whole wheat bread made with 3 tablespoons peanut butter and 2 teaspoons jam; Calories: 445 cals; Protein: 17 g; Carbohydrates: 41 g; Fat: 27 g; Sodium: 491 mg; Fiber: 6 g; Diabetic Exchange: Bread/Starch 2, Meat (High Fat) 1.5, Fat 2

tuna salad sandwich

What's in this for baby and me? Protein and fiber.

Light, fresh, and high in protein and fiber, this deli-style salad is perfect between two slices of whole wheat bread or on a bed of lettuce. Canned light tuna is a good source of DHA omega-3.

makes 2 sandwiches

One 6–6½-ounce can light tuna in spring water, drained, rinsed, and drained again

2 tablespoons thinly sliced scallions (green part only)

2 tablespoons finely diced celery (optional)

3 tablespoons light mayonnaise, to taste

1 tablespoon freshly squeezed lemon juice, to taste

Salt and freshly ground pepper, to taste

4 slices hearty whole grain bread or calcium-enriched bread (such as Calcium Enriched Roman Meal)

1. Combine all of the ingredients except the bread in a bowl and mix until well blended. Cover and refrigerate any leftovers.
2. To make each sandwich, spread the salad on one of the slices of bread, top with the remaining bread, and cut in half.

▶ **Variation:** Add chopped fresh dill, parsley, or your favorite fresh herb, a few small capers (drained), or finely diced green peppers to the salad.

▶ **Complete Meal Ideas:** Serve this sandwich with:

A raw or cooked vegetable, vegetable soup, or tossed salad (you
    might want to try Romaine Lettuce with Olive Oil–Lemon
    Dressing, page 169, or raw vegetables with the Spinach Dip,
    page 177, or the Artichoke-Spinach Dip, page 178)
Reduced-fat 2% milk or low-fat yogurt
Fresh fruit

APPROXIMATE NUTRITIONAL INFORMATION: Serving size: 1 tuna salad sandwich on whole wheat bread; Calories: 415 cals; Protein: 29 g; Carbohydrates: 47 g; Fat: 15 g; Fiber: 6 g; Sodium: 1,141 mg; Diabetic Exchange: Bread/Starch 3, Fat 1, Meat (Medium Fat) 4

indigestion and heartburn

Indigestion and heartburn are very common complaints during pregnancy, especially during the first and third trimesters. During the first trimester, heartburn is caused by increased hormone levels and smooth muscle relaxation, which allow acids to reflux (come back up) more easily. During the third trimester, decreased stomach capacity limits the space for food and stomach juices, resulting in indigestion and heartburn.

TIPS FOR COPING

- Avoid greasy, fatty, spicy, or fried foods.

- Avoid gas-forming foods such as cabbage and beans.

- Avoid all caffeinated beverages and chocolate.

- Avoid all citrus fruits and juices.

- Sit down when you eat and try to relax.

- Eat slowly and chew thoroughly.

- Don't eat and drink at the same time. Wait thirty to sixty minutes after eating to drink a beverage.

- Don't lie down after eating. Take a walk instead.

- Try not to eat three hours prior to bedtime.

- Eat frequent smaller meals instead of three large ones.

- Sip a cup of plain hot water after meals.

- If indigestion keeps you awake at night, try to sleep propped up with pillows.

- Wear loose-fitting clothing, especially around the abdomen and waist.

- Avoid bending over at the waist. Bend at the knees.

- Never take any medication for heartburn without consulting your doctor or nurse.

- Avoid preparations containing sodium or sodium bicarbonate.

wraps and rolls

veggie cheese wrap

What's in this for baby and me? Protein, calcium, vitamins A and C, folic acid, and fiber.

A DELICIOUS WAY to get your protein, calcium, vitamins A and C, folic acid, and fiber, not to mention a good dose of B vitamins. Complete Meal Ideas for all of the following wraps and rolls include reduced-fat 2% milk or low-fat yogurt and fresh fruit.

makes 1 wrap

4 slices of provolone, Swiss, or any cheese
    that melts easily

1 burrito-size (10-inch) tortilla

3 tomato slices

2 strips jarred roasted red peppers (optional)

A couple of avocado slices

A handful of lettuce leaves

1 tablespoon salsa, or to taste

Arrange the cheese over the tortilla and microwave for a few seconds to melt the cheese. Top with the remaining ingredients, roll up, and slice in half.

APPROXIMATE NUTRITIONAL INFORMATION: Serving size: 1 veggie cheese wrap; Calories: 416 cals; Protein: 20 g; Carbohydrates: 36 g; Fat: 22 g; Fiber: 15 g; Sodium: 884 mg; Calcium: 476 mg; Vitamin A: 1,950 IU; Vitamin C: 22 mg; Folic Acid: 91 mcg; Diabetic Exchange: Bread/Starch 2, Fat 2, Meat (High Fat) 2

chicken caesar wrap

What's in this for baby and me? Protein, vitamins A and C, and fiber.

LOADED WITH PROTEIN, vitamins A and C, and fiber, this wrap is also a good source of calcium and folic acid. Use your favorite store-bought Caesar salad dressing or the Caesar Salad Dressing on page 168.

makes 1 wrap

½ cup diced cooked chicken, or 4 ounces
   (about 4 slices) sliced turkey breast
A handful of sliced romaine leaves
3 tomato slices

1 burrito-size (10-inch) tortilla
2 tablespoons grated Parmesan cheese, or to
   taste
1 tablespoon Caesar salad dressing

Distribute the chicken, lettuce, and tomato slices evenly over the tortilla. Top with the Parmesan cheese and salad dressing. Roll up and slice in half.

APPROXIMATE NUTRITIONAL INFORMATION: Serving size: 1 chicken Caesar wrap; Calories: 377 cals; Protein: 31 g; Carbohydrates: 29 g; Fat: 15 g; Fiber: 11 g; Sodium: 757 g; Vitamin A: 1,190 IU; Vitamin C: 18 mg; Diabetic Exchange: Bread/Starch 2, Fat 1, Meat (Medium Fat) 3

asian-style turkey wrap

What's in this for baby and me? Protein, vitamins A and C, and fiber.

A SMALL AMOUNT of hoisin and Thai peanut sauce is the secret of this yummy Asian-style turkey wrap, which is high in protein, vitamins A and C, and fiber, and a good source of folic acid. Fresh cilantro adds the perfect punch.

makes 1 wrap

1 teaspoon hoisin sauce
1 teaspoon Thai peanut sauce
1 burrito-size (10-inch) tortilla
4 ounces (about 4 slices) sliced turkey breast

2–3 strips of jarred roasted red peppers
   (optional)
A handful of lettuce leaves
A couple sprigs of fresh cilantro (optional)

Mix the hoisin and peanut sauces in a small dish. Spread evenly over the tortilla. Top with the turkey slices and the remaining ingredients, roll up, and slice in half.

APPROXIMATE NUTRITIONAL INFORMATION: Serving size: 1 Asian-style turkey wrap; Calories: 249 cals; Protein: 25 g; Carbohydrates: 31 g; Fat: 3 g; Fiber: 11 g; Sodium: 1,759 mg; Vitamin A: 2,003 IU; Vitamin C: 65 mg; Diabetic Exchange: Bread/Starch 2, Meat (Medium Fat) 3

hummus-tabbouleh roll

What's in this for baby and me? Protein, vitamins A and C, folic acid, and fiber.

ROLLS DON'T GET much better or healthier than this—an excellent source of protein, vitamins A and C, folic acid, and fiber, and a good source of iron. If you have the time and energy to make homemade hummus and tabbouleh, see the recipes on page 175 for Healthy Hummus and on page 151 for Best-Ever Tabbouleh Salad. If not, don't feel guilty—store-bought varieties work just as well.

makes one roll

⅓ cup hummus (any flavor)

1 burrito-size (10-inch) tortilla or large whole
    wheat pita round

⅓ cup tabbouleh salad

3 tomato slices

A few cucumber slices

A handful of lettuce leaves

A squeeze of fresh lemon juice

Spread the hummus on the tortilla or cut open one edge of the pita bread and spread the hummus inside. Top with the remaining ingredients, roll up, and slice in half.

APPROXIMATE NUTRITIONAL INFORMATION: Serving size: 1 hummus-tabbouleh roll; Calories: 345 cals; Protein: 10 g; Carbohydrates: 52 g; Fat: 12 g; Fiber: 16 g; Sodium: 928 mg; Vitamin A: 1,350 IU; Vitamin C: 39 mg; Folic Acid: 109 mcg; Diabetic Exchange: Bread/Starch 3.5, Fat 2

keep-it-simple lobster salad sandwich

What's in this for baby and me? Protein.

SUCCULENT LOBSTER, CRUNCHY celery, and the zing of fresh dill are all you need for the perfect lobster salad. This simple sandwich offers an excellent source of protein, a good source of calcium, folic acid, B vitamins, vitamin E, and a dose of DHA omega-3.

Serves 2 (Makes 1½ cups)

2½ pounds fresh lobsters in their shells (or about 8 ounces cooked lobster)

⅓ cup finely diced celery

1½ tablespoons light mayonnaise

1 tablespoon freshly squeezed lemon juice, to taste

1 tablespoon chopped fresh dill (optional)

Salt and freshly ground pepper, to taste

2 or more enriched hot dog rolls with the slit at the top

1. If using fresh lobsters, boil or steam them for 12 to 17 minutes, depending on the size of the lobsters and the strength of the heat source. In general, 1½ pound lobsters will take about 15 minutes to cook. Allow the lobsters to cool, then shell them and cut the meat into a small dice. (You should have about 1 heaping cup diced lobster meat.)
2. Combine the lobster meat and the remaining ingredients in a bowl and mix well. Adjust the seasoning. Refrigerate if not serving immediately.
3. Open the rolls and lightly brown them under a broiler. Fill with the lobster salad and serve.

▶ *Timesaving Tip:* If you are short on time, ask your fishmonger to steam the lobsters for you. This will also save on clean-up at home. Packaged cooked lobster meat is also available in some stores.

▶ *Storage Tip:* This salad will keep for 1 day refrigerated.

▶ *Complete Meal Ideas:* Serve this sandwich with:
Soup (you might want to try the Creamy Asparagus-Artichoke Soup, page 90)
Reduced-fat 2% milk or low-fat yogurt
Fresh fruit

APPROXIMATE NUTRITIONAL INFORMATION: Serving size: 1 lobster sandwich; Calories: 273 cals; Protein: 27 g; Carbohydrates: 25 g; Fat: 6 g; Fiber: 1 g; Sodium: 739 mg; Diabetic Exchange: Bread/Starch 1, Meat (Lean) 3, Vegetable 2

listeriosis warning

Listeriosis is a food-borne illness that is caused by a bacterium called *Listeria monocytogenes*, found in soil and water. The bacteria are very resistant to common food preservation agents such as heat, nitrites, nitrates, and acids, and they can continue to multiply in refrigerated foods. *Listeria* is often present in the intestines of seemingly healthy animals. The bacteria can contaminate milk and meat products from infected animals and can also contaminate vegetables fertilized with tainted manure. It is important to note that "contaminated food may not look, smell, or taste different from uncontaminated food" (U.S. Food and Drug Administration, July 1997).[4]

Healthy people are generally resistant to listeriosis, but pregnant women are about twenty times more likely than other healthy adults to get listeriosis. About one-third of listeriosis cases happen during pregnancy. Infected pregnant women may experience only a mild, flu-like illness (including fever or a stiff neck); however, infections during pregnancy can lead to premature delivery, infection of the newborn, or even stillbirth.[5] Because the symptoms of listeriosis can take a few days or even weeks to appear and can be mild, you may not even know you have it. That is why it is important to take appropriate food safety precautions during pregnancy. Following is a list of guidelines to prevent listeriosis infection provided by the USDA's Food Safety and Inspection Service and the U.S. Food and Drug Administration[5]:

▶ Do not eat hot dogs, luncheon meats, or deli meats unless they are reheated until steaming hot.

▶ Do not eat soft cheeses such as unpasteurized feta or unpasteurized fresh mozzarella, Brie, Camembert, blue-veined cheeses, and Mexican-style cheeses such as queso fresco (also called queso blanco) and asadero. Pasteurized hard cheeses, semi-soft cheeses (such as part-skim low-moisture mozzarella and feta), processed cheese slices and spreads, cream cheese, and cottage cheese can be consumed safely.

▶ Do not eat refrigerated pâté or meat spreads. Canned or shelf-stable pâté and meat spreads can be eaten.

▶ Do not eat refrigerated smoked seafood unless it is an ingredient in a cooked dish such as a casserole. Examples of refrigerated smoked seafood include salmon, trout, whitefish, cod, tuna, and mackerel, which are most often labeled as "nova-style," "lox," "kippered," "smoked," or "jerky." Canned fish such as salmon and light tuna or shelf-stable smoked seafood may be eaten safely.

▶ Do not drink raw (unpasteurized) milk or eat foods that contain unpasteurized milk.

▶ Use all perishable items that are precooked or ready-to-eat as soon as possible. Observe all expiration dates.

▶ Wash the insides of refrigerators regularly, and be sure to thoroughly clean liquid spills, such as spills from hot dog and luncheon meat packages.

▶ Use a refrigerator thermometer to make sure that your refrigerator always stays at 40°F or below.

▶ Wash all fruits and vegetables with water.

▶ After handling raw foods, wash your hands with warm, soapy water, and wash the utensils, cutting boards, and dishes you used with hot, soapy water before using them again.

▶ Cook foods to well-done temperatures (see Well-Done Temperature Guide, page 435).

salads and dips
for munching and crunching

～

SALADS

I F YOU LOVE salads, you're in luck. All types of salads, from simple greens and raw or cooked vegetables to grain- or pasta-based salads, provide vitamins and nutrients beneficial to pregnant women—and their families. Like soups, salads require no special skills to make and they allow loads of room for creativity. Salads can be eaten as a snack between meals or as a side dish, or, with a little imagination, they can become a well-balanced entrée for lunch or dinner. There are numerous ways to transform a simple salad into a healthy main course by adding a bit of protein and a grain. Following are some ideas to help you jazz up your own salads and boost their nutritional value.

Tips for Making Healthier Salads

▶ *Protein Suggestions*

Cooked (preferably baked, grilled, or broiled) poultry or meat, cooked or canned fish (such as light tuna or salmon), cooked shellfish, hard-boiled eggs, pasteurized hard cheese, part-skim cottage cheese, beans (such as kidney beans, edamame, chickpeas, or lima beans), tofu, or nuts and seeds (such as pumpkin or sesame seeds).

▶ *Grain Suggestions*

Enriched whole wheat bread, tortillas, wheat germ, rice, enriched pasta, kasha, quinoa, tabbouleh, bulgur, wheat berries, or whole wheat croutons.

▶ *Dairy Suggestions*

Low-fat or nonfat plain yogurt, grated or cubed pasteurized hard cheese, part-skim cottage or ricotta cheese, or any safe-for-pregnancy cheese of your choice. (See Listeriosis Warning, page 129, for more information on safe cheeses.)

▶ **Power Greens**

Romaine, Boston, Bibb, loose-leaf, spinach, arugula, beet greens, escarole, Belgian endive, sorrel, dandelion, mustard greens, or sliced cabbage.

Healthy Choices at the Salad Bar

Most grocery stores, restaurants, and even fast food chains offer salad bars or prepared salads (avoid those with preservatives), an easy way to pick up lunch, dinner, or a side dish without having to expend energy on washing greens and chopping vegetables. It's up to you to make healthy choices. Here are a few tips for navigating the salad bar.

- Scan the salad bar to check for cleanliness and a well-maintained general appearance.
- Avoid composed salads made with mayonnaise unless they are in well-chilled containers.
- Choose romaine, Boston, bibb, loose-leaf, or iceberg lettuce (in that order).
- Try to include a grain and a protein in your salad.
- Choose a low-fat or reduced-fat salad dressing that has been kept well chilled, especially if it is mayonnaise-based, or make your own oil and vinegar dressing.
- Top your salad with sesame seeds, pumpkin seeds, or nuts (unless you are on a low-sodium diet).
- Avoid bacon bits, whether real or artificial.
- Compose a plain fruit salad for dessert, breakfast, or snack.
- Avoid tofu unless it is stored in clean water and kept well chilled.
- Use salad dressing in moderation.

DIPS

ACCOMPANIED BY NUTRITIOUS whole grain crackers or breads, vegetables, or low-fat chips (preferably baked, not fried), dips make a great snack for pregnant women, especially those on bed rest or on the go. Dips are the perfect cocktail food for entertaining, and they work wonders as a hunger buffer when dinner is running late. Almost all of the dips in this section can be made in advance, with the exception of guacamole, which tends to lose its fresh green color quickly. Most dips keep for at least three days under refrigeration.

The desire to dip starts at a young age, with french fries dipped in ketchup (some kids eat more ketchup than french fries!). Try going one step healthier by introducing kids to peeled baby carrots with spinach dip, guacamole with chips, or their favorite crackers with hummus. You'd be surprised at what you can get away with by making food a little playful.

Grocery stores, gourmet food stores, and restaurants offer countless choices of dips, but many store-bought varieties contain high levels of sodium, MSG, and fat. Avoid those brands. As with store-bought salad dressings, moderation is the key. Experiment with dips by adding your favorite herbs, grated or diced vegetables, spices, and plain low-fat yogurt or pasteurized instant nonfat dry milk powder for extra calcium.

nuts and seeds

Nuts and seeds, excellent sources of plant protein, are rich in folic acid and other B vitamins, copper, potassium, magnesium, and fiber. Nut butters have the same nutritional advantages as nuts, minus the fiber. When choosing a nut butter, look for the ones that do not contain partially hydrogenated oil. This will eliminate most of the big-name brands, although some, like Smuckers, have an all-natural peanut butter that is excellent. Branch out and try cashew, almond, hazelnut, and soy nut butters. Don't be turned off by the oil that sometimes collects on the surface of natural nut butters, just blend it in. Also, natural butters are best refrigerated.

Portion Sizes and Nutritional Information for Popular Nuts

NUTS (1-OUNCE SERVING)	CALORIES	PROTEIN (G)	FAT (G)	FIBER (G)	CARBS (G)	NUTRIENTS
Almonds	169	6	15	3.0	5	Vitamin E, magnesium, manganese, calcium, phosphorus, copper
Cashews	163	4	13	.8	9	Copper, phosphorus, magnesium, zinc, manganese
English Walnuts	185	4	18	2	4	Copper, manganese, phosphorus, magnesium
Peanuts	166	7	14	2	6	Manganese, vitamin E, niacin, folate, copper, phosphorus, magnesium
Pistachios	162	6	13	3	8	Thiamin, vitamin B_6, phosphorus, manganese, copper

nuts and seeds (cont.)

Portion Sizes and Nutritional Information for Popular Seeds

SEEDS	CALORIES	PROTEIN (G)	FAT (G)	FIBER (G)	CARBS (G)	NUTRIENTS
Ground Flaxseed (1 table-spoon)	30	2	2	2	2	Calcium, iron, ALA omega-3
Sesame Seeds (1 table-spoon)	51	2	4	1	2	Calcium, iron, phosphorus, zinc, magnesium, copper, manganese
Pumpkin Seeds (3 table-spoons)	54	2	2	1	6	Iron, magnesium, zinc, copper, manganese
Sunflower Seeds (2 table-spoons)	103	4	10	1	2	Vitamin E, folic acid, pantothenic acid, phosphorus, magnesium, copper, zinc, manganese, selenium

BUYING, STORING, AND USING NUTS AND SEEDS

Try to purchase nuts and seeds from a source with a fast turnover, because their high fat content makes them prone to rancidity. Store shelled nuts and seeds in airtight containers away from direct light. Pine nuts and other nuts with a high oil content are best kept refrigerated or frozen at all times. All shelled nuts and seeds can be frozen for up to one year. Always taste them before you use them: If they are bitter or sour, or have lost their crunch, toss them.

salads and dips for munching and crunching

~

SALADS

Asian-Style Pasta and Vegetable Salad ▼

Best-Ever Tabbouleh Salad ▼

Quinoa Salad ▼

Pasta Salad with Basil Pesto

Noodles with Spinach, Red Peppers, and Sesame Dressing ▼

Couscous Salad with Chickpeas and Vegetables ▼

Kids' Favorite Three-Bean Salad ▼

Vegetables with Lemon, Olive Oil, and Fresh Herbs ▼

Pink Potato Salad

Tomato and Mozzarella Salad with Fresh Basil

Roasted Beets with Goat Cheese, Walnuts, and Baby Greens

Asparagus, Hearts of Palm, and Tomato Salad ▼

Spinach Salad with Mandarin Oranges and Toasted Almonds ▼

Four Delicious Homemade Salad Dressings

My Big Fat Greek Salad

Lemony Coleslaw with Fresh Dill

Cucumber-Tomato Yogurt Salad

DIPS

Homemade Guacamole ▼

Roasted Red Pepper and Cheese Dip

Healthy Hummus ▼

Spinach Dip

Artichoke-Spinach Dip

Black Bean Dip ▼

▼ Vegan recipe

RECIPE NOTES

SOME NOTES ABOUT the recipes in this chapter:

- Always use the freshest greens and vegetables you can find.
- Be sure to wash all greens and vegetables thoroughly (see Tips for Washing and Storing Greens, page 446).
- Be sure to refrigerate salad or salad dressings that contain mayonnaise.
- Choose enriched pastas and breads. Read labels for folic acid and iron content.
- Feel free to use any kind of olive oil, from extra-light to heavy, full-bodied Greek olive oils. Flavored oils are always welcome.
- When making any type of vinaigrette, for best results, combine all of the ingredients except the oil with the vinegar, whisk, then whisk in the oil until emulsified.
- Rinse all canned beans and other canned vegetables to remove excess salt.
- Use only pasteurized cheeses, particularly in the case of mozzarella, feta, or goat cheese.
- Use reduced-fat sour cream or yogurt, or a mixture of both, for dips and salads.
- If you are a vegan, you can substitute tofu-based sour cream or tofu-based mayonnaise for dairy products.

pantry items for salads and dips
for munching and crunching

SALAD PANTRY

Fresh Produce

Avocados
Baby greens
Baby spinach
Broccoli florets
Carrots
Cauliflower florets
Cherry or grape tomatoes
Fresh herbs: basil, cilantro, dill, mint,
   and parsley
Garlic
Ginger
Green asparagus
Green beans
Lemons
Limes
Oranges
Potatoes
Red beets
Red bell peppers
Romaine lettuce
Scallions
Tomatoes
Watercress
Zucchini

Dairy and Soy Products

Grade A large eggs
Parmesan cheese (grated)
Pasteurized feta cheese
Pasteurized goat cheese
Pasteurized part-skim low-moisture
   mozzarella cheese

Canned, Bottled, and Jarred Staples

Anchovy paste
Artichoke hearts packed in water or
   brine
Balsamic vinegar
Canola oil
Chickpeas
Deli-style dill pickles
Dijon mustard
Fat-free low-sodium stock (any kind)
Hearts of palm
Light mayonnaise
Mandarin oranges in light syrup
Olive oil
Olives (any kind)
Orange juice
Red kidney beans
Red or white wine vinegar
Reduced-fat smooth peanut butter
Rice vinegar (plain or seasoned)
Sesame oil (preferably toasted)
Soy sauce (regular or light)
Sun-dried tomatoes packed in oil
Worcestershire sauce

Dry Staples

Quinoa (such as Ancient Harvest
   brand)
Couscous
Shaped pasta (such as fusilli) and thin
   pasta (such as linguine or capellini)
Pine nuts
Sliced or slivered almonds
Tabbouleh mix

Udon noodles (brown rice or
  buckwheat)
Walnuts

Condiments, Herbs, and Spices

Basil pesto
Dried basil
Dried oregano
Dried tarragon
Ground cumin
Italian seasoning

From the Salad Bar

Artichoke hearts
Baby spinach
Broccoli florets
Cauliflower florets
Cooked red beets
Deli-style pickles
Hard-boiled eggs
Lettuce
Shredded or grated carrots
Sliced olives
Sliced red bell peppers
Sliced romaine lettuce
Sliced scallions

DIP PANTRY

Fresh Produce

Baby spinach
Fresh herbs: cilantro and parsley
Garlic

Hass avocados
Lemons
Limes
Red onions
Scallions
Tomatoes

Dairy and Soy Products

Parmesan cheese (grated)
Part-skim ricotta cheese
Pasteurized feta cheese
Reduced-fat sour cream

Canned, Bottled, and Jarred Staples

Anchovy paste or fillets
Artichoke hearts packed in water or
  brine (14-ounce can)
Black beans (15.5-ounce can)
Canola oil
Chickpeas (15-ounce can)
Light mayonnaise
Olive oil
Pimentos
Roasted red bell peppers
Tahini

Condiments

Ground cumin
Tabasco sauce

Frozen Staples

Chopped spinach (10-ounce package)

color counts in the produce section

The most colorful and healthy part of any grocery store is the fresh produce section, where vitamins and minerals abound. As a general rule, the more colorful the produce, inside and out, the more nutrients it contains.

THE HEALTHIEST FRUITS AND VEGETABLES FOR EVERYONE

Asparagus

Beets

Blackberries

Blueberries

Broccoli

Brussels sprouts

Cherries

Kale

Kiwifruit

Oranges

Pink grapefruit

Red peppers

Spinach

Strawberries

Sweet potatoes

choosing the right greens

All greens are not created equal. Here are four common greens listed in order of nutrients found in a 1-cup serving.

ROMAINE
8 cals
1,456 IU Vitamin A
13 mg Vitamin C
76 mcg Folic Acid

BOSTON, BIBB, OR BUTTERHEAD
7 cals
534 IU Vitamin A
4 mg Vitamin C
40 mcg Folic Acid

LOOSE-LEAF
10 cals
1,064 IU Vitamin A
10 mg Vitamin C
28 mcg Folic Acid

ICEBERG
7 cals
182 IU Vitamin A
2 mg Vitamin C
30 mcg Folic Acid

to buy or not to buy organic

In 2002, the Food Organics Act was passed to ensure that labels using the word *organic* follow organic and ecologically balanced methods of growing, harvesting, and packaging products. In simple terms, organic food is grown using methods that are beneficial to human health and the ecosystem. Foods that meet the organic criteria are free of synthetic pesticides and herbicides, genetically modified organisms (GMOs), irradiation (treatment by radiation), hormones, antibiotics, artificial ingredients, and trans fats.

Is the organic label really worth the extra dollars? Yes, especially if it doesn't break your budget. That said, studies have not yet proven that organic foods do, in fact, contain more nutrients. They do contain significantly fewer harmful chemicals, which is a good thing. Following are some other benefits of organic foods.

▶ Organic farming helps protect the environment by keeping the soil healthy and nutrient-rich through crop rotation, hand weeding, growing combo crops, and mulching. To be considered organic, crops must be grown in soil that has been pesticide- and herbicide-free for at least four years.

▶ According to the Environmental Working Group, the "dirty dozen," foods with the highest levels of pesticides are peaches, apples, sweet bell peppers, celery, nectarines, strawberries, cherries, pears, imported grapes, spinach, lettuce, and potatoes. All fruit, regardless of whether it is organic or not, should be washed carefully before it is eaten.[1]

▶ Organic meat, poultry, and eggs are hormone- and antibiotic-free.

▶ Wild-caught fish contain fewer PCBs (polychlorinated biphenyls) and dioxins than farm-raised fish.

▶ Organic practices are safer for farmers, field workers, wildlife, and communities that might otherwise be exposed to dangerous toxins from chemicals.

folic acid sources

FOOD	SERVING SIZE	FOLIC ACID (MCG)
All Bran cereal	½ cup	400
Cooked lentils	½ cup	179
Romaine lettuce	2 cups	152
Chickpeas	½ cup	141
Asparagus	½ cup	131
Cooked black beans	½ cup	128
Cooked spinach	½ cup	131
Brewer's yeast	1 teaspoon	104
Sunflower seeds	¼ cup	76
Orange juice	1 cup	74
Canned kidney beans	½ cup	64
Avocado	½ medium	56
Wheat germ	2 tablespoons	51
Tomato juice	1 cup	49
Calcium-fortified white bread	2 slices	48
Brussels sprouts	½ cup	47
Roasted peanuts	¼ cup	45
Oranges	1 medium	39
Cooked broccoli	½ cup	39

asian-style pasta and vegetable salad

What's in this for baby and me? Vitamins A and C.

FILLED WITH VITAMINS A and C, and a good source of protein, folic acid, and fiber, this tasty, colorful dish is sure to please the whole family. Sautéed tofu (see Instructions for Sautéing Tofu, page 228), or any source of protein (such as cooked scallops, shrimp, salmon, or chicken), can turn this salad into a main course. Consider omitting the scallions, ginger, red bell peppers, and cilantro for young eaters.

serves 8 (makes about 8 cups)

1 pound thin pasta (such as linguine or capellini)	1 tablespoon seasoned rice vinegar or freshly squeezed lime juice
1 tablespoon canola oil	1 teaspoon brown sugar
2 teaspoons sesame oil	1 cup shredded carrots
½ cup sliced scallions	½ cup finely diced red bell pepper
2 tablespoons grated fresh ginger	1½ cups broccoli florets, cooked until crisp-tender
¾ cup reduced-fat low-sodium stock	
¼ cup reduced-fat smooth peanut butter	¼ cup chopped fresh cilantro
¼ cup soy sauce	

1. Cook the pasta according to the package directions; drain and rinse quickly under cool water. Drain again, place in a large bowl and set aside.
2. Heat the canola oil and sesame oil, in a medium skillet over medium heat until hot. Add the scallions and ginger and sauté for 1 minute. Add the stock and peanut butter and stir until smooth, then add the soy sauce, rice vinegar, and brown sugar, and bring to a boil. Reduce the heat and simmer for 2 minutes.
3. Add the sauce to the pasta, along with the remaining ingredients. Stir and toss until well combined. Adjust the seasoning and serve cold or at room temperature.

▶ *Storage Tip:* This salad keeps for 3 days refrigerated.

▶ *Health Tip:* If your doctor has restricted your salt intake, use low-sodium soy sauce. If your fat intake has been restricted, go easy on the peanut butter and reduce the amount of canola oil to 1 teaspoon.

▶ *Diabetic Tip:* Reduce the portion size to ½ cup.

▶ **Complete Meal Ideas:** Serve this salad with:

> 3 ounces protein (you might want to try the Chicken with
> Homemade Barbecue Sauce, page 305, or the Sautéed Tofu and
> Portobello Mushrooms on a Bed of Greens, page 227)
> Green salad
> Reduced-fat 2% milk or low-fat yogurt
> Fresh fruit

APPROXIMATE NUTRITIONAL INFORMATION: Serving size: 1 cup Asian-style pasta and vegetable salad; Calories: 184 cals; Protein: 8 g; Carbohydrates: 25 g; Fat: 7 g; Fiber: 3 g; Sodium: 532 mg; Vitamin A: 7,366 IU; Vitamin C: 43 mg; Diabetic Exchange (values per ½ cup serving): Bread/Starch 1.5, Fat 1, Vegetable 1

quinoa salad

What's in this for baby and me? Vitamins A and C and iron.

Quinoa (pronounced KEEN-wah) is an easy-to-cook grain that has an earthy taste and pop-in-your-mouth texture (see important washing instruction below). This salad is a great source of vitamins A and C and iron, and a good source of protein and fiber. It is advisable to purchase boxed quinoa (such as Ancient Harvest Quinoa) rather than buy it in bulk because boxed grains tend to be larger, cleaner, sweeter, and more fluffy when cooked.

serves 4 to 6 (makes about 5 cups)

1 cup quinoa, thoroughly rinsed under hot
   water (see Cooking Tip below)
⅓ cup finely diced red bell pepper
½ cup shredded or grated carrots
½ cup sliced black olives
¼ cup thinly sliced scallions

¼ cup chopped fresh cilantro or 2 tablespoons
   finely chopped fresh mint
1 tablespoon grated orange zest
3 tablespoons freshly squeezed orange juice
2 tablespoons seasoned rice vinegar
2 tablespoons canola oil
Salt, to taste

1. Prepare the quinoa according to the package directions. (If you do not have package directions, combine the thoroughly rinsed quinoa with 2 cups water in a saucepan and bring it to a boil. Reduce the heat and simmer, covered, for 15 to 20 minutes, or until the grains look transparent and the spiral-like germ has separated. Remove from heat and let stand for 5 minutes, then fluff with a fork and transfer to a large bowl.

2. Add the remaining ingredients to the quinoa and mix gently until well incorporated. Adjust the seasoning and serve chilled or at room temperature.

▶ *Cooking Tip:* It is absolutely essential to rinse quinoa before cooking it to remove the bitter natural outer coating on each grain. Most of this coating is removed before sale; however, there may be a small residue left on the grain. Rinse the quinoa in a fine-mesh strainer under cold running water for about 1 minute, or place it in the saucepan you plan to cook it in, add water, and swish the grains with your hands for about 1 minute; drain.

▶ *Storage Tip:* This salad keeps for 2 days refrigerated.

► **Complete Meal Ideas:** Serve this salad with:

Salad or vegetable soup (you might want to try the Black
Bean Soup with Cilantro, page 100, or the Tomato,
Mozzarella, and Fresh Basil Salad, page 157)
Reduced-fat 2% milk or low-fat yogurt
Fresh fruit that contains vitamin C

APPROXIMATE NUTRITIONAL INFORMATION: Serving size: 1 cup quinoa salad; Calories: 260 cals; Protein:
6 g; Carbohydrates: 35 g; Fat: 11 g; Fiber: 4 g; Sodium: 162 mg; Vitamin A: 4,029 IU; Vitamin C: 22 mg; Diabetic
Exchange: Bread/Starch 2, Fat 2

pasta salad with basil pesto

What's in this for baby and me? Protein, calcium, and folic acid.

Rich in protein, calcium, and folic acid, and a good source of vitamin C, iron, B vitamins, and fiber, this pasta salad makes the perfect lunch or dinner.

serves 6 (makes about 8 cups)

4½ to 5 cups cooked fusilli or your favorite shaped pasta, rinsed briefly under cold water (Note: 2½ cups dry fusilli yields about 4½ cups cooked pasta)

1 vine-ripened tomato, cut into small wedges, or about 1 cup cherry or grape tomatoes

One 13.75-ounce can artichoke hearts, drained and cut into small wedges

8 ounces pasteurized mozzarella cheese (see Health Tip below), cubed (about 1½ cups)

½ cup olives (any kind)

½ cup Basil Pesto (recipe follows) or store-bought pesto, or to taste

Salt and freshly ground pepper, to taste

Combine all of the ingredients in a large bowl and toss gently until well combined. Adjust the seasoning and serve.

▶ *Variation:* Substitute your favorite cheese for the mozzarella, and use any vegetables or greens in place of the artichokes, such as steamed or sautéed broccoli or zucchini, or fresh spinach or arugula.

▶ *Storage Tip:* This salad keeps for 3 days refrigerated. The pesto will lose its bright green color, but the taste will remain unaffected.

▶ *Health Tip:* Do not use unpasteurized fresh mozzarella cheese stored in water (see Listeriosis Warning, page 129).

▶ *Complete Meal Ideas:* Serve this pasta salad with:
   Green salad or green vegetable (you might want to try the Vegetables with Lemon, Olive Oil, and Fresh Herbs, page 153, or romaine lettuce with the Caesar Salad Dressing, page 168)
   Reduced-fat 2% milk or low-fat yogurt
   Fresh fruit that contains vitamin C

APPROXIMATE NUTRITIONAL INFORMATION: Serving size: 1 cup pasta salad with basil pesto; Calories: 241 cals; Protein: 13 g; Carbohydrates: 32 g; Fat: 7 g; Fiber: 3 g; Sodium: 336 mg; Calcium: 219 mg; Folic Acid: 103 mcg; Diabetic Exchange: Bread/Starch 2, Fat .5, Meat (Medium Fat) 1

basil pesto

WATER IS SUBSTITUTED for some of the oil in this recipe, resulting in a superb, reduced-fat pesto that is scrumptious on hot linguine, fish, or poultry, as well as pasta salads. To preserve the bright green color of freshly made pesto, make sure that the plastic wrap is directly against the surface of the pesto.

makes about 1 cup

2 cups tightly packed fresh basil leaves (about
    2 ounces)
¼ cup plus 1 tablespoon olive oil or canola oil
3 tablespoons grated Parmesan cheese

⅓ cup pine nuts, toasted
1 large garlic clove, crushed
Salt and freshly ground pepper, to taste
2 tablespoons water

In a food processor pulse all of the ingredients until smooth, scraping down the sides of the bowl as necessary. Adjust the seasoning. Transfer to a bowl and cover the pesto with plastic wrap directly against the surface. Refrigerate until needed.

▶ *Storage Tip:* This pesto keeps for 5 days refrigerated, and it can be frozen for up to 1 month. Unless you plan to use it all at once, freeze it in portion-size servings in small or snack-size zip-lock bags.

APPROXIMATE NUTRITIONAL INFORMATION: Serving size: 2 tablespoons basil pesto; Calories: 24 cals; Protein: 1 g; Carbohydrates: .6 g; Fat: 2 g; Fiber: .2 g; Sodium: 54 mg; Diabetic Exchange: FREE

noodles with spinach, red bell peppers, and sesame dressing

What's in this for baby and me? Vitamins A and C, and folic acid.

THIS NOODLE SALAD is an excellent source of vitamins A and C and folic acid, and a good source of protein, iron, B vitamins, and fiber. Feel free to add your favorite ingredients, including grated carrots or broccoli florets or zucchini slices cooked until crisp-tender. This salad can be made a day ahead, but, in that case, the spinach should be added just before serving. If serving to children, omit the red pepper and possibly the garlic.

serves 4 (makes about 4½ cups)

8 ounces linguine or udon noodles

2 tablespoons toasted sesame oil

2 tablespoons soy sauce, or to taste

1 tablespoon seasoned rice vinegar, or to taste

½ cup thinly sliced red bell pepper

1½ cups tightly packed baby spinach leaves or 1 bunch watercress leaves, trimmed (use top leafy part only), washed, and dried

1 very small garlic clove, crushed

1. Cook the noodles according to the package directions. Drain and rinse quickly under cold water. Drain again, then place in a large bowl.
2. Add the sesame oil, soy sauce, and rice vinegar to the noodles and toss to coat. Add the remaining ingredients and toss gently until well combined. Adjust the seasoning and serve.

▶ *Storage Tip:* This salad keeps for 3 days refrigerated, although the spinach will wilt.

▶ *Complete Meal Ideas:* Serve these noodles with:
  3 ounces protein (you might want to try the Asian-Style Turkey Wrap, page 126, or the Old Bay Tofu Cakes with Cocktail Sauce, page 225.)
  Reduced-fat 2% milk or low-fat yogurt
  Fresh fruit that contains vitamin C

APPROXIMATE NUTRITIONAL INFORMATION: Serving size: 1 cup noodles with sesame dressing; Calories: 253 cals; Protein: 8 g; Carbohydrates: 39 g; Fat: 7 g; Fiber: 3 g; Sodium: 438 mg; Vitamin A: 1,880 IU; Vitamin C: 30 mg; Diabetic Exchange: Bread/Starch 2.5, Fat 1.5, Vegetable 1

couscous salad with chickpeas and vegetables

What's in this for baby and me? Protein, iron, vitamin C, folic acid, and fiber.

Couscous salad makes an easy and delicious side dish for just about any main course, and provides an excellent source of protein, iron, vitamin C, folic acid, and fiber, and a good source of vitamin A and B vitamins. Any small-grained pasta, such as orzo, acini di pepe, or quinoa (see instructions for cooking quinoa on page 187), can be used in place of the couscous.

serves 4 (makes about 4 cups)

3 cups cooked couscous (about ¾ cup uncooked couscous)

2 tablespoons wine vinegar

1 small garlic clove, crushed (optional)

½ teaspoon Dijon mustard (optional)

3 tablespoons olive oil or canola oil

1 vine-ripened tomato, cut into wedges, or 12 cherry or grape tomatoes, halved

½ cup diced red bell pepper (optional)

⅔ cup (one 7¾-ounce can) chickpeas

⅔ cup canned or jarred artichoke hearts, quartered

½ cup olives (any kind)

⅓ cup pine nuts, toasted

¼ cup chopped fresh parsley

¼ cup finely sliced scallions

Fresh lemon juice, to taste

Salt and freshly ground pepper, to taste

1. Cook the couscous according to the package directions. In general, about ¾ cup of couscous and 1¼ cups of water yield 3 cups cooked couscous. Transfer the couscous to a large bowl and allow to cool. Then fluff with a fork or your hands to separate the grains.
2. In a small bowl, mix the vinegar and garlic and mustard until well blended. Add the olive oil, mix well, and set aside.
3. Add the remaining ingredients except the lemon juice and salt and pepper to the couscous, then add the dressing and mix gently until all of the ingredients are well combined. Add lemon juice to taste, adjust the seasoning, and serve.

▶ *Timesaving Tip:* Pick up your favorite cleaned and ready-cut vegetables, such as grated carrots, peppers, zucchini, broccoli florets, cucumbers, tomatoes, or chickpeas, from a salad bar and add them to the couscous salad.

▶ *Storage Tip:* This salad keeps for 3 days refrigerated.

► **Health Tip:** If your doctor has restricted your salt or fat intake, use less olive oil and omit the olives, pine nuts, and salt.

► **Diabetic Tip:** Reduce the portion size to ½ cup.

► **Complete Meal Ideas:** Serve this couscous salad with:
  3 ounces protein (you might want to try the Healthy Hummus, page 175, or the Marinated Grilled or Broiled Lamb Chops, page 313)
  Reduced-fat 2% milk or low-fat yogurt
  Fresh fruit that contains vitamin C

APPROXIMATE NUTRITIONAL INFORMATION: Serving size: 1 cup couscous salad with chickpeas and vegetables; Calories: 397 cals; Protein: 12 g; Carbohydrates: 47 g; Fat: 19 g; Fiber: 9 g; Sodium: 364 mg; Vitamin C: 36 mg; Folic Acid: 115 mcg; Iron: 4 mg; Diabetic Exchange (values per ½ cup serving): Bread/Starch 1.5, Fat 2, Vegetable .5

best-ever tabbouleh salad

What's in this for baby and me? Vitamins A and C.

TABBOULEH IS A super-healthy Middle Eastern dish made from bulgur wheat and vegetables. This salad is an excellent source of vitamins A and C, and a good source of protein, iron, folic acid, and fiber. Packaged tabbouleh mixes are convenient and tasty, and a good starting point for adding other ingredients, such as brown rice, wheat berries, grated carrots, or cucumbers.

serves 4 to 6 (makes about 4 cups)

One 6-ounce package tabbouleh (Middle Eastern wheat salad mix)

2 tablespoons freshly squeezed lemon juice, or to taste

3 tablespoons olive oil or canola oil

2 vine-ripened tomatoes, cut into small dice

⅔ cup finely diced red bell pepper (½ red bell pepper)

½ cup chickpeas or your favorite canned beans, rinsed

½ cup pine nuts, toasted

Salt and freshly ground pepper, to taste

1. Place the contents of the tabbouleh package in a medium bowl and add boiling water (not cold water) in the amount stated on the package. Stir, then cover with foil and let sit for 20 minutes.
2. Add the remaining ingredients and mix thoroughly. Adjust the seasoning and serve.

▶ **Storage Tip:** This salad keeps for 2 days refrigerated.

▶ **Diabetic Tip:** Reduce the portion size to ½ cup.

▶ **Complete Meal Ideas:** Serve this salad with:
3 ounces protein (you might want to try the Healthy Hummus, page 175, or the Marinated Grilled or Broiled Lamb Chops, page 313)
Whole wheat pita bread and cheese, or cheese toasts
Reduced-fat 2% milk or low-fat yogurt
Fresh fruit that contains vitamin C

APPROXIMATE NUTRITIONAL INFORMATION: Serving size: 1 cup tabbouleh salad; Calories: 259 cals; Protein: 6 g; Carbohydrates: 16 g; Fat: 21 g; Fiber: 4 g; Sodium: 220 mg; Vitamin A: 1,424 IU; Vitamin C: 52 mg; Diabetic Exchange (values per ½ cup serving): Bread/Starch .5, Fat 2, Vegetable .5

kids' favorite three-bean salad

What's in this for baby and me? Vitamin C, folic acid, and fiber.

Don't tell your kids that their favorite three-bean salad is packed with vitamin C, folic acid, and fiber and is a good source of protein, vitamin A, and iron—they might reject it simply because it's too healthy! Chickpeas and kidney beans are called for in this recipe because they seem to be the most readily available in small ("salad topper" 7.5-ounce) can sizes. However, feel free to add your family's favorites, from black-eyed peas to cannellini beans.

serves 4 (makes about 4 cups)

8 ounces green beans, washed, ends trimmed, cut into ½-inch pieces, and cooked until crisp-tender

⅔ cup (one 7.5-ounce can) red kidney beans, rinsed and drained

⅔ cup (one 7.5-ounce can) chickpeas, rinsed and drained

½ cup cherry or grape tomatoes, sliced in half

¼ cup chopped fresh cilantro

2 tablespoons olive oil or canola oil

1 tablespoon freshly squeezed lime or lemon juice, or to taste

A dash of ground cumin

Salt and freshly ground pepper, to taste

Combine all of the ingredients in a bowl and mix well. Adjust the seasoning and serve.

▶ *Timesaving Tip:* Omit the olive oil, lime juice, and cumin and use your favorite bottled dressing. Use frozen green beans instead of fresh; cook them according to package directions.

▶ *Storage Tip:* This salad keeps 4 days refrigerated. The lime juice will cause a slight discoloration of the green beans and cilantro, but this does not affect the taste.

▶ *Complete Meal Ideas:* Serve this with:
    3 ounces protein (you might want to try the Chicken Caesar Wrap,
        page 126, or the Spinach and Cheese Quesadillas, page 224.)
    Reduced-fat 2% milk or low-fat yogurt
    Fresh fruit that contains vitamin C

APPROXIMATE NUTRITIONAL INFORMATION: Serving size: 1 cup three-bean salad; Calories: 180 cals; Protein: 7 g; Carbohydrates: 22 g; Fat: 8 g; Fiber: 8 g; Sodium: 334 mg; Vitamin C: 18 mg; Folic Acid: 100 mcg; Diabetic Exchange: Bread/Starch 1.5, Fat 1

vegetables with lemon, olive oil, and fresh herbs

~

What's in this for baby and me? Vitamins A and C, folic acid, and fiber.

THIS VEGETABLE SIDE dish, which can be served warm or at room temperature, goes well with any main course. Cauliflower, broccoli, green beans, or zucchini—all high in vitamins, folic acid, and fiber—work well in this recipe. You can serve one vegetable or a mixture. Be sure to drain the vegetables well and blot them dry with paper towels before adding the dressing. The fresh herbs really add to this dish, so don't leave them out.

serves 4 (makes about 4 cups)

12–16 ounces fresh vegetables, washed (see below)

2 tablespoons olive oil

2 tablespoons freshly squeezed lemon juice, or to taste

Salt and freshly ground pepper, to taste

2 tablespoons chopped fresh parsley, cilantro, or your favorite fresh herb

▶ *Cauliflower or Broccoli* (12 to 16 ounces equals about 5 cups broccoli florets and about 6 cups cauliflower florets)

Boil, steam, or microwave the florets until crisp-tender. Drain well and blot dry with paper towels. Put in a bowl, add the olive oil, and toss gently. Add the remaining ingredients and toss again. Adjust the seasoning and serve.

APPROXIMATE NUTRITIONAL INFORMATION: Serving size: 1 cup cauliflower florets; Calories: 116 cals; Protein: 6 g; Carbohydrates: 11 g; Fat: 8 g; Fiber: 6 g; Sodium: 197 mg; Vitamin A: 2,807 IU; Vitamin C: 152 mg; Folic Acid: 101 mcg; Diabetic Exchange: Fat 1.5, Vegetable 2

APPROXIMATE NUTRITIONAL INFORMATION: Serving size: 1 cup broccoli florets; Calories: 116 cals; Protein: 6 g; Carbohydrates: 11g; Fat: 7 g; Fiber: 6 g; Sodium: 197 mg; Vitamin A: 2,807 IU; Vitamin C: 152 mg; Diabetic Exchange: Fat 1, Vegetable 2

▶ *Green Beans* (16 ounces equals about 4 cups)

Trim the ends of the beans, then boil, steam, or microwave them until crisp-tender. Drain well and blot dry with paper towels. Put in a bowl, add the olive oil, and toss gently. Add the remaining ingredients and toss again. Adjust the seasoning and serve.

APPROXIMATE NUTRITIONAL INFORMATION: Serving size: 1 cup green beans; Calories: 102 cals; Protein: 2 g; Carbohydrates: 10 g; Fat: 7 g; Fiber: 4 g; Sodium: 150 mg; Diabetic Exchange: Fat 1, Vegetable 2

▶ **Zucchini** (16 ounces equals about 3 small zucchini. Note: It is important to use young, small zucchini rather than the large overgrown squash that are abundant at the end of the summer.)

1. Cook the whole zucchini in boiling salted water for about 6 to 8 minutes, or until tender. Check tenderness by piercing the middle of a zucchini with the tip of a knife. (See Cooking Tip 2 for microwave instructions.)
2. Drain carefully (the zucchini skin tears easily) and cool slightly. When cool enough to handle, trim the ends, then cut the zucchini into ¼-inch slices and place in a serving bowl. Add the olive oil and toss gently, then add the remaining ingredients and toss again. Adjust the seasoning and serve.

APPROXIMATE NUTRITIONAL INFORMATION: Serving size: 1 cup zucchini; Calories: 80 cals; Protein: .8 g; Carbohydrates: 5 g; Fat: 7 g; Fiber: 2 g; Sodium: 150 mg; Diabetic Exchange: Fat 1, Vegetable 1

▶ **Cooking Tip 1:** The lemon will cause a slight discoloration of the broccoli, zucchini skin, green beans, and parsley. This does not affect the taste.

▶ **Cooking Tip 2:** To microwave the zucchini, cut in half, place in a microwaveable container with about 2 tablespoons water, and microwave on high. Cooking time will be around 5 to 7 minutes, depending on your microwave.

▶ **Storage Tip:** This salad keeps for 2 days refrigerated.

▶ **Complete Meal Ideas:** Serve these vegetables with:
   3 ounces protein (you might want to try the Tilapia Mediterranean-
      Style, page 329, or the Vegetarian Omelet for One, page 229)
   Reduced-fat 2% milk or low-fat yogurt
   Fresh fruit that contains vitamin C

pink potato salad

~

What's in this for baby and me? Vitamins A and C.

Beets make this potato salad healthier and prettier than traditional potato salad. High in vitamins A and C, and a good source of folic acid and fiber, it is delicious served on a bed of lettuce or alongside a sandwich. The pickles and chopped dill give the salad a playful bite and may just satisfy your pickle craving.

serves 4 to 6 (makes about 4 cups)

2 medium red beets, scrubbed (see
   Timesaving Tip below)
1 large potato, scrubbed
3 large carrots, scrubbed
1–2 hard-boiled eggs, chopped

1 large deli-style kosher dill pickle, cut into
   small dice, or to taste
⅓ cup light mayonnaise, or to taste
Salt and freshly ground pepper, to taste
3 tablespoons chopped fresh parsley or dill

1. Place the beets, potato, and carrots in a large saucepan, cover with water, and bring to a boil. Cook until tender (pierce the vegetables with a knife to check for doneness), about 20 to 25 minutes for the potato and the carrots, 30 to 40 minutes for the beets. Drain and cool.
2. Peel the beets, potatoes, and carrots and cut into ¼-inch cubes (see Cooking Tip 2 for advice on peeling the carrots). Place in a large bowl.
3. Add the remaining ingredients and gently mix. Cover with plastic wrap and refrigerate until well chilled, about 2 hours. Adjust the seasoning and serve.

▶ *Timesaving Tip:* In a pinch, you can substitute canned or jarred beets, or plain cooked beets from a salad bar, for the fresh beets. Drain them well. (Note: If using canned or jarred beets, the pink color of the salad will probably not be as intense.) Buy pre-sliced sandwich dill pickles to save a bit of time on the chopping.

▶ *Cooking Tip 1:* You can boil the eggs in the same saucepan as the vegetables. The eggshells will turn a grayish color from the beets, but the eggs will not be affected.

▶ *Cooking Tip 2:* To peel the cooked carrots, using a paring knife, remove the skin from around the carrot, rather than using a top-to-bottom peeling motion.

▶ *Storage Tip:* This salad keeps for 3 days refrigerated. The intensity of the pink color will increase with time.

► **Complete Meal Ideas:** Serve this salad with:

    3 ounces protein (you might want to try the Tuna Salad Sandwich,
        page 123, or the Spice-Rubbed Pork Chops, page 311)
    Green salad or vegetable
    Reduced-fat 2% milk or low-fat yogurt
    Fresh fruit

APPROXIMATE NUTRITIONAL INFORMATION: Serving size: ¾ cup pink potato salad; Calories: 150 cals; Protein: 3 g; Carbohydrates: 18 g; Fat: 8 g; Fiber: 3 g; Sodium: 671 mg; Vitamin A: 13,149 IU; Vitamin C: 14 mg; Diabetic Exchange: Bread/Starch 1, Fat 1.5, Vegetable .5

tomato and mozzarella salad
with fresh basil

What's in this for baby and me? Protein, calcium, and vitamin C.

IF YOU GROW tomatoes in your garden, you probably already know what a joy this salad is during the summer months. High in protein, calcium, and vitamin C, and a good source of vitamin A, this simple-to-prepare salad can't be beat!

serves 4 (makes about 4 cups)

2 large vine-ripened tomatoes, cubed, or about 1¾ cups halved cherry or grape tomatoes

8 ounces pasteurized part-skim low-moisture mozzarella cheese (see Health Tip below), cut into ½-inch cubes (about 1½ cups)

⅓ cup thinly sliced fresh basil leaves

1 tablespoon red or white wine vinegar, or to taste

A couple of drops of balsamic vinegar (optional)

2 tablespoons olive oil, or to taste

Salt and freshly ground pepper, to taste

Combine all of the ingredients in a bowl, mix gently, and serve. (Refrigerate any leftovers.)

▶ *Health Tip:* Use only pasteurized mozzarella cheese. Do not use unpasteurized fresh mozzarella cheese stored in water (see Listeriosis Warning, page 129).

▶ *Storage Tip:* This salad is best eaten the day it is made.

▶ *Complete Meal Ideas:* Serve this salad with:
   Whole wheat bread or roll
   Green salad, green vegetable, or green soup (you might want to try the Creamy Asparagus-Artichoke Soup, page 90, or the Artichoke-Spinach Dip, page 178, with whole wheat bread or crackers)
   Reduced-fat 2% milk or low-fat yogurt
   Fresh fruit

APPROXIMATE NUTRITIONAL INFORMATION: Serving size: 1 cup tomato and mozzarella salad; Calories: 234 cals; Protein: 16 g; Carbohydrates: 5 g; Fat: 17 g; Fiber: .8 g; Sodium: 451 mg; Vitamin C: 12 mg; Calcium: 423 mg; Diabetic Exchange: Fat 1.5, Meat (Medium Fat) 2, Vegetable 1

roasted beets with goat cheese, walnuts, and baby greens

What's in this for baby and me? Protein, calcium, vitamin A, and folic acid.

Hᴵɢʜ ɪɴ ᴘʀᴏᴛᴇɪɴ, calcium, vitamin A, and folic acid, and a good source of vitamin C and fiber, this salad is designed for beet lovers. The recipe calls for roasting the beets, but you can boil them, if you prefer. In a pinch, canned or jarred beets also work. Toasting the walnuts is optional, but it does enhance their flavor.

serves 2 to 3

3 beets, leaves and roots trimmed, scrubbed

1 tablespoon red wine vinegar

½ teaspoon Dijon mustard

2 tablespoons olive oil or canola oil

3 to 4 cups baby greens, washed and dried

2.5 ounces pasteurized goat cheese (see Health Tip below), broken into small chunks

2 tablespoons walnuts

Salt and freshly ground pepper, to taste

1. Preheat the oven to 425°F. Line a baking dish with foil.
2. Place the beets in the dish and bake for 45 minutes to 1 hour, or until tender. Check for tenderness by inserting the tip of a knife into the middle of a beet. Let cool slightly.
3. When cool enough to handle, remove the skin from the beets. Slice the beets into matchsticks and place them in a bowl (be careful not to stain your clothing with the beet juice).
4. Mix the vinegar with the mustard in a small bowl, then whisk in the olive oil. Set aside.
5. Arrange the baby greens in a serving bowl or on a platter. Place the beets on top of the greens. Drizzle the dressing evenly over the top, then garnish with the goat cheese and walnuts. Sprinkle with salt and pepper and serve immediately.

▶ *Health Tip:* Use only pasteurized goat cheese (see Listeriosis Warning, page 129).
▶ *Complete Meal Ideas:* Serve this salad with:
    Whole wheat bread or roll
    Reduced-fat 2% milk or low-fat yogurt
    Fresh fruit

APPROXIMATE NUTRITIONAL INFORMATION: Serving size: half of the beet salad (without the dressing); Calories: 243 cals; Protein: 15 g; Carbohydrates: 9 g; Fat: 17 g; Fiber: 3 g; Sodium: 174 mg; Vitamin A: 1,500 IU; Diabetic Exchange: Fat 3.5, Vegetable 2

APPROXIMATE NUTRITIONAL INFORMATION: Serving size: 1 tablespoon salad dressing; Calories: 82 cals; Protein: 0 g; Carbohydrates: 0 g; Fat: 9 g; Fiber: 0 g; Sodium: 5 mg; Diabetic Exchange: Fat 2, Meat (Medium Fat) 2, Vegetable 2

asparagus, hearts of palm, and tomato salad

~

What's in this for the baby and me? Vitamins A and C and folic acid.

A TASTY SALAD loaded with vitamins A and C and folic acid, and it is also a good source of protein, iron, and fiber. Canned or jarred hearts of palm are found in the canned vegetable or international food section of most grocery stores. This salad is best eaten the day it is made.

serves 4 (makes about 4 cups)

1 pound asparagus, washed, tough ends trimmed, and cut into 1½-inch pieces
One 14-ounce can hearts of palm, drained and cut into ½-inch slices
1–2 vine-ripened tomatoes, diced

4 cups baby greens, washed and dried (optional)
2 tablespoons red wine vinegar
½ teaspoon Dijon mustard
¼ cup olive oil or canola oil
Salt and freshly ground pepper, to taste

1. Boil, steam, or microwave the asparagus until crisp-tender. The cooking time will depend on the cooking method, but the average cooking time is about 5 minutes. Drain, place in a bowl, and cool.
2. Add the hearts of palm and tomatoes to the asparagus; set aside. Arrange the baby greens on a serving platter; set aside.
3. In a small bowl, mix the vinegar and mustard. Add the olive oil and mix until well blended. Add most of the dressing to the salad and toss gently. Adjust the seasoning. Drizzle the remaining dressing evenly over the baby greens, place the asparagus salad in the center, and serve immediately.

▶ *Timesaving Tip:* Use presliced "salad cut" hearts of palm if available. Frozen, canned, or jarred asparagus can be substituted for the fresh (follow package directions for preparation)—although the texture and taste will not equal that of the fresh.

▶ *Diabetic Tip:* Reduce the portion size to ½ cup.

▶ **_Complete Meal Ideas:_** Serve this salad with:

> 3 ounces protein (you might want to try the Pr-egg-o Salad Sandwich, page 118, or the Flank Steak with Salsa Verde, page 290)
>
> Whole wheat bread
>
> Reduced-fat 2% milk or low-fat yogurt
>
> Fresh fruit that contains vitamin C

APPROXIMATE NUTRITIONAL INFORMATION: Serving size: 1 cup asparagus, hearts of palm, and tomato salad; Calories: 176 cals; Protein: 5 g; Carbohydrates: 10 g; Fat: 14 g; Fiber: 4 g; Sodium: 252 mg; Vitamin A: 1,314 IU; Vitamin C: 26 mg; Folic Acid: 115 mcg; Diabetic Exchange (values per ½ cup serving): Fat 1.5, Vegetable 1

travel tips

Whether you are traveling near or far, it is important to use common sense and advance planning during pregnancy. Be sure to inform your doctor of your travel plans. While traveling in an airplane is almost always safe during pregnancy, it is not recommended for women who have obstetrical medical conditions that could result in an emergency. Some complications include pregnancy-induced hypertension, poorly controlled diabetes, sickle cell disease, a history of premature labor, placental abnormalities, or weakened cardiovascular systems.[2]

PLANNING AHEAD

▶ Ask your doctor if it is safe for you to travel and if you should carry a copy of your medical records with you.

▶ Ask your doctor about immunizations (some are safe, others are not) and what types of medications to include in your first-aid kit, especially those for diarrhea and constipation.

▶ Preferably before you leave, or as soon as you arrive, determine the hospitals, doctors, and pharmacies that would be available should you require medical care.

▶ Check with your airline for travel restrictions during pregnancy, and order special meals (such as vegetarian, low-sodium, diabetic, or kosher) if your diet requires one.

PACKING YOUR BAG

▶ Carry all medications and important items in your carry-on luggage.

▶ Take along favorite foods that may be hard to find.

▶ Carry emergency snacks—crackers, cookies, fruit (fresh or dried), fruit cups, sliced vegetables, juice boxes, peanut butter, energy bars, cereal, and granola bars.

▶ Carry bottled water if the tap water is unsafe or if bottled water is unavailable in stores. Don't forget to include enough water for brushing your teeth.

▶ Pack loose clothing and comfortable shoes. Wear support hose if possible.

▶ Take powdered milk, long-life milk, or calcium supplements if you foresee a problem meeting your calcium needs.

▶ Pack sun block if you are headed to a sunny destination. Avoid prolonged exposure to the sun, which may lead to dizziness, fainting, dehydration, heat stroke, and sunburn (not to mention skin cancer).

GETTING THERE

▶ Wear loose travel clothing and comfortable shoes (preferably slip-ons, so you don't have to bend over), which allow your feet to swell.

▶ During long flights, train trips, or car rides, be sure to stretch your legs at least every two hours. This is important during the later stages of pregnancy, when blood clots are more likely.

▶ Be sure to drink plenty of (bottled) water throughout your journey.

▶ Don't hold it in—find a bathroom, or go behind a bush if you have to. The last thing you need is a urinary tract infection.

▶ Don't lift heavy bags. Hire a porter if necessary.

SAFE EATING

▶ Make sure you can identify everything you eat and that it is cooked well-done. Do not eat any raw meat (such as beef carpaccio or salmon gravlax) or raw fish (such as sushi or sashimi).

▶ If you are traveling to a less-developed country, eat only fruits or vegetables with a peel—apples, oranges, bananas, pineapples, mangoes, papayas, tangerines, etc.—and wash all fruit before you peel it.

▶ Stay hydrated. If the water is unsafe, drink only bottled water. If safe water is unavailable, drink canned or bottled fruit juice or other beverages. Do not drink sodas, beer, or any other beverages from a tap.

▶ Do not use ice cubes if the drinking water is unsafe.

▶ Brush your teeth with bottled water if the drinking water is unsafe.

▶ Follow the Tips for Eating in Restaurants (page 275) when dining out.

▶ Explain your dietary needs to your waiter. Most restaurants will fix a special dish following your dietary restrictions.

▶ If you think you may have food poisoning (severe vomiting or diarrhea), seek medical help immediately. Do not wait until you are dehydrated.

spinach salad with mandarin oranges and toasted almonds

~

What's in this for baby and me? Vitamins A and C and fiber.

A WINNING COMBINATION! This spinach salad is packed with vitamins A and C and fiber, and it is a good source of protein and iron. The Asian-style dressing complements the sweet oranges.

serves 2 to 3

DRESSING

1 teaspoon soy sauce

1 tablespoon seasoned rice vinegar

3 tablespoons canola oil

A few drops of toasted sesame oil

1 very small garlic clove, crushed

Freshly ground pepper, to taste

SPINACH SALAD

2 cups packed baby spinach (one 6-ounce bag), washed and dried (see Timesaving Tip)

⅓ cup sliced or slivered almonds, toasted (see Cooking Tip)

½ cup mandarin oranges in juice (no added sugar), drained

1. To make the salad dressing, combine all of the ingredients in a small bowl and mix well. Set aside.
2. To make the salad, combine the spinach, almonds, and mandarin oranges in a salad bowl. Add the dressing, toss gently, and serve immediately.

▶ *Cooking Tip:* To toast the almonds, place them in a small nonstick skillet over medium heat and stir until golden brown. Or, place the almonds on a baking sheet under a broiler for a minute or two—watch them carefully, because they tend to burn quickly.

▶ *Diabetic Tip:* Omit the almonds and use only one-quarter of the dressing.

▶ *Complete Meal Ideas:* Serve this salad with:

    3 ounces protein (you might want to try the Sautéed Shrimp with Pasta,
        page 315, or the Homemade Tofu-Bean Burritos, page 222)
    Whole wheat bread
    Reduced-fat 2% milk or low-fat yogurt
    Fresh fruit that contains vitamin C

APPROXIMATE NUTRITIONAL INFORMATION: Serving size: half of the spinach salad; Calories: 170 cals; Protein: 6 g; Carbohydrates: 15 g; Fat: 11 g; Fiber: 6 g; Sodium: 42 mg; Vitamin A: 2,222 IU; Vitamin C: 20 mg; Diabetic Exchange: Fat 2, Vegetable 3

APPROXIMATE NUTRITIONAL INFORMATION: Serving size: half of the dressing; Calories: 187 cals; Protein: .3 g; Carbohydrates: .4 g; Fat: 20 g; Fiber: 0; Sodium: 154 mg; Diabetic Exchange (values per one-quarter of the salad dressing): Fat 2

homemade croutons

Fat-free homemade croutons are a wonderful snack any time of day. They are perfect "dippers" and a welcome addition to almost any soup. Any type of bread (fresh or stale) can be used to make croutons. French baguettes make light, delicate croutons, while hearty country, sourdough, rosemary, olive, and whole wheat breads make more robust, flavorful croutons.

To make croutons, preheat the oven to 350°F. Cut bread into cubes. Distribute the bread cubes evenly on a baking sheet and bake for 20 minutes. Turn the croutons, and continue baking for 5 to 10 minutes, or until hard and light golden brown. Cool, then store in an airtight container or zip-lock bag.

four delicious
homemade salad dressings

~

Having a supply of washed and chilled lettuce on hand, along with a jar of home-made salad dressing, makes creating a fabulous salad an effortless task. Once you've tried these homemade dressings you will find it hard to go back to the store-bought bottled stuff. The Tarragon Vinaigrette has the longest shelf life of these dressings, about three weeks, so you can make it in a large batch. Shake or mix well before dressing your salad.

french-style tarragon vinaigrette

The red wine vinegar can be replaced with sherry vinegar, rice vinegar, or any other flavored vinegar. Balsamic vinegar adds a rich, sweet flavor to dressings, but it should be used sparingly so as not to overpower the vinaigrette. The garlic can be replaced with minced shallots, the sugar with some honey, and the oil with plain or flavored oil.

makes about ⅔ cup

2 teaspoons Dijon mustard, or to taste

1 small garlic clove, smashed

¼ cup red wine vinegar

½ teaspoon dried tarragon, basil, or oregano (optional)

¼ teaspoon salt

Pinch of sugar

Freshly ground pepper, to taste

¼ cup canola oil

¼ cup olive oil

Combine the mustard, garlic, if using, vinegar, tarragon, if using, salt, sugar, and pepper in a jar with a lid or in a small bowl and shake or whisk until well blended. Add the canola oil and olive oil and shake or whisk until emulsified.

▶ **Cooking Tip:** This recipe can easily be doubled.

▶ **Storage Tip:** This dressing will keep refrigerated for up to 3 weeks.

APPROXIMATE NUTRITIONAL INFORMATION: Serving size: 1 tablespoon French-style tarragon vinaigrette; Calories: 99 cals; Protein: 0 g; Carbohydrates: 0 g; Fat: 11 g; Fiber: 0 g; Sodium: 64 mg; Diabetic Exchange: Fat 2

sun-dried tomato and basil dressing

THIS DRESSING IS great on boiled or steamed vegetables (especially potatoes), on a firm-leaved green salad (such as sliced romaine leaves), or on a pasta salad with chunks of pasteurized feta or pasteurized goat cheese. It also makes a delicious sandwich spread. For a thicker sauce that is mouthwatering with fish, crab cakes, hamburgers, veggie burgers, or tofu cakes (see Old Bay Tofu Cakes, page 225), add 1 tablespoon light mayonnaise and reduce the water to ¼ cup.

makes about ¾ cup

⅓ cup sun-dried tomatoes packed in oil

2 teaspoons red wine vinegar

2 teaspoons balsamic vinegar

¼ cup canola oil

¼ cup plus 3–4 tablespoons boiling water

½ teaspoon dried oregano or Italian
   seasoning

Salt and freshly ground pepper, to taste

Combine all of the ingredients in a blender or food processor and process until smooth. The dressing can be thinned with additional hot water, 3 to 4 tablespoons, if desired.

▶ *Health Tip:* If your doctor has restricted your fat intake, use less oil and more water.

APPROXIMATE NUTRITIONAL INFORMATION: Serving size: 1 tablespoon sun-dried tomato and basil dressing; Calories: 48 cals; Protein: 0 g; Carbohydrates: 0 g; Fat: 5 g; Fiber: .2 g; Sodium: 8 mg; Diabetic Exchange: Fat 1

caesar salad dressing

Who can resist a really good Caesar salad? This recipe uses a tablespoon of light mayonnaise instead of the traditional uncooked eggs, which are dangerous to eat during pregnancy (see Eggs and *Salmonella enteritidis*, page 79). Toss this salad with romaine lettuce and croutons followed by a generous dusting of Parmesan cheese.

makes about ½ cup

1 tablespoon light mayonnaise

2 tablespoons freshly squeezed lemon juice,
   or to taste

1 teaspoon Worcestershire sauce

1 small garlic clove, squeezed through a garlic
   press or minced

½ teaspoon anchovy paste (optional)

¼ teaspoon salt

Freshly ground pepper, to taste

⅓ cup olive oil

2 tablespoons canola oil

Combine all of the ingredients except the olive oil and canola oil in a small bowl and whisk until smooth. Gradually add the olive oil and canola oil, whisking until emulsified.

▶ *Cooking Tip:* This salad dressing will separate as it sits. Whisk or shake it to re-emulsify it.

▶ *Storage Tip:* This dressing will keep refrigerated for up to 3 days.

APPROXIMATE NUTRITIONAL INFORMATION: Serving size: 1 tablespoon Caesar salad dressing: Calories: 117 cals; Protein: 0 g; Carbohydrates: 0 g; Fat: 13 g; Fiber: 0 g; Sodium: 96 mg; Diabetic Exchange: Fat 2.5

What's in this for baby and me? Vitamins A and C, folic acid, and fiber.

Rich in vitamins A and C, folic acid, and fiber, and a good source of protein and calcium, this power-packed salad is surprisingly quick and easy to assemble. The order in which you add the ingredients is vital to the success of this salad. Adding the olive oil first coats the leaves so they are not "burned" by the acid of the lemon juice.

serves 2

4 cups washed and sliced romaine lettuce

¼ cup grated Parmesan cheese

1 ripe avocado, peeled, pitted, and sliced

1½ tablespoons olive oil, or to taste

Juice of ½ a fresh lemon, or to taste

Salt and freshly ground pepper, to taste

Place the romaine lettuce, Parmesan cheese, and avocado in a salad bowl. Drizzle the olive oil evenly over the top, then toss gently. Add the lemon juice and salt and pepper and toss gently again. Serve immediately.

▶ *Diabetic Tip:* Reduce the portion size to 1 cup salad.

APPROXIMATE NUTRITIONAL INFORMATION: Serving size: half of this salad; Calories: 304 cals; Protein: 8 g; Carbohydrates: 10 g; Fat: 28 g; Fiber: 6 g; Sodium: 205 mg; Vitamin A: 3,504 IU; Vitamin C: 41 mg; Folic Acid: 211 mcg; Diabetic Exchange (values per 1 cup serving of salad): Fat 3, Vegetable 1

my big fat greek salad

*What's in this for baby and me? Vitamins A and C,
folic acid, calcium, iron, and fiber.*

THE GREEKS HAVE a natural gift when it comes to making healthy and delicious salads.
Loaded with vitamins A and C, folic acid, calcium, iron, and fiber, this salad is also a
good source of protein and B vitamins.

Serves 2

**4 artichoke hearts (canned), drained, and cut
  into wedges**

**1 large vine-ripened tomato, diced, or 12
  cherry or grape tomatoes, halved**

⅓ cup crumbled pasteurized feta cheese

12 pitted black or green olives

**¼ cup sliced red onions (optional, see
  Cooking Tip)**

3 tablespoons olive oil

1 tablespoon vinegar (any kind)

**2 teaspoons freshly squeezed lemon juice, to
  taste**

Dash of dried oregano

Salt and freshly ground pepper, to taste

4 cups mixed greens, for garnish

1. Combine all of the ingredients *except 1 tablespoon of the olive oil and the mixed
   greens* in a bowl and toss gently.
2. Arrange the mixed greens on two plates, and drizzle the remaining 1 tablespoon of
   olive oil on top of them. Divide the Greek salad in half and arrange it on top of the
   greens. Serve promptly. Refrigerate leftovers.

▶ *Cooking Tip:* If you like the taste of raw onions but not the gas they sometimes cause,
just soak the sliced onions in cold water for 10 minutes, drain, and pat dry.

▶ *Health Tip:* Use only pasteurized feta cheese (see Listeriosis Warning, page 129).

▶ *Complete Meal Ideas:* Serve this salad with:
  A soup (such as Greek-Style Chicken, Lemon, and Egg Soup, page 98)
  A whole wheat pita or a whole wheat roll
  Reduced-fat 2% milk or low-fat yogurt
  Fresh fruit

APPROXIMATE NUTRITIONAL INFORMATION: Serving size: half of the Greek salad; Calories: 368 cals;
Protein: 10 g; Carbohydrates: 22 g; Fat: 29 g; Fiber: 5 g; Sodium: 1,001 mg; Vitamin A: 1,745 IU; Vitamin C: 27
mg; Folic Acid: 98 mcg; Calcium: 196 mg; Iron: 4 mg; Diabetic Exchange: Fat 5, Vegetable 5

lemony coleslaw with fresh dill

What's in this for baby and me? Vitamins A and C.

PACKED WITH VITAMINS A and C, this coleslaw is a great sidekick for anything from grilled hamburgers to lasagna. To save time, buy a packaged coleslaw mix, or pick up the shredded cabbage and carrots from a grocery store salad bar. Jicama, fennel bulb, and radishes are crunchy additions. Dress the slaw at the last minute.

Serves 4

LEMON DRESSING
1 tablespoon olive oil or canola oil
1½ tablespoons freshly squeezed lemon juice,
    to taste
1 tablespoon light mayonnaise
Salt and freshly ground pepper to taste

8 ounces (about 4 cups) thinly sliced white or
    red cabbage, or a mix of both,
    or an 8-ounce packaged coleslaw mix
¼ cup grated carrots
¼ chopped celery
2 tablespoons chopped fresh dill

1. To make the lemon dressing, combine all of the ingredients in a small bowl and whisk until emulsified. Refrigerate until ready to use.
2. Combine the cabbage, carrots, celery, and dill in a large bowl and toss gently. Dress the slaw and adjust the seasoning before serving. Refrigerate leftovers.

▶ **Complete Meal Ideas:** Serve this coleslaw with:
   3 ounces of protein (you might want to try Spice-Rubbed Pork Chops,
       page 311, or the Crispy Fried Tofu with Sesame-Soy Sauce, page 259)
   Brown rice or a whole grain
   Reduced-fat 2% milk or low-fat yogurt
   Fresh fruit

APPROXIMATE NUTRITIONAL INFORMATION: Serving size: one-quarter of the lemony coleslaw; Calories: 64 cals; Protein: 1 g; Carbohydrates: 5 g; Fat: 5 g; Fiber: 2 g; Sodium: 52 mg; Vitamin A: 1,078 IU; Vitamin C: 26 mg; Diabetic Exchange: Fat 1, Vegetable 1

cucumber-tomato yogurt salad

What's in this for baby and me? Calcium.

THIS HIGH-CALCIUM INDIAN salad, also known as *raita*, is commonly eaten as a cooling accompaniment to hot curries. A good source of protein, vitamin A, and B vitamins, it is delicious as a side dish for grilled foods and stews. You can use reduced-fat yogurt, but the salad won't be as creamy and thick.

Makes 2½ cups

2 cups plain full-fat yogurt

1 garlic clove, crushed

½ teaspoon ground cumin

1 tablespoon thinly sliced fresh mint leaves

1 tablespoon chopped fresh cilantro

1 cup peeled, seeded, and grated cucumber, the juice gently squeezed out

½ cup vine-ripened tomatoes, seeded and cut into a small dice

Salt and freshly ground pepper, to taste

Combine all of the ingredients in a bowl and stir. Refrigerate for 1 hour before serving to allow the flavors to develop.

▶ *Variation:* 2 tablespoons of fresh mint or coriander leaves can be used instead of a tablespoon of each.

▶ *Storage Tip:* This salad keeps for 2 days refrigerated.

▶ *Complete Meal Ideas:* Serve this salad with:
   Any curry or richly flavored main course (you might
      want to try Vegetarian Curry, page 206)
   Brown basmati rice or rice noodles
   Green salad or vegetable
   Fresh fruit

APPROXIMATE NUTRITIONAL INFORMATION: Serving size: ½ cup cucumber-tomato yogurt salad; Calories: 95 cals; Protein: 7 g; Carbohydrates: 13 g; Fat: 2 g; Fiber: 0 g; Sodium: 90 mg; Calcium: 240 mg; Diabetic Exchange: Milk 1

homemade guacamole

What's in this for baby and me? Vitamin C.

Hᴵɢʜ ɪɴ ᴠɪᴛᴀᴍɪɴ C and a good source of folic acid and fiber, homemade guacamole is delicious served as a dip for sliced fresh vegetables and baked tortilla chips, or with fajitas, quesadillas, tacos, or any grilled main course. It is also wonderful spread on sandwiches instead of mayonnaise.

makes 2½ cups

3 ripe avocados, preferably Hass

3 tablespoons very finely chopped red onion or sweet white onion (such as Vidalia)

1 large vine-ripened tomato, cut into small dice

2 tablespoons freshly squeezed lime juice, or to taste

3 tablespoons chopped fresh cilantro (optional)

1 small garlic clove, crushed

Dash of Tabasco sauce or freshly ground pepper to taste

Salt, to taste

1. Cut the avocados in half and remove the pits. Cut the halves into quarters, then peel them and place in a small bowl. Using the back of a fork, mash the avocados to a chunky consistency. (Do not use a food processor or blender.)
2. Add the remaining ingredients and mix until well combined. Season to taste, cover with the plastic wrap placed flush against the surface of the guacamole, and refrigerate a couple hours before serving.

▶ *Storage Tip:* This dip keeps refrigerated for 1 day. Some discoloration will occur, but the taste will not be affected.

▶ *Diabetic Tip:* Reduce the portion size to 2 tablespoons.

APPROXIMATE NUTRITIONAL INFORMATION: Serving size: ¼ cup guacamole; Calories: 158 cals; Protein: 2 g; Carbohydrates: 8 g; Fat: 15 g; Fiber: 4 g; Sodium: 12 mg; Vitamin C: 13 mg; Diabetic Exchange (values per 2 tablespoon serving): Fat 1.5

roasted red pepper and cheese dip

What's in this for baby and me? Vitamin C.

Tasty and easy to prepare, this dip makes a perfect snack or sandwich spread. It is a great source of vitamin C and a good source of protein, calcium, and vitamin A. The feta cheese gives the dip a great consistency and the perfect tang. Serve with your favorite raw vegetables or whole wheat crackers for a vitamin and fiber fix.

makes about 1 cup

⅓ cup part-skim ricotta cheese

⅔ cup (about 4 ounces) crumbled pasteurized feta cheese (see Health Tip below)

⅓ cup sliced jarred roasted red peppers

Salt and freshly ground pepper, to taste

Combine all of the ingredients in the bowl of a food processor and pulse, scraping down the sides of the bowl as needed, until smooth and creamy. Do not overmix, or the dip will be runny. Refrigerate any leftovers.

▶ *Health Tip:* Use only pasteurized feta cheese (see Listeriosis Warning, page 129).

▶ *Storage Tip:* This dip keeps for 3 days refrigerated.

APPROXIMATE NUTRITIONAL INFORMATION: Serving size: ¼ cup roasted red pepper and cheese dip; Calories: 105 cals; Protein: 6 g; Carbohydrates: 3 g; Fat: 8 g; Fiber: .1 g; Sodium: 388 mg; Vitamin C: 19 mg; Diabetic Exchange: Fat 1, Meat (Medium Fat) 1

healthy hummus

What's in this for baby and me? Protein, folic acid, and fiber.

An excellent source of protein, folic acid, and fiber, and a good source of vitamin C and iron, hummus is a wonderful addition to any pregnant woman's diet, and many kids love it. Serve hummus with toasted whole wheat pita bread, Melba toast, whole wheat crackers, or sliced fresh vegetables. For a delicious vegetarian sandwich, see the Hummus-Tabbouleh Roll on page 127. If your dietary needs call for extra calories, or if you are serving small children who don't need to watch their fat intake, feel free to substitute additional olive oil or canola oil for the water.

makes about 2 cups

One 15-ounce can chickpeas, rinsed and
    drained
1 small garlic clove, crushed
½ teaspoon ground cumin
¼ cup freshly squeezed lemon juice, or to
    taste

2 tablespoons canola oil or olive oil
1 tablespoon tahini
A few drops of Tabasco sauce (optional)
2–3 tablespoons water (add more or less to
    desired consistency)
Salt, to taste

Combine all of the ingredients in the bowl of a food processor or blender and process until completely smooth, scraping down the sides of the bowl as needed. Season and serve; refrigerate leftovers.

▶ **Cooking Tip 1:** For a slightly higher yield, use a 19-ounce can of chickpeas and increase the following ingredients: 2 small garlic cloves, 3 tablespoons canola oil or olive oil, 2 tablespoons tahini, and ¼ cup water.

▶ **Cooking Tip 2:** If serving this hummus as an appetizer, garnish it with 2 tablespoons chopped fresh parsley and a dash of cayenne pepper. Or, dribble extra olive oil on top and sprinkle with olives or toasted pine nuts.

▶ **Storage Tip:** This dip keeps for 3 days refrigerated.

▶ **Health Tip:** If your doctor has restricted your fat intake, substitute water for the olive oil.

APPROXIMATE NUTRITIONAL INFORMATION: Serving size: ½ cup homemade hummus; Calories: 261 cals; Protein: 10 g; Carbohydrates: 31 g; Fat: 12 g; Fiber: 8 g; Sodium: 154 mg; Folic Acid: 189 mcg; Diabetic Exchange: Bread/Starch 2, Fat 2.5, Meat (Lean) .5

constipation

Constipation is a common problem for pregnant women. Like indigestion and heart-burn, it usually occurs during the first and third trimesters. During the first trimester, increased hormonal levels tend to cause constipation, while during the third trimester, smooth-muscle relaxation and cramped and compressed abdominal space slow down waste elimination. It is important to include high-fiber foods in your diet and to drink plenty of fluids, including water, milk, and (some) fruit juice.

TIPS FOR COPING

▶ Increase high-fiber foods in your diet, such as whole grain cereals and breads, beans, lentils, peas, raw fruits and vegetables, and dried fruit. A good fiber intake is about 25 to 30 g per day.

▶ Increase fluids—drink at least 8 glasses of water per day, and ideally a total of 12 cups of fluid per day.

▶ With permission from your doctor, get regular exercise, which helps get your intestines moving.

▶ Go for walks after meals.

▶ Try a glass of prune juice or some prunes in the morning.

▶ Iron supplements cause constipation in some women. Try taking your supplement at different times of the day.

▶ While sitting on the toilet, massage the sides of your back, starting at the base of your ribs, in a downward motion.

▶ Do not take any form of laxative, bulk-forming supplemental fiber (such as psyllium and methylcellulose), or mineral oil without the consent of your doctor.

spinach dip

What's in this for baby and me? Vitamin A.

This spinach dip is high in vitamin A and a good source of vitamin C, calcium, and folic acid. Fresh vegetables for dipping provide additional vitamins and fiber. This recipe can be cut in half to serve fewer people or doubled to feed a crowd. If your kids like dip, this one could be a winner—but you might want to leave out the anchovy paste.

makes about 2 cups

One 10-ounce package frozen chopped spinach, thawed, drained, and squeezed dry
¼ cup sliced scallions
¼ cup fresh parsley leaves
1½ teaspoons anchovy paste, or to taste (optional)

3 tablespoons freshly squeezed lemon juice, or to taste
⅓ cup part-skim ricotta cheese
½ cup reduced-fat sour cream
2 tablespoons light mayonnaise
Salt and freshly ground pepper, to taste

Combine the spinach, scallions, parsley, anchovy paste, if using, and lemon juice in the bowl of a food processor and process until fairly smooth. Add the ricotta cheese, sour cream, and mayonnaise and pulse just until blended. Season and serve; refrigerate leftovers.

▶ **Variation:** Use about 12 ounces of fresh spinach in place of the frozen spinach. Cook the spinach (sauté, steam, microwave, or boil), drain, and squeeze out as much liquid as possible before proceeding with the recipe.

▶ **Storage Tip:** This dip keeps for 2 days refrigerated. The spinach will lose its bright green color from the acid of the lemon juice, but the taste is unaffected.

▶ **Health Tip:** If your doctor has restricted your salt intake, omit the anchovy paste and go easy on the salt. If you need to reduce your fat intake, omit the mayonnaise and use low-fat ricotta cheese and nonfat yogurt or nonfat sour cream instead of reduced-fat sour cream. Yogurt produces a less creamy dip.

APPROXIMATE NUTRITIONAL INFORMATION: Serving size: ¼ cup spinach dip; Calories: 61 cals; Protein: 3 g; Carbohydrates: 4 g; Fat: 4 g; Fiber: 1 g; Sodium: 87 mg; Vitamin A: 2,982 IU; Diabetic Exchange: Fat 1, Vegetable 1

artichoke-spinach dip

What's in this for baby and me? Vitamins C and A and folic acid.

An EXCELLENT SOURCE of vitamins C and A and folic acid and a fine source of calcium and fiber, this dip is a great snack any time of day.

makes about 1 ½ cups

2 tightly packed cups baby spinach (one
    6-ounce bag)
One 14-ounce can artichoke hearts, drained
1 scallion, trimmed and sliced
¼ cup grated Parmesan cheese

¼ cup jarred roasted red bell peppers
    (optional)
2 tablespoons light mayonnaise
Salt and freshly ground pepper, to taste
Squeeze of fresh lemon juice

1. Microwave, boil, or steam the spinach just until wilted, about 1 minute. Drain and squeeze as much liquid from the spinach as possible.
2. Place the cooked spinach, artichoke hearts, scallion, Parmesan cheese, bell peppers, if using, and mayonnaise in the bowl of a food processor and pulse to the desired consistency. Season with salt, pepper, and lemon juice. Refrigerate any leftovers.

▶ *Storage Tip:* This dip keeps for 2 days refrigerated.

APPROXIMATE NUTRITIONAL INFORMATION: Serving size: ¼ cup artichoke-spinach dip; Calories: 72 cals; Protein: 5 g; Carbohydrates: 9 g; Fat: 3 g; Fiber: 4 g; Sodium: 185 mg; Vitamin A: 5,246 IU; Vitamin C: 23 g; Diabetic Exchange: Fat 1, Vegetable 1.5

black bean dip

What's in this for baby and me? Vitamin C, folic acid, and fiber.

Here's a bean dip that's rich in vitamin C, folic acid, and fiber, and is a good source of protein. It goes deliciously with whole wheat crackers, vegetables, and, of course, baked corn tortilla chips.

makes about 1¾ cups

One 15.5-ounce can black beans, rinsed and drained

2 tablespoons chopped jarred roasted red peppers or pimentos

2 tablespoons water

1 tablespoon canola oil or olive oil

1½ tablespoons freshly squeezed lime juice, or to taste

2 tablespoons chopped fresh cilantro

½ teaspoon minced garlic

½ teaspoon ground cumin, or to taste

½ teaspoon salt, or to taste

A couple of drops of Tabasco

Combine all of the ingredients in the bowl of a food processor or blender and process until completely smooth, scraping down the sides of the bowl as needed. Adjust seasoning and serve; refrigerate leftovers.

▶ *Storage Tip:* This dip keeps for 2 days refrigerated.

APPROXIMATE NUTRITIONAL INFORMATION: Serving size: ½ cup black bean dip; Calories: 146 cals; Protein: 7 g; Carbohydrates: 20 g; Fat: 5 g; Fiber: 7 g; Sodium: 359 mg; Vitamin C: 12 mg; Folic Acid: 120 mcg; Diabetic Exchange: Bread/Starch 1.5, Fat 1

vegetarian and vegan delights

～

Despite the title, this chapter really is for *everyone*. The recipes and information will benefit *all* diets, and eating more vegetables and vegetable-based proteins is just plain healthy, no matter what age or gender you are.

For starters, please don't let anyone tell you that a vegetarian or vegan cannot have a perfectly healthy pregnancy and a healthy baby, or babies. Most pregnant vegetarians do not need to drastically change their lifestyle or eating habits unless they were unhealthy to begin with. The general guidelines for nutrition during pregnancy are the same for vegetarians and non-vegetarians, but there are a couple of adjustments to note.

The Institute of Medicine has established a higher iron RDA for vegetarians—48.6 milligrams per day, an increase from 27 milligrams per day for non-vegetarians. This is admittedly difficult to achieve without supplements.[1] The reason for this increase is because vegetarians consume non-heme iron from plant sources, which is not as easily absorbed by the body as heme iron from meat.

Also, while the Institute of Medicine has not specified a zinc RDA for vegetarians, it *suggests* that the requirement should be as much as 50 percent higher than 11 milligrams per day for omnivores. This would increase the vegetarian zinc recommendation to 16.5 milligrams per day.[2]

To optimize nutritional benefits, both vegetarians and non-vegetarians should eat balanced meals that include a variety of foods. Eating a mix of healthy foods maximizes the body's ability to absorb nutrients, particularly calcium, iron, and zinc. Depending on one's eating habits and any special situations, some vegetarians and vegans may find it challenging to meet the requirements for protein, calcium, vitamin D, iron, vitamin B_{12}, zinc, and iodine.

Vegetarians and vegans are encouraged to read *Eating for Pregnancy* from cover to cover so as not to miss any of the health information or tips. Tell your health care provider that you are a vegetarian or vegan, describe your dietary habits, and address any concerns regarding your pregnancy. Inquire about vegetarian prenatal vitamins and vegetarian supplements; there are many varieties on the market.

VEGETARIAN FOOD GROUPS

A PREGNANT VEGETARIAN will need to consume the following amounts from the basic food groups. (To give you an idea of portion sizes, see Food Groups and Serving Sizes for Pregnant Women, page 37.) If inadequate weight gain is a problem, try eating more frequent snacks that contain protein; try to include more unsaturated oils (such as olive, walnut, soybean, and sesame oils) in your cooking; and incorporate more dairy products. Vegetarians and vegans rarely have a problem with gaining too much weight during pregnancy.

FOOD GROUPS FOR A VEGETARIAN PREGNANCY[3]

Grain Group = 9 or more servings per day

Fruits = 4 or more servings per day

Vegetables = 3 or more servings per day

Protein Group = 3 servings per day

Milk and Dairy Group = 4 or more servings per day

Others (Fats and Sweets) = use sparingly

PROTEIN

MEETING THE PROTEIN requirements of pregnancy is usually not a problem for most vegetarians, although vegans who do not eat any dairy products might be challenged. Some vegetarian sources of protein include pasteurized cheese, low-fat cottage cheese, milk, low-fat yogurt, tofu (plain and enriched), tempeh, eggs, enriched soy beverages, cooked beans, soybeans, nuts, and nut butters (see Protein Sources, page 280, for a more complete list). Consult your doctor or a registered dietitian if you feel you cannot meet your increased protein requirements during pregnancy, or if you are considering a protein supplement.

CALCIUM AND VITAMIN D

VEGETARIANS WHO EAT dairy products can fulfill their calcium and vitamin D requirements from milk, yogurt, and pasteurized cheeses. If your vegetarian diet excludes all dairy products, a calcium and vitamin D supplement will likely be advised. (For a list of Nondairy Calcium Sources, see page 185.) To ensure vitamin D production, vegans should try to get at least twenty minutes of direct sunlight on their hands and faces two to three times a week. Some good news is that vegetarians tend to absorb and retain more calcium from foods than non-vegetarians. However, calcium bioavailability, or the body's ability to absorb calcium, may be reduced by oxalic acid (oxalates) and phytic acid (phytates), found in certain plants and vegetables, and unrefined cereals.[4] This information is important to note because some vegetarian diets rely on large amounts of leafy greens and green vegetables for calcium intake.

IRON

IRON IS ESSENTIAL throughout pregnancy, and iron deficiency occurs in vegetarian and non-vegetarian pregnancies alike. To help reach your 48.6 milligram daily goal, consume blackstrap molasses, iron-fortified cereals, cooked beans (especially lima beans and soybeans), green leafy vegetables (such as spinach, Swiss chard, kale, and beet greens), lentils, whole and enriched grains, baked potatoes (with skin on), tempeh, meat analogs, seeds, prune juice, and dried fruit (see Iron Sources, page 38, for a more complete list).

The tannins in leaf tea, coffee, calcium supplements, and certain foods high in phytic acid can limit iron absorption. To maximize iron absorption, vegetarians should try to consume iron-rich foods with foods high in vitamin C. Also, vegetarians should opt for iron- and zinc-fortified soy products to minimize the inhibitory effect of phytic acid contained in certain soy products, such as soy flour, soy protein isolate, and tofu processed with calcium sulfate. (See Recommendations for Optimizing Iron and Zinc Bioavailability in Vegetarians, page 230, and Sample Menus for Optimizing Iron and Zinc Bioavailability, page 231.)

VITAMIN B$_{12}$

BECAUSE PLANTS DO not contain vitamin B$_{12}$, vegans may need to supplement their diets to ensure an adequate intake of B$_{12}$. Vegetarians who include eggs and dairy products in their diets are seldom at risk for a vitamin B$_{12}$ deficiency. Some good sources of vitamin B$_{12}$ include fortified soy beverages, milk products, fortified tofu and other fortified soy products, meat analogs, enriched breakfast cereals, and brewer's yeast.

ZINC

DAIRY PRODUCTS ARE among the best dietary sources of zinc for vegetarians. Vegans can obtain zinc from other sources such as whole grains, legumes, brown rice, spinach, nuts, seeds, tofu, tempeh, fortified cereals, and wheat germ. As with iron, your body's ability to absorb zinc may be reduced by the presence of phytates, oxalates, fiber, calcium supplements, and soy proteins containing phytic acid. (See Recommendations for Optimizing Iron and Zinc Bioavailability in Vegetarians, page 230.) Try to consume 16.5 milligrams per day.

IODINE

PLANT-BASED DIETS tend to be low in iodine, which can put some vegetarian women at risk for iodine deficiency. Using iodized salt in cooking and on the table is the answer for most diets: ¾ teaspoon used in cooking and at the table will provide enough iodine to meet the RDA for pregnancy of 220 micrograms per day. Seaweed such as nori and hiziki is high in iodine.

OMEGA-3 FATTY ACIDS

THE BEST SOURCE of brain- and retina-building DHA and EPA omega-3 fatty acids is fish. Is this bad news for vegetarians and vegans? Not necessarily, but they may have to work harder to get DHA into their diets. Here are a few good options: consume DHA-enriched products (see Omega-3-Enriched Products to Add to Your Breakfast Line-Up, page 40), increase consumption of foods high in ALA, or take vegetarian supplements containing microalgae-derived DHA either in liquid form, vegicaps, or vegan capsules. Consult with your doctor before taking any supplements.

As previously mentioned, the conversion of ALA to EPA and DHA is limited, but it may be somewhat higher during pregnancy. Studies have shown that certain factors listed below can strip essential fatty acids from the body.

- Excessive consumption of saturated fats, hydrogenated fats, and trans fats (partially hydrogenated oils)
- A lack of zinc, magnesium, or vitamins B_3, B_6, or C
- Viral infections and the presence of hormones released in response to stress
- Alcohol
- Smoking[5]

RECIPE NOTES

IF YOU ARE a vegetarian, you are sure to have fun with these vegetarian recipes and the thirty-five vegan recipes throughout this book. (Vegan recipes are designated by the ▼ symbol.) Most of the recipes are quick and easy, and are designed to put a healthy twist on some old favorites. There are a few exceptions that are a bit more time-consuming and labor intensive—such as the Light and Healthy Vegetable Ragout, the Best-Ever Vegetarian Lasagna, and the Vegetarian Pad Thai, but the extra time and effort you put into these creations are well worth it. As with all cooking, choose the best fresh produce and ingredients you can find in your local grocery store, whole food store, health food store, or farmers' market. This is especially true for vegetarians who rely on fresh produce for the bulk of their diet.

Some notes about the recipes in this chapter:

- Most dairy products can be replaced with soy products, from soy milk to soy sour cream, and margarine can be substituted for butter. A few exceptions are mentioned in the recipes.
- Reduced-fat 2% milk can be substituted for whole milk.
- If you need to increase your calcium intake, choose calcium-fortified cheeses, including packaged grated cheddar cheese and Monterey Jack.
- If you need to watch your fat intake, use low-fat cheeses or those made with 2% milk, and use reduced-fat 2% milk.
- Check the expiration date on all packages of tofu and tempeh, and make sure that they are properly packaged. Try to avoid tofu sold out of tubs with water.
- Wash all greens and vegetables thoroughly, even if the package claims that they are prewashed (see Tips for Cleaning Fresh Produce, page 445).
- Use MSG-free vegetarian bouillon cubes to add extra flavor (unless you need to watch your sodium intake).

protein in soy foods

Pregnant vegetarians can often feel challenged to fulfill their daily protein needs. While the required 60 grams of protein may seem like a lot, the math can, in fact, be fairly simple, even for vegans.

PROTEIN CONTENTS FOR SOY PRODUCTS

½ cup tempeh = 19.5 g

¼ cup of roasted soy nuts = 19 g

½ cup edamame = 17 g

1 soy protein bar = 14 g

4 ounces of firm tofu = 13 g

1 soy burger = 10 to 12 g

8 ounces plain soy milk = 10 g

1 veggie dog = 8 g

2 tablespoons soy nut butter = 7 g

1 soy sausage link = 6 g

8 ounces soy yogurt = 5 g

- To save time, pick up as many ingredients as possible from a salad bar, including shredded carrots, chopped onions, sliced mushrooms, and sliced red bell peppers.
- Try to avoid overcooking vegetables, a common mistake, especially when stir-frying. Keep in mind that the vegetables will continue to cook once removed from the heat.
- Don't be afraid to experiment and modify the recipes to suit your family's needs and tastes.

nondairy calcium sources

FOOD	SERVING SIZE	CALCIUM (MG)
Calcium-fortified orange juice	8 ounces	350
Blackstrap molasses	2 tablespoons	344
Enriched soy beverage	8 ounces	300
Calcium-fortified bread	2 slices	160
All-Bran cereal	½ cup	150
Cooked spinach	½ cup	122
Canned salmon (bone-in)	2 ounces	121
Cooked turnip greens	½ cup	99
Tempeh	½ cup	92
Almonds, dry roasted	¼ cup	92
Corn tortillas	2 tortillas	91
Cooked soybeans	½ cup	88
Almond butter	2 tablespoons	86
Molasses	2 tablespoons	82
Flour tortillas	2 tortillas	80
Cooked bok choy	½ cup	79
Tofu (not fortified)	4 ounces	75
Dried figs	¼ cup	72
Vegetarian baked beans	½ cup	64
Plain bagel	1 bagel	53
Cooked mustard greens	½ cup	52
Cooked okra	½ cup	50
Cooked kale	½ cup	47
Baked acorn squash	½ cup	45
Baked butternut squash	½ cup	42
Fresh orange	1 medium	42
Cooked pinto beans	½ cup	41
Cooked chickpeas	½ cup	40
Collard greens	½ cup	40

a guide to cooking healthy grains

Barley (Hulled or Pearled)

USES: Soups, casseroles, side dishes, salads, hot cereals, stuffing

BASIC COOKING INSTRUCTIONS: Add directly to soups. If using barley as a cooked product in salads or side dishes, bring 3 cups of water to a boil, add ½ cup barley, and simmer, uncovered, for 45 minutes, or until the grains are soft. Drain, rinse under cold running water, and drain again. (Note: One-half cup of raw barley makes about 2 cups of cooked barley.)

TIPS: Quick-cooking barley, such as Quaker Oats' Mother's Quick Cooking Barley, cooks in about 10 minutes. Barley flakes, which resemble rolled oats, can be made into hot cereal. Barley grits, a fine grind of the grain, are used for hot cereal.

Brown Rice

USES: Side dishes, salads, soups, risottos, pilafs, stuffing

BASIC COOKING INSTRUCTIONS: Ratio: 2 cups water to 1 cup rice. Stove-top cooking method: Bring the water to a boil in a large saucepan. Add the rice, return to a boil, reduce heat to a simmer, cover, and cook for about 45 minutes, or until the grains are tender and the water has evaporated. (Note: The grains will not be as soft as white rice, but they should not be too hard either.) Oven method: Preheat the oven to 400° F. Bring the water to a boil and set aside. Place the rice in an 8-inch Pyrex dish, add the water, cover with foil, and bake for 45 minutes, or until the grains are tender.

TIPS: Brown rice comes in short, medium, or long grains, or basmati rice. The outer hull, or bran, is left on the brown rice grain, adding twice as much fiber as that of white rice, in addition to vitamin E. Lundberg Family Farms produces fabulous brown rice in an assortment of varieties and mixtures.

Buckwheat Groats (also known as kasha)

USES: Side dishes, breakfast cereals, pilafs, stuffing

BASIC COOKING INSTRUCTIONS: Ratio: 2 cups water to 1 cup kasha. Bring the water to a boil and set aside. In a medium-size nonstick saucepan, heat 2 teaspoons canola oil over medium-high heat. Add the kasha and stir until the grains are slightly toasted and aromatic, about 3 minutes. Add the reserved water, stir, return to a boil, then reduce heat to a simmer, cover and cook for 10 to 12 minutes (cooking time depends on the grind, see below), or until the grains are tender and the water is absorbed.

TIPS: Whole or coarse buckwheat groats best retain their shape when cooked. The fine or medium grains have a shorter cooking time and they tend to get a bit mushy when cooked.

Bulgur Wheat (also known as tabbouleh, also spelled tabouleh, taboule, or tabouli)

USES: Salads, pita pockets sandwiches with hummus, stuffing

BASIC COOKING INSTRUCTIONS: Ratio: 1½ cups water to 1 cup grains. (The amount of water will depend on the size of the grain. Drain off any water that is not absorbed after 25 minutes of soaking.). Bulgur grains are softened not cooked. Bring the water to a boil. Place the grains in a heatproof bowl, add the boiling hot water, stir, cover with plastic wrap, and let sit at room temperature for 20 to 25 minutes, or until the grains are soft and all of the water is absorbed.

TIPS: Boxed tabouleh mixes that contain the spices are quick and easy to prepare. The best brand is Near East Taboule Mix Wheat Salad—it seems to have the perfect balance of spices to grains.

Quinoa

USES: Salads, side dishes, stuffing

BASIC COOKING INSTRUCTIONS: Ratio: 2 cups water to 1 cup quinoa. Rinse the quinoa in a fine-mesh strainer under cold running water for about 1 minute, then drain. Combine the rinsed quinoa with water in a saucepan and bring to a boil. Reduce heat and simmer, covered, for 15 to 20 minutes, or until the grains look transparent and the spiral-like germ has separated. Remove from heat and let stand for 5 minutes, then fluff with a fork.

TIPS: It is advisable to purchase boxed quinoa (such as Ancient Harvest Quinoa) rather than to buy it in bulk from bins. Boxed grains tend to be larger, cleaner, sweeter, and fluffier when cooked. It is absolutely essential to rinse quinoa before cooking it to remove the bitter natural outer coating on each grain. Most of this coating is removed before sale, but, there may be a small residue left on the grain. This grain is a complete protein, comparable to the protein found in meat and eggs.

Whole Wheat Couscous

USES: Salads, side dishes, stuffing

BASIC COOKING INSTRUCTIONS: Ratio: 1½ cups water or stock to 1 cup couscous. Bring the water to a boil in a saucepan. Add the couscous, stir, return to a boil, cover, and remove from heat. Let sit, covered, for 7 minutes. Fluff with a fork.

TIPS: Whole wheat couscous contains more fiber and iron than regular couscous. Israeli, Mediterranean, or Middle Eastern couscous (all the same thing) are perfectly round grains of toasted pasta that have no fiber or iron, but they make a fun salad. (Kids might like these tiny balls in their salad.)

welcome to the world of soy

TOFU: Tofu, or soybean curd, is a high-protein, low-fat staple in many Asian diets. Making tofu is similar to making cheese. First, soybeans are partially cooked, then pureed. Soy milk is extracted from the puree, poured into shaping containers, and solidified with one of two natural coagulants—nigari (magnesium chloride from seawater) or calcium sulphate. The texture of tofu varies from silky (almost liquid . . . good for smoothies) to extra firm. Tofu is sold in regular or plain, lower-fat, seasoned, marinated, and baked varieties. Tofu can be used in endless ways, depending on its consistency and flavor. It is an excellent substitute for meat in dishes such as hamburgers, lasagna, meatballs, stir-fries, casseroles, and taco filling.

TEMPEH: Tempeh is a firm, nubby, soy-based brick that is high in protein and fiber, low in fat, and a good source of calcium, iron, phosphorus, vitamin A, and the B vitamins. To make tempeh, cooked and hulled soybeans (or a combination of soybeans and a grain such as brown rice, barley, wheat, or quinoa) are spread out on trays and inoculated with a beneficial mold culture called *Rhisopus oligosporous*. This mold causes a fermentation process to occur during which the soybean-grain mixture is bound together. Tempeh can be sautéed and used in salads, soups, stews, or with vegetable side dishes. It can be seasoned, pan-fried, and added to sandwiches in place of deli meats; breaded and pan-fried as cutlets and served with a sauce; or crumbled, cooked, and used in fillings in place of ground beef.

SOY MILK: Soy milk is expressed from soybeans that have been soaked and boiled. The flavor varies from brand to brand, but in general it has a nutty and a slightly sweet flavor. Compared to cow's milk, soy milk has about the same amount of protein, half the calories and fat, and one-fifth the calcium. It is lactose-free. Soy milk is often enriched with calcium or protein, and other vitamins, including A, D, and B_{12}. Beverages made from a soy milk base include soy smoothies and shakes; soy milk coffee creamer lattes, mochas, and chai made with soy milk; and soy energy drinks. Soy milk comes in a variety of flavors—vanilla, carob, strawberry, and chocolate—sweetened or unsweetened, non-fat, low-fat, or 1% fat, and organic or non-organic. Soy milk can be consumed straight, or it can be used as a substitute for dairy milk in cooking and baking.

SOY CHEESE, CREAM CHEESE, SOUR CREAM, YOGURT, AND COFFEE CREAMER: All of these products are excellent low-fat, cholesterol-free, lactose-free alternatives to their corresponding dairy products.

SOY NUTS: Soy nuts are whole soy beans that have been partially cooked, split, and dry-roasted. They come in all sorts of flavors including barbeque, wasabi, and Cajun. They can be eaten as a high-protein snack or tossed in salads and soups.

SOY NUT BUTTER: Soy nut butter is made from ground soy nuts. It comes in a variety of textures (from pasty to creamy) and degrees of sweetness, depending on the brand.

MISO: Miso is a salty, fermented soybean paste with a texture of natural peanut butter. Naturally aged miso ferments for a couple of weeks or up to three years, depending on the type. The ingredient list on packages of naturally aged miso should include only soybeans (plus a grain), salt, water, and *Aspergillis orzyae* (a friendly mold). The three most commonly available types of miso are: soybean miso (also called Hatcho miso; dark brown color; strong flavor), soybean and rice miso (this is the most popular miso; white, red, and brown colors; sweet and mild flavors), and soybean and barley miso (also called mugi miso; yellow or brown color; nubby texture; balanced, earthy flavor).

In most grocery stores, miso can be found near the tofu in resealable plastic tubs. It is best known as a base for simple, broth-type soups, but it can be used in sauces, marinades, dips, and dressings. Miso acts as a salt or soy sauce substitute—so a little goes a long way. The fermentation process makes miso easily digestible, and the lactic-acid bacteria and enzymes that it contains aid in general digestion (much like the cultures in yogurt do). When cooking with miso, do not boil it, as this destroys the beneficial enzymes.

Sodium Note: One tablespoon of Hatcho or soybean miso contains 750 milligrams of sodium.

FRESH GREEN SOY BEANS (EDAMAME): Bright green, fresh soy beans are usually sold whole or shelled, and frozen, but they can also be found cooked in their fuzzy green pods, usually in the take-out sushi section of a grocery store or whole foods store. The flavor of the beans is slightly sweet and nutty—a cross between fresh green peas and lima beans. Fresh soy beans are high in protein, vitamin C, thiamine, and vitamin A. They can be served as a side dish (with a dash of soy sauce) or in salads, soups, stir-fries, and pasta dishes, or used as a substitute for green peas in recipes.

DRY WHOLE SOY BEANS: Rich in polyunsaturated oils, soybeans are the only legume with a complete protein. Look for smooth beans with an even creamy-white color and no surface blemishes, such as holes or cracks. Dry whole soy beans have a very long cooking time, over three hours, and they tend to produce a lot of foam during cooking. For convenience, use canned cooked soy beans, usually available in the bean aisle or health food section of grocery stores. Cooked beans can be used in the following ways: mashed coarsely as a substitute for ground meat in chili, stews, and Mexican dishes (such as taco filling); ground for soy burgers or veggie patties; processed until smooth for a hummus-type dip; left whole for bean salads, stir-fries, soups, and other dishes calling for beans.

SOY FLAKES: Soy flakes are made from soybeans that have been dry-roasted, split, and tilled in a roller mill, then dehydrated. Soy flakes do not require presoaking, but they do take 30 to 40 minutes to cook. Soy flakes can be added to grains (such as brown rice or pearl barley), soups, stews, chilies, stuffings, and vegetable burgers.

SOY GRANULES: Soy granules are made from precooked, defatted, and dehydrated soybeans. They do not need to be soaked or precooked before being added to hot cereals, casseroles, soups, or stews. They can also be added to baked goods in place of nuts.

SOY GRITS: Soy grits are made from whole, dry soybeans that are sometimes lightly toasted, then cracked into several pieces. They do not require presoaking and take about 40 minutes to cook (follow package directions as cooking times vary). Cooked soy grits can be combined with other cooked or prepared grains such as rice, barley, quinoa, or tabbouleh, or included in pilafs, stuffings, or stews.

SOY POWDER: Soy powder comes from ground, cooked, dehydrated soybeans. It is similar to soy flour but contains less hull material, and unlike flour it dissolves in liquid. Soy powder can be added to shakes or blender drinks for extra protein, or to baked goods, pancakes, and other breakfast food batters.

TEXTURIZED VEGETABLE PROTEIN (TVP): TVP is a processed soy food made from high-protein defatted soy flour that is exposed to heat and pressure to form granules or small fibrous chunks. It is the main ingredient in meat analog products such as burgers, sausages, bacon, and bacon bits. Keep in mind that although these soy products are high in protein, many also contain high amounts of fat. Packaged TVP sold in whole and health food stores can be reconstituted and added to tacos, burritos, bean stews, and sloppy joes.

vegetarian delights

Light and Healthy Vegetable Ragout ▼
Three-Bean Vegetarian Chili ▼
Vegetarian Curry
Best-Ever Vegetarian Lasagna
Spaghetti with Herbed Tofu Balls and Tomato Sauce
Pasta with Tomatoes, Herbs, and Pasteurized Goat Cheese
Spinach-Cheese Quiche
Grilled or Roasted Marinated Vegetables ▼
Vegetarian Pad Thai
Homemade Tofu-Bean Burritos ▼
Cheese and Spinach Quesadillas
Old Bay Tofu Cakes with Cocktail Sauce
Sautéed Tofu and Portobello Mushrooms on a Bed of Greens ▼
Vegetarian Omelet for One
Lentil, Brown Rice, and Mushroom Pilaf
Swiss Chard or Spinach with Garlicky Soy Dressing ▼
Lima Beans with Artichoke Hearts and Dill
Okra and Tomatoes ▼
Classic Creamed Spinach
Simple and Tasty Brussels Sprouts ▼
Southern-Style Sweet Potato Casserole
Baked Acorn Squash with Molasses ▼
Annie Mozer's Greens ▼
Twenty-Minute Tomato Sauce ▼
Edamame, Corn, and Bean Salad ▼
Brown Rice and Lentil Salad ▼
Asian-Style Pickled Sesame Cabbage ▼
Tofu with Vegetables and Coconut Milk ▼
Quick Broccoli and Red Bell Pepper Frittata
Miso Soup with Tofu and Rice Noodles ▼
Tofu with Soba Noodles, Carrots, Cucumbers, and Sesame Sauce ▼
Crispy Fried Tofu with Sesame-Soy Sauce ▼
Veggie Burgers
Very Simple Fried Rice with Vegetables
Spinach Risotto
Roasted New Potatoes with Garlic and Rosemary ▼
Savory Corn Cakes with Cilantro
Spinach Paneer
Kshama Vyas's Indian Dal ▼

▼ Vegan recipe

seven 2,000-calorie sample menus for vegetarian and vegan pregnancies

Think of these menus as blueprints. Mix and match, and make any adjustments to these menus to fit your eating plans.

Day One Vegetarian

Breakfast
2 enriched whole wheat waffles
2 tablespoons maple syrup
1 cup calcium-fortified orange juice
1 banana

Snack
1 cup mango smoothie (see Super Fruit Smoothies, page 76)

Lunch
1 quesadilla with cheese and vegetables (see Cheese and Spinach Quesadillas, page 224)
3 tablespoons salsa
2 cups mixed greens with ½ avocado (or ⅓ cup guacamole, see Homemade Guacamole, page 173)
2 tablespoons salad dressing (see Four Delicious Homemade Salad Dressings, page 166)
1 apple
1 cup enriched soy milk

Snack
6 ounces soy yogurt
⅓ cup granola (see Fruit-Filled Granola, page 370)
½ cup berries

Dinner

One serving vegetable lasagna (see Best-Ever Vegetarian Lasagna, page 208)
8 asparagus spears
1 whole wheat roll
1 teaspoon tub margarine
½ cup frozen yogurt

Nutrition Information for Day One Vegetarian

Calories: 2,010 cals
Fat: 65 g
Carbohydrates: 313 g
Protein: 51 g
Fiber: 39 g
Iron: 18 mg
Calcium: 1,157 mg
Folic Acid: 421 mcg

Day Two Vegetarian

Breakfast
2 eggs, scrambled
2 slices whole wheat bread, toasted
2 teaspoons tub margarine
1 cup calcium-fortified orange juice

Snack
1 almond granola bar
6 ounces low-fat soy fruit yogurt

Lunch
¾ cup bean salad (see Kid's Favorite Three-Bean Salad, page 152, or Edamame,
Corn, and Bean Salad, page 247)
2 cups mixed greens with 5 cherry tomatoes and 5 cucumber slices
2 tablespoons salad dressing (see Four Delicious Homemade Salad Dressings,
page 166)
½ cup low-fat 2% cottage cheese
5 whole wheat crackers
1 cup enriched soy milk

Dinner
1½ cups whole wheat spaghetti with ½ cup tomato sauce and 3 ounces sautéed
tofu (see Spaghetti with Herbed Tofu Balls and Tomato Sauce, page 210)
½ cup broccoli florets
¾ cup mango sorbet

Nutrition Information for Day Two Vegetarian
Calories: 2,103 cals
Fat: 65 g
Carbohydrates: 306 g
Protein: 93 g
Fiber: 35 g
Iron: 17 mg
Calcium: 1,632 mg
Folic Acid: 419 mcg

Day Three Vegetarian

Breakfast
2 slices French toast (see French Toast Banana Sandwich, page 55)
1 cup calcium-fortified orange juice
6 ounces low-fat soy fruit yogurt

Snack
1 banana
2 tablespoons peanut butter
2 brown rice cakes

Lunch
1 cup squash or carrot soup (see Butternut Squash–Carrot Soup with Ginger, page 96)
½ cup egg salad (see Pr-egg-o Salad Sandwich, page 118)
2 slices whole wheat bread
1 cup enriched soy milk
½ cup (4 ounces) mandarin orange slices in light syrup

Dinner
1 serving tofu cakes (see Old Bay Tofu Cakes with Cocktail Sauce, page 225)
½ cup tabbouleh salad (see Best-Ever Tabbouleh Salad, page 151)
½ cup broccoli
1 cup mixed greens
1 tablespoon salad dressing (see Four Delicious Homemade Salad Dressings, page 166)
½ cup raspberry sorbet

Nutrition Information for Day Three Vegetarian

Calories: 2,060 cals	Fat: 62 g
Carbohydrates: 324 g	Protein: 66 g
Fiber: 23 g	Iron: 13 mg
Calcium: 1,382 mg	Folic Acid: 363 mcg

Day Four Vegan

Breakfast
1 cup fortified whole grain breakfast cereal
1 cup enriched soy milk
1 banana
1 cup calcium-fortified orange juice

Snack
1 medium whole wheat bagel
2 slices vegan cheese
¼ cup roasted, salted soy nuts

Lunch
1 vegan burger
1 whole wheat bun
Salad Bar Salad made with 1½ cups romaine lettuce, 5 cherry tomatoes, ¼ cup shredded carrots
2 tablespoons salad dressing (see Four Delicious Homemade Salad Dressings, page 166)
6 ounces low-fat soy fruit yogurt

Dinner
3 ounces sautéed tofu with ½ cup bok choy and sesame seeds
1 cup brown rice
½ cup soy pudding
2 vegan oatmeal cookies
1 cup enriched soy milk

Nutrition Information for Day Four Vegan

Calories: 2,048 cals	Fat: 56 g
Carbohydrates: 324 g	Protein: 85 g
Fiber: 49 g	Iron: 43 mg
Calcium: 1,192 mg	Folic Acid: 911 mcg

Day Five Vegan

Breakfast
1 cup oatmeal
1 tablespoon molasses
1 cup enriched soy or rice milk
½ grapefruit

Snack
1 medium whole wheat bagel
2 slices vegan turkey
1 peanut butter vegan granola bar

Lunch
1 vegan burrito (See Home-Made Tofu Bean Burritos, page 222)
2 cups mixed greens, ½ cut seasoned croutons, ¼ cup shredded carrots
2 tablespoons salad dressing (see Four Delicious Homemade Salad Dressings, page 166)
1 cup tomato juice
1 banana

Dinner
3 ounces tofu sautéed with a spice packet (see Crispy Fried Tofu with Sesame-Soy Sauce, page 259)
½ cup cooked spinach (see Swiss Chard or Spinach with Garlicky Soy Dressing, page 233)
1 cup whole wheat couscous with ⅓ cup roasted cashew nuts, 1 tablespoon chopped parsley
1 soy ice cream sandwich
½ cup blueberries

Nutrition Information for Day Five Vegan
Calories: 2,063 cals
Carbohydrates: 300 g
Fiber: 39 g
Calcium: 1,010 mg
Fat: 67 g
Protein: 78 g
Iron: 23 mg
Folic Acid: 490 mcg

Day Six Vegan

Breakfast
2 whole wheat vegan waffles
3 tablespoons maple syrup or fruit syrup (see Diabetic-Friendly Strawberry-
Raspberry Syrup, page 59)
1 cup strawberries (if not using fresh fruit syrup)
1 cup calcium-fortified orange juice

Snack
⅓ cup hummus (see Healthy Hummus, page 175)
1 whole wheat pita
8 baby carrots

Lunch
1½ cups lentil soup (see Lentil Soup with Brown Rice and Spinach, page 102)
1 slice sprouted spelt bread
1 vegetable and bean vegan tamale
1 cup enriched soy milk
1 apple

Dinner
1 cup vegetable ragout (see Light and Healthy Vegetable Ragout, page 202)
1½ cups whole wheat ziti
2 cups mixed greens with ⅓ cup roasted walnuts and 2 tablespoons dried
cranberries
2 tablespoons balsamic salad dressing (see Four Delicious Homemade Salad
Dressings, page 166)
½ cup peach sorbet
½ cup blueberries

Nutrition Information for Day Six Vegan

Calories: 2,028 cals	Fat: 39 g
Carbohydrates: 378 g	Protein: 61 g
Fiber: 48 g	Iron: 23 mg
Calcium: 1,071 mg	Folic Acid: 615 mcg

Day Seven Vegan

Breakfast
1 cup fortified whole grain breakfast cereal
1 cup enriched soy milk
½ cup blueberries
1 slice whole wheat bread, toasted
1 tablespoon almond butter

Snack
½ cup black bean dip (see Black Bean Dip, page 179)
10 whole wheat crackers
¼ cup roasted mixed nuts
8 baby carrots

Lunch
1½ cups miso soup with tofu and greens (see Miso Soup with Tofu and Rice
Noodles, page 255)
7 pieces vegetable maki (take-out) with 1 teaspoon soy sauce, pickled ginger,
and wasabi
½ cup seaweed salad
1 orange
1 cup enriched soy milk

Dinner
2 cups fried brown rice with tofu and vegetables (see Very Simple Fried Rice
with Vegetables and substitute the egg with tofu, page 263)
8 asparagus spears
½ cup frozen soy ice cream
½ cup fresh raspberries or fruit sauce (see Rhubarb Sauce, page 373)

Nutrition Information for Day Seven Vegan
Calories: 2,010 cals	Fat: 68 g
Carbohydrates: 315 g	Protein: 61 g
Fiber: 56 g	Iron: 44 mg
Calcium: 1,191 mg	Folic Acid: 1,028 mcg

vegetarian staples to have on hand

Try to keep your pantry and freezer stocked with the following items:

- ▶ Whole grain iron-, B_{12}-, and folic acid–fortified breakfast cereals
- ▶ Wheat germ
- ▶ Quick-cooking whole grain cereals
- ▶ Molasses
- ▶ Milk powder
- ▶ Whole wheat crackers
- ▶ Whole grains (such as barley, brown rice, bulgur wheat, and quinoa)
- ▶ Enriched pastas
- ▶ Tortillas
- ▶ Canned beans (pinto beans, kidney beans, soybeans, and chickpeas)
- ▶ Prepared vegetable soups
- ▶ Jarred or bottled tomato sauce
- ▶ V-8 juice, tomato juice, or other vegetable juices
- ▶ Calcium-fortified orange juice
- ▶ Nut spreads (including peanut butter and soy butter)
- ▶ Nuts and seeds
- ▶ Dried fruits
- ▶ Canned fruits in light syrup
- ▶ Frozen fruits or sorbets
- ▶ Frozen vegetables
- ▶ Frozen fruit juice concentrates
- ▶ Frozen fortified waffles (preferably whole wheat)
- ▶ Main-course frozen foods, such as burritos, enchiladas, tamales, veggie burgers, pizza, and spinach lasagna
- ▶ Seaweed
- ▶ Ground flaxseed and flaxseed oil

pantry items for vegetarian delights

Fresh Produce
Acorn squash
Baby greens or lettuce
Baby spinach
Bok choy and baby bok choy
Broccoli florets
Brussels sprouts
Carrots: regular and peeled baby
   carrots
Celery
Collard greens
Cucumbers
Fresh herbs: basil, cilantro, dill, mint,
   oregano, parsley, and rosemary
Garlic
Ginger
Green asparagus
Green beans
Green cabbage
Kale
Lemons
Limes
Mushrooms: button, cremini,
   portobello, and shiitake
Mustard greens
New potatoes
Okra
Onions: sweet (such as Vidalia),
   yellow, and red
Purple eggplant
Radishes
Red bell peppers
Red sweet potatoes
Shittake mushrooms
Scallions
Spinach
Swiss chard
Tomatoes
Zucchini

Dairy and Soy Products
Cheddar cheese (grated)
Extra-firm tofu (15-ounce package
   drained weight)
Fontina cheese
Grade A large eggs
Gruyère cheese
Half-and-half (preferably ultra-
   pasteurized)
Heavy cream
Low-fat buttermilk
Milk: whole, reduced-fat 2% milk, or
   enriched plain soy beverages
Monterey Jack cheese (grated)
Paneer
Parmesan cheese (grated)
Pasteurized feta cheese
Pasteurized goat cheese
Pasteurized part-skim low-moisture
   mozzarella cheese
Unsalted butter

Canned, Bottled, and Jarred Staples
Artichoke hearts packed in water or
   brine (14-ounce can)
Balsamic vinegar
Black beans (15.5-ounce can)
Black-eyed peas (15.5-ounce can)
Black olives (preferably pitted)
Canola oil
Canola oil cooking spray
Cocktail sauce
Coconut milk
Corn
Crushed tomatoes (28-ounce can)
Dijon mustard
Fat-free low-sodium stock (any kind)
Hoisin sauce

Ketchup

Light or regular coconut milk (14-ounce can)

Light skim evaporated milk

Molasses

Olive oil

Peanut butter

Peeled and diced tomatoes (14.5-ounce can)

Red kidney beans (16-ounce can)

Red wine vinegar

Reduced-fat stock (any flavor)

Refried beans

Rice vinegar (preferably seasoned)

Rice wine

Roasted red bell peppers

Salsa

Sesame oil (preferably toasted)

Soybeans (15-ounce can)

Soy sauce (regular or light)

Tomato juice or V-8 juice

Tomato puree

White vinegar

Herbs and Spices

Basil

Chili powder

Cumin

Dried oregano

Dried thyme

Garam masala

Ground allspice, cinnamon, or cloves

Ground cumin

Ground nutmeg

Italian seasoning

Mild curry powder

Old Bay seasoning

Roasted sesame seeds

Turmeric

Dry Staples

Bread crumbs (plain or seasoned)

Brown sugar

Burrito-size tortillas (10-inch tortillas)

Chinese rice noodles

Cornmeal

Dried cranberries

Fajita-size tortillas (6-inch tortillas)

Flour: unbleached all-purpose, whole wheat, quick-dissolving

No-boil lasagna noodles

Lentils, green and red

Nuts: peanuts, walnuts, pecans

Pad Thai rice noodles

Pasteurized instant nonfat dry milk

Rice: brown and/or white, Arborio, basmati

Rice vermicelli noodles

Somen or soba noodles

Thin spaghetti, capellini, or linguine

Whole wheat buns

Frozen Staples

9-inch pie crusts (preferably whole wheat)

Artichoke hearts

Corn

Chopped spinach

Edamame

Lima beans

From the Salad Bar

Broccoli florets

Cauliflower florets

Diced onions

Roasted red bell peppers

Shredded carrots

Sliced mushrooms

Sliced red bell peppers

light and healthy vegetable ragout

What's in this for baby and me? Vitamins A and C.

THIS VERSATILE RAGOUT works as a side dish; burrito filling with beans, rice, and cheese; in a sandwich; or over pasta or couscous with lots of fresh herbs and grated Parmesan cheese. It is an excellent source of vitamins A and C and a good source of fiber. Thinned with some tomato sauce or crushed tomatoes, it turns into a fabulous sauce for vegetarian lasagna. Slow Cooker Instructions follow.

serves 6 (makes about 8 cups)

⅓ cup olive oil or canola oil

1 medium onion, finely chopped

2 garlic cloves, minced

1 tablespoon dried oregano

2 large carrots, peeled and coarsely grated or shredded (about 1½ cups)

1 red bell pepper, cored, seeded, and cut into ¼-inch dice

1 medium (about 1 pound) purple eggplant, peeled and cut into ¼-inch dice (see Cooking Tip below)

Two 14.5-ounce cans diced tomatoes, drained

1¼ cups tomato juice or V-8 juice

1½ teaspoons sugar

1 medium zucchini, washed and cut into ¼-inch dice (optional)

One 14-ounce can quartered artichoke hearts (optional)

¼ cup chopped fresh basil or cilantro (optional)

Salt and freshly ground pepper, to taste

1. Heat the oil in a 6-quart non-reactive saucepan over medium-high heat. Add the onion and sauté for 3 minutes. Add the garlic, oregano, carrots, and red bell pepper and continue to sauté for 3 minutes, stirring frequently.
2. Add the eggplant and cook, stirring constantly, for 3 minutes. Add the tomatoes, tomato juice, and sugar, and stir, then reduce the heat and gently simmer, uncovered, for 15 minutes, stirring occasionally. Add the optional zucchini and artichoke hearts, stir, and cook for about 25 minutes, or until the vegetables are tender and the sauce has reached the desired consistency.
3. Add the basil, if desired, and season with salt and pepper. Serve immediately.

▶ *Timesaving Tip:* Because this recipe calls for a lot of chopped vegetables, see which ones you can pick up at a salad bar.

▶ **Cooking Tip:** Removing the moisture from the eggplant with salt is an optional step that requires 20 minutes to 1 hour. The advantage of this is that eggplant will not absorb as much oil, and it should also remove any bitterness. Place the diced eggplant in a colander on a large plate with a rim, sprinkle with 2 teaspoons salt, and toss gently. Allow the eggplant to stand for at least 20 minutes, or up to 1 hour. Rinse the eggplant quickly under cold water, then spread it out on a double thickness of paper towels. Cover with more paper towels and press firmly to extract as much water as possible.

▶ **Storage Tip:** This ragout keeps for 3 days refrigerated, and it can be frozen for up to 1 month.

▶ **Slow Cooker Instructions:**
1. Follow Step 1, then add the eggplant and cook, stirring constantly, for 3 minutes.
2. Transfer the contents of the skillet to the slow cooker and add the tomatoes, tomato juice, sugar, and optional zucchini. Cover and cook on high for 5 hours. Note: If you prefer a slightly thicker sauce, add 2 tablespoons quick-dissolving flour during the last 15 minutes of cooking. Finish the ragout as directed in Step 3.

▶ **Complete Meal Ideas:** Serve this ragout with:
　　Pasta, rice, couscous, or any other grain
　　3 ounces protein (you might want to make the Old Bay Tofu Cakes, page
　　　　225, and use the vegetable ragout instead of the cocktail sauce)
　　Reduced-fat 2% milk or low-fat yogurt
　　Fresh fruit

APPROXIMATE NUTRITIONAL INFORMATION: Serving size: 1 cup vegetable ragout; Calories: 146 cals; Protein: 3 g; Carbohydrates: 15 g; Fat: 9 g; Fiber: 4 g; Sodium: 553 mg; Vitamin A: 7,958 IU; Vitamin C: 60 mg; Diabetic Exchange: Fat 2, Vegetable 3

three-bean vegetarian chili

*What's in this for baby and me? Protein, iron,
vitamins A and C, folic acid, and fiber.*

This chili is an excellent source of protein, iron, vitamins A and C, folic acid, and fiber, and a good source of calcium and B vitamins. For extra protein, add tofu sautéed with a dash of chili powder, or add frozen ground soy burger (see Variation below). Some garnishes to pass at the table include grated cheddar or Monterey Jack cheese, thinly sliced romaine lettuce, scallions, and black olives. Slow Cooker Instructions follow.

serves 6 (makes about 7 cups)

2 tablespoons olive oil or canola oil

1 small red onion, finely chopped

1 garlic clove, minced

1 tablespoon chili powder

2 teaspoons ground cumin

1 teaspoon dried oregano

1 red bell pepper, cored, seeded, and cut into
 small dice (optional)

8 ounces mushrooms (any kind), washed and
 thinly sliced (optional)

One 15.5-ounce can black beans, rinsed and
 drained

One 15.5-ounce can red kidney beans, rinsed
 and drained

One 15-ounce can soybeans (do not drain), or
 any other canned bean, rinsed and drained

One 14.5-ounce can diced tomatoes (do not
 drain)

1 cup water or low-sodium vegetable stock

A sprinkle or two of quick-dissolving flour,
 such as Wondra (optional)

1½ tablespoons balsamic vinegar, or to taste
 (optional)

½ cup chopped fresh cilantro, for garnish

1. Heat the olive oil in a 6-quart saucepan over medium-high heat. Add the onion and sauté for 3 minutes. Add the garlic, chili powder, cumin, and oregano and sauté for 30 seconds. Add the optional red bell pepper and mushrooms and sauté for 3 minutes.

2. Add the black beans, red kidney beans, soybeans, diced tomatoes, and water and bring to a boil. Reduce the heat to a gentle simmer and cook for 30 minutes, or until slightly thickened. If the chili is not thick enough for your taste after 30 minutes of cooking, add a dash or two of quick-dissolving flour and cook for 2 minutes longer.

3. Add the balsamic vinegar, if using, adjust the seasoning, and garnish with the cilantro. Serve immediately with the accompaniments of your choice.

▶ **Variation:** Cut one 15-ounce package (drained weight) extra-firm tofu into ½-inch cubes and blot dry with paper towels. Sauté according to the instructions on page 228. Cover the sautéed tofu with foil and set aside. Add the tofu during the last 5 minutes of cooking in Step 2. You can also add frozen ground soy burger in Step 2 along with the beans. Feel free to add or substitute your favorite vegetables in Step 1.

▶ **Storage Tip:** This chili keeps for 5 days refrigerated, and it can be frozen for 1 month. Freeze in single-meal-size portions in zip-lock bags or plastic containers for lunch or dinner.

▶ **Slow Cooker Instructions:** Use 1½ cups of water or vegetable stock instead of 1 cup.
1. Follow Step 1 using a skillet instead of a saucepan.
2. Transfer the contents of the skillet to the slow cooker and add the black beans, kidney beans, soybeans, tomatoes, and water. Cover and cook on high for 5 hours. Add 2 tablespoons of quick-dissolving flour during the last 30 minutes of cooking. Finish the chili as directed in step 3.

▶ **Complete Meal Ideas:** Serve this chili with:
　　Brown rice, tortilla, or a whole wheat roll
　　Tossed salad (you might want to try romaine lettuce
　　　with the Caesar Salad Dressing, page 168)
　　Reduced-fat 2% milk or low-fat yogurt
　　Fresh fruit that contains vitamin C

APPROXIMATE NUTRITIONAL INFORMATION: Serving size: 1 cup three-bean chili; Calories: 267 cals; Protein: 17 g; Carbohydrates: 34 g; Fat: 8 g; Fiber: 11 g; Sodium: 790 mg; Vitamin A: 1,820 IU; Vitamin C: 68 mg; Folic Acid: 151 mcg; Iron: 5 mg; Diabetic Exchange: Bread/Starch 1.5, Meat (Medium Fat) 1.5, Vegetable 2

vegetarian curry

What's in this for baby and me? Protein, iron, vitamins A and C, and folic acid.

THIS CURRY IS an excellent source of protein, iron, vitamins A and C, and folic acid, and a good source of calcium and fiber. Have all of your ingredients ready (along with cooked rice or noodles) before you begin. A surprising number of kids like a mild curry flavor and might enjoy this dish. By all means, use your family's favorite vegetables and consider omitting the cilantro and peanuts from the children's portions.

serves 4 (makes about 7 cups)

2 tablespoons canola oil

2 tablespoons minced or grated fresh ginger, or to taste

1 garlic clove, minced

1 cup sliced baby carrots or shredded regular carrots

½ red bell pepper, quartered and thinly sliced

1 medium zucchini, washed, halved lengthwise, and thinly sliced

12–16 ounces asparagus, washed, tough ends trimmed, and cut into ½-inch slices (about 2 cups sliced asparagus), or broccoli florets, washed and ends trimmed

One 15-ounce package (drained weight) extra-firm tofu, drained, cut into ½-inch cubes, and blotted dry with paper towels

½ cup thinly sliced scallions

1 tablespoon plus 1 teaspoon mild curry powder, or to taste

One 14-ounce can light or regular coconut milk

1 tablespoon quick-dissolving flour (such as Wondra), to desired consistency

⅓ cup chopped fresh cilantro or basil

Juice of 1 lime, or to taste

Salt, to taste

½ cup dry-roasted peanuts or cashew nuts, coarsely chopped (optional)

1. In a large nonstick skillet or large wok, heat 1 tablespoon of the canola oil over medium-high heat. Add the ginger and garlic and cook for 30 seconds. Add the carrots, bell pepper, zucchini, and asparagus and sauté for 3 minutes. Transfer the cooked vegetables to a serving dish, cover with foil, and set aside.
2. Add the remaining 1 tablespoon canola oil to the skillet and heat over medium-high heat. Add the tofu, scallions, and curry powder and sauté for 3 minutes. Add the coconut milk and cook for 3 minutes, or until hot. Sprinkle in the quick-dissolving flour and stir to mix. Add the reserved vegetables and mix gently, then stir in the cilantro and lime juice. Adjust the seasoning.
3. Transfer the curry to a serving bowl, garnish with the peanuts, if desired, and serve immediately.

▶ *Cooking Tip:* Regular coconut milk produces a creamier sauce.

▶ *Advance Preparation:* The curry can be made a day in advance. Reduce the cooking time of the vegetables to 2 minutes if the curry will be reheated in a microwave oven later. (The accompanying rice can be made up to 3 days in advance, or the rice noodles up to 1 day in advance.)

▶ *Timesaving Tip:* Pick up shredded carrots and other prepared vegetables from a salad bar. Convenient fresh vegetable stir-fry packs are available in some grocery stores. They usually come in 12-ounce packages and can be supplemented with your favorite vegetables. Sixteen-ounce bags of frozen stir-fry vegetables are also available in most grocery stores. Follow the package directions for stir-frying vegetables in oil.

▶ *Variation:* Non-vegetarians can substitute poultry, shrimp, seafood, or meat for the tofu; adjust the cooking time as necessary.

▶ *Diabetic Tip:* Omit the peanuts, to reduce the fat.

▶ *Complete Meal Ideas:* Serve this curry with:
    Brown rice, rice noodles, or quinoa
    Reduced-fat 2% milk or low-fat yogurt
    Fresh fruit that contains vitamin C

APPROXIMATE NUTRITIONAL INFORMATION: SERVING SIZE: 1¾ cups vegetarian curry; Calories: 422 cals; Protein: 19 g; Carbohydrates: 19 g; Fat: 31 g; Fiber: 5 g; Sodium: 465 mg; Vitamin A: 10,049 IU; Vitamin C: 52 mg; Folic Acid: 120 mcg; Iron: 7 mg; Diabetic Exchange: Fat 4, Meat (Medium Fat) 2, Vegetable 3

best-ever vegetarian lasagna

What's in this for baby and me? Protein, calcium, iron, vitamins A and C, folic acid, and fiber.

Wʜɪʟᴇ ᴛʜᴇʀᴇ ᴀʀᴇ ways to make this family favorite less of a hassle (see Timesaving Tip below), the fact remains that it takes time to assemble and bake any lasagna—but the results are definitely worth the effort. This lasagna is an excellent source of protein, calcium, iron, vitamins A and C, folic acid, and fiber, and a good source of B vitamins. Do not use the tofu if you plan to freeze the lasagna before baking.

serves 8

Tᴏᴍᴀᴛᴏ Sᴀᴜᴄᴇ (makes 4 cups)

2 tablespoons olive oil

1 medium onion, finely chopped

1 garlic clove, minced

1 tablespoon dried basil or Italian seasoning

1 tablespoon dried oregano

One 28-ounce can crushed tomatoes

2 tablespoons chopped fresh basil, oregano, or dill, or a combination

Vᴇɢᴇᴛᴀʙʟᴇs

1 tablespoon olive oil or canola oil

1 pound mushrooms, preferably cremini, washed, trimmed, and thinly sliced

10 ounces baby spinach leaves, washed, or one 10-ounce package frozen chopped spinach, thawed and drained well

Enough no-boil (or oven-ready) lasagna noodles to fill a 13 x 9 x 2-inch pan

One 15-ounce package (drained weight) firm tofu, thinly sliced and pressed (see Cooking Tip below) (optional)

4 cups shredded pasteurized part-skim low-moisture mozzarella cheese or Fontina cheese (about 1 pound)

6 tablespoons grated Parmesan cheese (optional)

1. To make the sauce, heat the olive oil in a large saucepan over medium-high heat. Add the onion and sauté for 3 minutes. Add the garlic, basil, and oregano and continue to sauté for 2 minutes. Add the crushed tomatoes, stir, and bring to a boil, then reduce the heat and simmer, uncovered, for 10 minutes. Stir in the fresh herbs and remove from the heat. The sauce should yield 4 cups; if not, add water (or tomato juice) to make 4 cups. Set aside.

2. To cook the vegetables, heat the olive oil in a large nonstick skillet over medium-high heat. Add the mushrooms and sauté for 5 minutes. Using a slotted spoon, transfer the mushrooms to a bowl, leaving behind any juices in the skillet. If using fresh spinach, add it to the skillet, in batches if necessary, and sauté until just wilted, about 3 minutes. Add the spinach to the mushrooms and set aside. (If using frozen spinach, add it directly to the mushrooms.)

3. To assemble the lasagna, spread ¾ cup sauce over the bottom of an ungreased 13 x 9 x 2-inch pan. Place 3 or 4 no-boil lasagna noodles over the sauce (follow the instruc-

tions on your lasagna box—different brands require different preparation methods). Spread about one-third of the vegetables evenly over the noodles, followed by one-third of the tofu slices, if using, ¾ cup of the sauce, 1 cup of the mozzarella cheese, and 2 tablespoons of the Parmesan cheese (if using). Repeat the layering process of noodles, vegetables, tofu, sauce, and cheeses two more times. For the last layer, place 3 or 4 noodles on top of the cheese, then add the remaining sauce to cover the noodles, and top with the remaining mozzarella cheese. (See Advance Preparation below for make-ahead and freezing instructions at this point.)

4. To bake, adjust an oven rack to the middle position and preheat the oven to 375°F. Cover the pan with foil (lightly greased or sprayed with cooking oil spray) and bake for 45 minutes.

5. Remove the foil and bake for 15 minutes more, or until the top is nicely browned and a knife inserted into the middle of the lasagna indicates soft noodles. Remove the lasagna from the oven and let cool for 10 minutes before slicing.

▶ **Cooking Tip:** If adding tofu to this lasagna, drain it well, then slice it into ½-inch slices. Line a large plate with a triple thickness of paper towels, place the tofu slices on the plate, then using a second bunch of paper towels, blot the tofu to remove excess water. Repeat for the remaining slices.

▶ **Timesaving Tip:** Use frozen spinach or purchase fresh spinach in a microwaveable bag. After microwaving, drain the spinach and squeeze gently. Use presliced mushrooms from a package or a salad bar. Use store-bought high-quality pasta sauce (you will need 4 cups sauce).

▶ **Advance Preparation:** The sauce can be made up to 3 days in advance, covered, and refrigerated. After completing Step 3, the lasagna can be wrapped with plastic wrap and refrigerated overnight, or it can be frozen for up to 1 month. The frozen lasagna can be placed directly in the oven, but the cooking time will increase by about 15 to 20 minutes.

▶ **Storage Tip:** The cooked lasagna will keep for 3 days refrigerated and it can be frozen for up to 1 month. Use a microwave or conventional oven to reheat.

▶ **Complete Meal Ideas:** Serve this lasagna with:
Tossed salad or a green vegetable (you might want to try the Vegetables with Lemon, Olive Oil, and Fresh Herbs, page 153.)
Reduced-fat 2% milk or low-fat yogurt
Fresh fruit that contains vitamin C

APPROXIMATE NUTRITIONAL INFORMATION: Serving size: one-eighth vegetarian lasagna; Calories: 371 cals; Protein: 24 g; Carbohydrates: 34 g; Fat: 16 g; Fiber: 7 g; Sodium: 526 mg; Vitamin A: 2,944 IU; Vitamin C: 19 mg; Folic Acid: 83 mcg; Calcium: 480 mg; Iron: 5 mg; Diabetic Exchange: Bread/Starch 2, Fat 1, Meat (Medium Fat) 2, Vegetable 1

spaghetti with herbed tofu balls and tomato sauce

What's in this for baby and me? Protein, calcium, iron,
vitamins A and C, folic acid, and fiber.

A VEGETARIAN TWIST on meatballs, this spaghetti with tofu balls and tomato sauce provides an excellent source of protein, calcium, iron, vitamins A and C, folic acid, and fiber.

serves 4 (makes about 25 tofu balls and about 3½ cups tomato sauce)

12 to 16 ounces enriched thin spaghetti or
    linguine
½ tablespoon unsalted butter
HERBED TOFU BALLS
    One 15-ounce package (drained weight)
        extra-firm tofu, drained, finely crumbled
        (use your hands or a fork), and blotted
        with paper towels
    ½ cup plain or seasoned breadcrumbs
    ⅓ cup finely grated Parmesan cheese
    3 large eggs, lightly beaten
    ¼ cup chopped fresh cilantro
    ¼ cup chopped fresh parsley

    ½ cup thinly sliced scallions
    ½ teaspoon salt
    Freshly ground pepper, to taste
    1 tablespoon canola oil
TOMATO SAUCE
    1 tablespoon canola oil or olive oil
    1 garlic clove, minced
    1 teaspoon dried oregano
    1 teaspoon Italian seasoning
    One 28-ounce can crushed tomatoes
    Additional chopped fresh cilantro and parsley,
        for garnish (optional)
    Grated Parmesan cheese, for the table

1. Cook the pasta according to the package directions; drain and return to the pot. Add the butter, stir, cover, and set aside in a warm place.
2. To make the herbed tofu balls, combine all of the ingredients except the oil in a bowl and mix until well blended. Using a rounded measuring tablespoon, scoop out mounds of the tofu mixture and place on 2 large plates, then form each portion into a ball.
3. Heat the canola oil in a large nonstick skillet over medium-high heat. Add half the tofu balls and sauté, turning several times, for about 7 minutes, or until light golden brown and heated through. Repeat with the remaining tofu balls. Transfer the tofu balls to a clean plate lined with a paper towel. Cover with foil to keep warm. (Do not rinse the skillet.)
4. To make the tomato sauce, heat the canola oil in the same skillet over medium heat. Add the garlic, oregano, and Italian seasoning and cook for 30 seconds. Add

the crushed tomatoes, stir, and simmer for 10 minutes, or until slightly thickened. Adjust the seasoning before serving.

5. To serve, place some of the pasta in a bowl, top with some of the tofu balls, and cover with sauce and chopped fresh herbs. Serve with Parmesan cheese.

▶ *Advance Preparation:* *Variation:* The tofu balls can be formed up to 4 hours in advance and refrigerated. The sauce can be made up to 2 days in advance, covered, and refrigerated. Add any fresh herbs at the last minute.

▶ *Timesaving Tip:* Use your favorite store-bought spaghetti sauce and fresh pasta, which has a shorter cooking time.

▶ *Variation:* You can doctor up this simple tomato sauce by sautéing the following in Step 3: ½ cup finely chopped onions, 8 ounces sliced cremini or button mushrooms, or ½ cup chopped red bell pepper before adding the garlic. You can also add sliced olives, caper berries, or fresh herbs to the finished sauce.

▶ *Complete Meal Ideas:* Serve this spaghetti with:
    Tossed salad or a green vegetable (you might want to try a tossed
        salad with the French-Style Tarragon Vinaigrette, page 166)
    Reduced-fat 2% milk or low-fat yogurt
    Fresh fruit that contains vitamin C

APPROXIMATE NUTRITIONAL INFORMATION: Serving size: one-fifth serving or 5 herbed tofu balls; Calories: 207 cals; Protein: 17 g; Carbohydrates: 12 g; Fat: 10 g; Fiber: .7 g; Sodium: 467 mg; Calcium: 188 mg; Diabetic Exchange: Bread/Starch 1, Meat (Medium Fat) 2

APPROXIMATE NUTRITIONAL INFORMATION: Serving size: 1¼ cups cooked spaghetti with ¾ cup tomato sauce; Calories: 355 cals; Protein: 12 g; Carbohydrates: 64 g; Fat: 7 g; Fiber: 7 g; Sodium: 555 mg; Vitamin A: 14,445 IU; Vitamin C: 18 mg; Folic Acid: 148 mcg; Iron: 5 mg; Diabetic Exchange: Bread/Starch 4, Fat 1.5

pasta with tomatoes, herbs, and pasteurized goat cheese

What's in this for baby and me? Protein, calcium, iron, vitamins A and C, and folic acid.

THIS NO-FUSS DISH, which is a high source of protein, calcium, iron, vitamins A and C, and folic acid, and a good source of fiber, is especially delicious in tomato season. The secret is adding a no-cook sauce to piping-hot pasta. For young eaters, substitute Parmesan cheese for the goat cheese.

serves 3 to 4

FRESH TOMATO SAUCE

2 large vine-ripened tomatoes, cut into small dice

3 tablespoons chopped fresh dill

3 tablespoons thinly sliced fresh basil

1 tablespoon olive oil, or to taste

2 teaspoons freshly squeezed lemon juice, or to taste

Salt and freshly ground pepper, to taste

8 ounces thin pasta, such as capellini or thin spaghetti

4 ounces pasteurized goat cheese, crumbled, or to taste (see Health Tip below)

1. Bring a large pot of water for cooking the pasta to a boil.
2. To make the sauce, combine all of the ingredients in a bowl and mix gently with a spoon. Adjust the seasoning and set aside.
3. Cook the pasta, drain, and immediately place it in individual serving bowls. Add the sauce and cheese and toss gently with two large forks until the sauce is well incorporated. Serve immediately.

▶ *Health Tip:* Use only pasteurized feta cheese (see Listeriosis Warning, page 129).

▶ *Complete Meal Ideas:* Serve this pasta with:
Tossed salad or a green vegetable (you might want to try the Spinach Salad with Mandarin Oranges and Toasted Almonds, page 163)
Reduced-fat 2% milk or low-fat yogurt
Fresh fruit

APPROXIMATE NUTRITIONAL INFORMATION: Serving size: one-third pasta dish (served over 1½ cups enriched cooked spaghetti); Calories: 527 cals; Protein: 22 g; Carbohydrates: 65 g; Fat: 20 g; Fiber: 5 g; Sodium: 141 mg; Vitamin A: 1,319 IU; Vitamin C: 18 mg; Folic Acid: 165 mcg; Diabetic Exchange: Bread/Starch 4, Fat 1, Meat (Medium Fat) 1.5

traditional classification of vegetarian diets

LACTO-OVO VEGETARIAN

Foods included: **Fruits, grains, legumes, nuts, seeds, vegetables, milk and milk products, eggs**

Foods excluded: **Meat, poultry, fish**

LACTO VEGETARIAN

Foods included: **Fruits, grains, legumes, nuts, seeds, vegetables, milk and milk products**

Foods excluded: **Meat, poultry, fish, eggs**

OVO VEGETARIAN

Foods included: **Fruits, grains, legumes, nuts, seeds, vegetables, eggs**

Foods excluded: **Meat, poultry, fish, milk and milk products**

VEGAN

Foods included: **Fruits, grains, legumes, nuts, seeds, vegetables**

Foods excluded: **Meat, poultry, fish, eggs, milk, milk products, honey, gelatin**

spinach-cheese quiche

What's in this for baby and me? Protein, calcium, and vitamin A.

Packed with protein, calcium, and vitamin A, and a good source of iron, this quiche is ideal for breakfast, lunch, or dinner. You can play around with the filling, but try to avoid ending up with a hodgepodge of flavors.

serves 4 to 6

One 9-inch piecrust, frozen or Homemade
Whole Wheat Piecrust (recipe follows)
Spinach-Cheese Filling
1¾ cups whole milk, soy beverage, half-and-
half, or light skim evaporated milk
2 large eggs plus 2 large egg yolks
1 teaspoon Dijon mustard (optional)
½ teaspoon salt
Freshly ground pepper, to taste

4 ounces (1 cup) grated cheddar, Monterey
Jack, or Gruyère cheese
8 ounces frozen chopped spinach, thawed and
squeezed dry, or fresh spinach (see
Cooking Tip below for preparation
instructions)
2 tablespoons thinly sliced scallions (optional)
2 tablespoons chopped fresh dill or parsley
(optional)

1. Preheat the oven to 375°F. If using a store-bought piecrust, use the middle rack and prebake the crust according to package directions. If using the homemade piecrust, adjust oven rack to the lowest rung.
2. To make the filling, combine the milk, eggs, yolks, mustard, if using, salt, and pepper in a bowl and whisk until well blended.
3. Place half of the cheese in the bottom of the piecrust and top with half the spinach, half the scallions, and half the fresh herbs. Add half of the milk-egg mixture, then repeat this layering procedure with the remaining ingredients and the rest of the milk-egg mixture. (Note: If you are using bulky ingredients in your filling, you may not have room for all of the milk-egg mixture. Discard any extra mixture; do not overfill your quiche, or it may overflow in the oven.)
4. Bake a prebaked piecrust quiche for 25 to 30 minutes, or a homemade piecrust quiche for 50 to 60 minutes, or until the middle of the quiche is set. The quiche is done when the tip of a knife inserted in the center of comes out clean and an instant-read thermometer reads 160°F. Remove the quiche from the oven and allow it to cool for 10 minutes on a cooling rack before serving. (Leftovers should be refrigerated and reheated in a microwave or conventional oven. Reheating in a microwave oven will cause the crust to become slightly soggy.)

homemade whole wheat piecrust

makes one 9-inch piecrust

¾ cup unbleached all-purpose flour

¾ cup whole wheat flour

¼ teaspoon salt

8 tablespoons (1 stick) unsalted butter, cut
  into small pieces

1 large egg, slightly beaten

1. Combine both flours and the salt in a large bowl. Add the butter and rub in with your fingertips, or use a pastry blender, until the dough resembles small crumbs. Add the egg and stir with a fork until the dough holds together.
2. Flour your hands, then gather the dough and knead for a minute, or until it is smooth and soft. (Do not overwork the dough, or it will lose its flakiness. It is better to undermix than to overmix.) Form the dough into a thick disk, cover with plastic wrap, and refrigerate for 20 minutes, or up to 2 days.
3. Roll out the dough on a piece of lightly floured parchment paper or plastic wrap (this prevents sticking). Transfer the dough to an ungreased 9-inch pie pan and crimp the edges or decorate with a fork. Prick the bottom of the pie with a fork and refrigerate for at least 15 minutes, or freeze for 10 minutes, before filling and baking.

▶ *Calcium Boost:* In a measuring cup combine ⅓ cup pasteurized instant nonfat dry milk with the whole milk. Mix until the milk powder has dissolved, then follow directions in Step 2.

▶ *Advance Preparation:* The egg mixture for the filling can be made 1 day in advance and refrigerated. The dough for the piecrust can be made up to 2 days in advance and refrigerated, or it can be frozen for up to 2 months. Thaw slightly before use; the dough should be cold.

▶ *Cooking Tip:* If using fresh spinach, remove the stems, wash the leaves, and then microwave, steam, or boil the spinach just until wilted. (Some grocery stores sell spinach packaged in microwaveable bags.) Drain, cool, and squeeze out as much liquid as possible, then coarsely chop.

▶ *Variation:* In addition to the cheese, use about 1 cup of a single filling or a mixture of any of these fillings per quiche. To prevent a soggy crust, be sure to thoroughly drain or dry all filling ingredients.

Asparagus: Cook until crisp-tender, drain well, and chop into ¼-inch pieces.

Broccoli florets: Cook until crisp-tender, drain well,
   pat dry with a paper towel, and chop.

Summer squash or zucchini: Quarter, thinly slice,

and sauté; drain on paper towels.

Swiss chard or leeks: Thoroughly wash, slice, and boil,
steam, or sauté until wilted and tender.

▶ *Health Tip:* If your doctor has restricted your fat intake, use low-fat cheddar cheese and reduced-fat 2% milk, "lite" skim evaporated milk, or nonfat dry milk for the filling.

▶ *Complete Meal Ideas:* Serve this quiche with:

Tossed salad, a vegetable, or vegetable soup (you might
want to try the Gazpacho, page 112, or the Asparagus,
Hearts of Palm, and Tomato Salad, page 159)
Reduced-fat 2% milk or low-fat yogurt
Fresh fruit, V-8 juice, or another source of vitamin C

APPROXIMATE NUTRITIONAL INFORMATION: Serving size: 1 slice (one-eighth) spinach cheese quiche (with a store-bought pie crust); Calories: 254 cals; Protein: 10 g; Carbohydrates: 16 g; Fat: 17 g; Fiber: 1 g; Sodium: 430 mg; Vitamin A: 2,639 IU; Calcium: 224 mg; Diabetic Exchange: Bread/Starch 1, Fat 2, Meat (High Fat) 1

APPROXIMATE NUTRITIONAL INFORMATION: Serving size: 1 slice (one-eighth) spinach cheese quiche with homemade whole wheat pie crust; Calories: 329 cals; Protein: 12 g; Carbohydrates: 21 g; Fat: 22 g; Fiber: 2 g; Sodium: 384 g; Vitamin A: 3,253 IU; Calcium: 231 mg; Diabetic Exchange: Bread/Starch 1.5, Fat 3, Meat (High Fat) 1

APPROXIMATE NUTRITIONAL INFORMATION: Serving size: 1 slice (one-eighth) homemade whole wheat pie crust (crust only); Calories: 198 cals; Protein: 4 g; Carbohydrates: 17 g; Fat: 13 g; Fiber: 2 g; Sodium: 83 mg; Diabetic Exchange: Bread/Starch 1, Fat 2.5

healthy additions to vegetarian cooking

Hard cheese (see Listeriosis Warning, page 129, for safe cheeses)

Low-fat cottage cheese

Part-skim ricotta cheese

Soy nuts

Tofu (enriched)

Canned beans and peas

Hard-boiled eggs

Shredded carrots

Plain low-fat yogurt or soy yogurt

Dried apricots and other dried fruits

Molasses

Sesame and pumpkin seeds

Nuts

Nut butters

V-8 or tomato juice

Diced or sliced red bell peppers

Enriched pasta

Seaweed

Ground flaxseed

Brewer's yeast

grilled or roasted marinated vegetables

What's in this for baby and me? Vitamins A and C.

HIGH IN VITAMINS A and C and a good source of fiber, these roasted vegetables are delicious as a side dish or main course. Sautéing the onion and garlic separately brings out their sweetness more than grilling them does, but you can do either.

serves 6 (makes about 4 cups)

1 medium red bell pepper, washed, cored, seeded, and quartered

1 medium (about 8 ounces) purple eggplant, washed and cut into ½-inch slices (see Cooking Tip below)

2 medium (about 8 ounces) zucchini, washed and cut into ½-inch slices on the diagonal

8 ounces large button mushrooms or other large mushrooms, such as shiitake or portobello, washed and stems trimmed

1 tablespoon dried oregano

1 tablespoon dried basil or Italian seasoning

1 teaspoon salt

Freshly ground pepper, to taste

1 tablespoon freshly squeezed lemon juice

⅓ cup plus 2 tablespoons olive oil

1 medium sweet onion (preferably Vidalia), finely diced

2 garlic cloves, minced

One 14.5-ounce can diced tomatoes, drained

¼ cup chopped fresh basil or cilantro leaves, for garnish (optional)

1. Place the bell pepper, eggplant, zucchini, and mushrooms in a very large bowl (or in a large roasting pan if roasting). Add the oregano, basil, salt, pepper, lemon juice, and ⅓ cup of the olive oil, then gently toss until all the vegetables are well coated. Allow the vegetables to marinate at room temperature for 10 to 20 minutes.

2. Heat the remaining 2 tablespoons olive oil in a small nonstick skillet over medium-high heat. Add the onion and sauté, stirring occasionally, for 5 to 7 minutes, or until light golden. Add the garlic and sauté for 1 more minute. Add the canned tomatoes and cook just until heated; set aside. Cover to keep warm.

3. Preheat the grill (or see Roasting Instructions below). Grill the vegetables over medium-high heat for about 15 minutes, or until nicely browned and cooked through. Turn and move the vegetables around on the grill as necessary to promote even cooking and to avoid scorching.

4. Discard the marinade, then return the grilled vegetables to the bowl in which they were marinated. While they are still warm, chop the cooked vegetables into small dice.

5. Place the diced vegetables in a serving bowl, add the reserved tomato mixture and the basil, and mix gently. Serve immediately.

▶ **Cooking Tip:** Removing the moisture from the eggplant with salt is an optional step that requires 20 minutes to 1 hour. The advantage of this is that it should remove any bitterness, and the eggplant will not absorb as much oil. Place the sliced eggplant in a colander on a large plate with a rim, sprinkle it with 2 teaspoons salt, and toss gently. Allow the eggplant to stand for at least 20 minutes, or up to 1 hour. Rinse the eggplant quickly under cold water, then spread it out on a double thickness of paper towels. Cover with more paper towels and press firmly to extract as much water as possible.

▶ **Roasting Instructions:** To roast the vegetables, preheat the oven to 475°F. Meanwhile, combine the prepared vegetables in a large roasting pan and marinate them as in Step 1. Roast the vegetables for 20 to 30 minutes, stirring them after 15 minutes of cooking. The vegetables are done when the eggplant and bell peppers are soft. Meanwhile, prepare the tomato mixture following the instructions in Step 2. Finish the vegetables as in Step 4.

▶ **Complete Meal Ideas:** Serve these vegetables with:
Enriched pasta, brown rice, couscous, or a whole wheat roll
3 ounces protein (you might want to try the Old Bay Tofu Cakes with Cocktail Sauce, page 225, or Crispy Fried Tofu with Sesame-Soy Sauce, page 259)
Reduced-fat 2% milk or low-fat yogurt
Fresh fruit

APPROXIMATE NUTRITIONAL INFORMATION: Serving size: ⅔ cup grilled or roasted vegetables; Calories: 196 cals; Protein: 3 g; Carbohydrates: 12 g; Fat: 16 g; Fiber: 3 g; Sodium: 620 mg; Vitamin A: 1,716 IU; Vitamin C: 67 mg; Diabetic Exchange: Fat 3, Vegetable 2

vegetarian pad thai

What's in this for baby and me? Protein, iron, vitamins A and C, folic acid, and fiber.

THIS THAI-STYLE stir-fry is packed with protein, iron, vitamins A and C, folic acid, and fiber, and it is a good source of calcium. Non-vegetarians can add a source of protein, such as shrimp or chicken. One large nonstick skillet will be used three times in this recipe; it does not need to be rinsed after each use. If a little sticking occurs, gently scrape the bottom of the pan using a wooden spoon and wipe with paper towels.

serves 4

6 ounces Pad Thai rice noodles

SAUCE

   2 tablespoons hoisin sauce

   ¼ cup ketchup

   ¼ cup soy sauce

   ¼ cup warm water

   2 tablespoons seasoned rice vinegar

   2 tablespoons freshly squeezed lime juice

   2 tablespoons sugar

STIR-FRY

   2 tablespoons canola oil

   1 cup thinly sliced or shredded carrots

   12–16 ounces asparagus, washed, tough ends trimmed, and cut into 1-inch

   pieces (about 2 cups sliced asparagus)

2 cups broccoli florets, washed and cut into very small florets

One 15-ounce package (drained-weight) extra-firm tofu, drained, cut into ½-inch cubes, and blotted dry with paper towels

½ cup thinly sliced scallions

3 large eggs, lightly beaten

GARNISHES

   ⅓ cup chopped fresh cilantro

   ⅓ cup chopped fresh mint

   ½ cup roasted peanuts, crushed or coarsely chopped

   1 lime, cut into wedges

1. Cook the noodles according to the package directions. Drain the cooked noodles, run them under cold water, drain again, and set aside.
2. To make the sauce, whisk together all of the ingredients in a small bowl. Set aside.
3. To make the stir-fry, heat 1 tablespoon of the canola oil in a large nonstick skillet over medium-high heat. Add the carrots, asparagus, and broccoli and sauté for 3 minutes. (Do not overcook; the vegetables will continue to cook off the heat.) Transfer the vegetables to a bowl, cover with foil, and set aside. (Do not rinse the skillet.)
4. Add 1½ teaspoons canola oil to the skillet and heat over medium-high heat. Add the tofu and sauté for 5 minutes, or until heated through and light golden brown. Add half of the sauce and all the scallions to the skillet, stir, and cook for 1 minute,

or until slightly thickened. Transfer to a bowl, cover with foil, and set aside. (Do not rinse the skillet.)

5. Add the remaining 1½ teaspoons canola oil to the skillet and heat over medium-high heat. Add the eggs and cook, stirring constantly, for 1 minute, or until set. (They will resemble scrambled eggs.) Add the remaining sauce and the reserved cooked noodles to the skillet, stir, and cook for 2 minutes.

6. To serve, transfer the noodles to individual serving bowls or a large serving dish. For individual servings, divide the reserved tofu and vegetables, then add the garnishes to each bowl. Or, make a bed of noodles in a large dish, and top with the tofu and the vegetables, followed by the garnishes. Serve immediately.

▶ *Advance Preparation: Variation:* The sauce can be made up to 3 days in advance. The whole dish may be made up to 12 hours in advance and reheated in a microwave just before serving.

▶ *Timesaving Tip:* Pick up shredded carrots, broccoli florets, and other prepared vegetables from a salad bar.

▶ *Health Tip:* If your doctor has restricted your sodium intake, use low-sodium or light soy sauce and go easy on the salt.

▶ *Complete Meal Ideas:* Serve this Pad Thai with:
Reduced-fat 2% milk or low-fat yogurt
Fresh fruit

APPROXIMATE NUTRITIONAL INFORMATION: Serving size: one-fourth vegetarian Pad Thai; Calories: 407 cals; Protein: 22 g; Carbohydrates: 41 g; Fat: 18 g; Fiber: 5 g; Sodium: 1,311 mg; Vitamin A: 10,044 IU; Vitamin C: 60 mg; Folic Acid: 153 mcg; Iron: 4 mg; Diabetic Exchange: Bread/Starch 2.5, Fat 1, Meat (Medium Fat) 2.5

homemade tofu-bean burritos

What's in this for baby and me? Protein, calcium, folic acid, and fiber.

THESE TOFU-BEAN burritos are an excellent source of protein, calcium, folic acid, and fiber, and a good source of iron. Add your favorite ingredients and serve with salsa, avocados, or Homemade Guacamole (page 173), sliced lettuce, reduced-fat sour cream, and/or jalapeño peppers.

serves 4 to 6 (makes about 4 cups filling)

1½ tablespoons canola oil

1 small onion, finely chopped

1 small garlic clove, minced

1½ teaspoons ground cumin

1½ teaspoons chili powder, or to taste

1½ teaspoons dried oregano

One 15-ounce package (drained weight) extra-firm tofu, cut into ½-inch cubes and blotted

dry with paper towels

One 15.5-ounce can black beans, rinsed and drained

6 large burrito-size (10-inch) tortillas

1½ cups (about 6 ounces) grated cheddar cheese, or Monterey Jack cheese, or a mixture

½ cup chopped fresh cilantro

1. Heat the canola oil in a large nonstick skillet over medium-high heat. Add the onion and sauté for 3 minutes, or until light golden. Add the garlic, cumin, chili powder, and oregano and sauté for 30 seconds longer.
2. Add the tofu and sauté for 3 minutes. Add the beans and sauté until heated through, about 3 minutes more. Cover with foil to keep warm and set aside.
3. To assemble the burritos, heat a large nonstick skillet over medium-high heat. Place a tortilla in the skillet and heat for 30 seconds on each side, or just until heated but not crisp. Place the warm tortilla on a work surface. Place ⅔ cup of the tofu-bean filling on the bottom third of the tortilla, and top with 3 tablespoons of the cheese and 1½ tablespoons cilantro. Make sure that the filling is neatly stacked and compressed, then fold the bottom edge over the filling, tuck in the sides, and roll up. Repeat with the remaining ingredients. Serve with your favorite garnishes.

► *Advance Preparation: Variation:* The filling can be made up to 2 days in advance. The burritos can be assembled up to 8 hours in advance. Place them on a plate, cover with a slightly dampened paper towel followed by plastic wrap and refrigerate. Reheat in a microwave oven before serving.

► *Complete Meal Ideas:* Serve these burritos with:
Lettuce and tomato, as part of the filling or as a side salad
Reduced-fat 2% milk or low-fat yogurt
Fresh fruit

APPROXIMATE NUTRITIONAL INFORMATION: Serving size: one tofu-bean burrito; Calories: 412 cals; Protein: 23 g; Carbohydrates: 40 g; Fat: 18 g; Fiber: 15 g; Sodium: 528 mg; Folic Acid: 86 mcg; Calcium: 304 mg; Diabetic Exchange: Bread/Starch 2.5, Fat 1, Meat (Medium Fat) 2

gas and tips for coping

Excess gas is a normal part of almost all pregnancies. It can be uncomfortable, and even embarrassing. Here are a few tips to help reduce gas:

► Eliminate gas-producing foods in your diet as much as possible. Some common culprits include beans, raw cucumber, raw peppers, raw cabbage, raw onion, cauliflower, and dried fruit.

► Get your body moving! Go for a walk after meals, or whenever you can. This will help keep your digestive tract functioning smoothly.

► Eat smaller meals more frequently.

► Chew foods well.

► Eat slowly.

cheese and spinach quesadillas

What's in this for baby and me? Protein and calcium.

LOADED WITH PROTEIN and calcium, and a good source of vitamin A, iron, and fiber, quesadillas are as much fun to make as they are to eat. Serve with salsa, guacamole (recipe page 173) or avocado slices, or reduced-fat sour cream.

makes 1 quesadilla

2 fajita-size 6-inch tortillas (any flavor)

A heaping ⅓ cup grated cheddar cheese, Monterey Jack, or any other good melting cheese (see Health Tip below)

½ cup lightly packed baby spinach, washed

and stems trimmed, or ⅓ cup chopped frozen spinach, thawed, drained, and squeezed

1 tablespoon thinly sliced scallions (optional)

1 tablespoon chopped fresh cilantro (optional)

1. Place 1 tortilla in a nonstick skillet over medium-high heat and heat until hot. Flip it over, and distribute the cheese, spinach, and optional ingredients evenly on top. Cover it with the second tortilla. Cook the quesadilla until the cheese begins to melt and the bottom is light golden, about 2 minutes, then flip and cook the other side until light golden.
2. Cut the quesadilla into quarters and serve with your favorite toppings.

▶ *Cooking Tip:* For a child-size portion, use one tortilla, add the desired amount of cheese (and any other fillings your child likes), and cook over medium-high heat until the cheese melts and the tortilla is light golden, then fold the tortilla in half, remove it from the skillet, and serve.

▶ *Variation:* Feel free to add your favorite ingredients to these quesadillas—olives, chopped jarred roasted red peppers, chopped cooked broccoli florets, or chopped cooked asparagus tips.

▶ *Health Tip:* Do not use soft Mexican cheese, such as queso fresco and asadero (see Listeriosis Warning, page 129).

▶ *Complete Meal Ideas:* Serve these quesadillas with:
    Tossed salad, tomato salad, or vegetable soup (you might want to try
        the Gazpacho, page 112, or My Big Fat Greek Salad, page 170)
    Reduced-fat 2% milk or low-fat yogurt
    Fresh fruit, V-8 juice, or a source of vitamin C

APPROXIMATE NUTRITIONAL INFORMATION: Serving size: 1 cheese and spinach quesadilla; Calories: 257 cals; Protein: 12 g; Carbohydrates: 19 g; Fat: 15 g; Fiber: 2 g; Sodium: 393 mg; Diabetic Exchange: Bread/Starch 1, Fat 2, Meat (Medium Fat) 1

old bay tofu cakes with cocktail sauce

What's in this for baby and me? Protein and vitamin C.

OLD BAY SEASONING isn't just for crab cakes anymore! These tofu cakes are a fabulous way to get protein and vitamin C into your diet, as well as a good amount of vitamin A, calcium, and iron. They double as delicious burgers on whole wheat buns with lettuce, sliced tomatoes, and pickles. If serving to children, you may want to replace the Old Bay seasoning with a milder spice—and don't forget to replace the cocktail sauce with ketchup!

serves 6 (makes about 10 cakes)

One 15-ounce package (drained weight) extra-firm tofu, drained, finely crumbled (use your hands or a fork), and blotted dry with paper towels

½ cup plain or seasoned bread crumbs

3 large eggs, lightly beaten

2 teaspoons Old Bay seasoning, or to taste

⅓ cup grated Parmesan cheese

⅓ cup chopped fresh cilantro, basil, or dill

¼ cup diced jarred roasted red peppers (optional)

1 tablespoon canola oil

Cocktail sauce, for the table

1. To make the tofu cakes, combine all of the ingredients except the oil (and cocktail sauce) in a bowl and mix until well blended. Using a ⅓-cup measuring cup, place portion sizes of the mixture on two large plates, then form each portion into a patty.
2. Heat the canola oil in a large nonstick skillet over medium-high heat. Add the cakes, in batches, and cook for about 3 to 4 minutes on each side, or until golden brown and heated through. If they begin browning too quickly, reduce the heat. Serve hot with cocktail sauce.

▶ ***Advance Preparation:*** *Variation:* The tofu cakes can be shaped, covered, and refrigerated for up to 24 hours. Do not freeze them.

▶ *Complete Meal Ideas:* Serve these tofu cakes with:

  Tossed salad, a green vegetable, or coleslaw (you might want to try
      romaine lettuce with the Caesar Salad Dressing, page 168)
  Corn bread, a whole wheat roll, or pasta salad
  Reduced-fat 2% milk or low-fat yogurt
  Fresh fruit that contains vitamin C

APPROXIMATE NUTRITIONAL INFORMATION: Serving size: 2 tofu cakes; Calories: 229 cals; Protein: 16 g; Carbohydrates: 11 g; Fat: 13 g; Fiber: .5 g; Sodium: 232 mg; Vitamin C: 17 mg; Diabetic Exchange: Bread/Starch 1, Fat 1, Meat (Medium Fat) 2

sautéed tofu and portobello mushrooms on a bed of greens

What's in this for baby and me? Protein.

THIS SALAD IS an excellent source of protein, and a good source of calcium, iron, vitamins A and C, folic acid, and fiber. Use your favorite bottled dressing, or make the French-Style Tarragon Vinaigrette on page 166. The tofu can be replaced with tempeh, sautéed as directed in Step 2. Serve this salad with hearty bread to mop up the dressing.

serves 2 to 3

1½ tablespoons canola oil

8 ounces portobellos, washed, trimmed, and thinly sliced (see Variation below)

1 small garlic clove, minced

Salt and freshly ground pepper, to taste

15 ounce package (drained weight) extra-firm tofu, drained, cut into strips, and blotted dry with paper towels

1 teaspoon dried oregano, to taste

2 tablespoons balsamic vinegar, to taste

One 10-ounce bag baby salad greens, washed and dried

¼ cup crumbled pasteurized feta cheese or pasteurized goat cheese (see Health Tip below), to taste (optional)

¼ cup salad dressing, to taste

1. Heat 1 tablespoon of the canola oil in a large nonstick skillet over medium-high heat. Add the mushrooms and sauté for 5 minutes. Add the garlic, season with salt and pepper, and sauté 1 minute longer. Transfer the mushrooms to a bowl and set aside.
2. Add the remaining 1½ teaspoons canola oil to the skillet and heat over medium-high heat. Add the tofu and oregano and sauté for 5 minutes. Add the balsamic vinegar and sauté for 1 minute longer. Return the reserved mushrooms to the skillet and sauté for 1 minute. Remove from the heat.
3. Place the salad greens in a serving bowl or on individual plates. Add the tofu-mushroom mixture and feta cheese, then drizzle the salad dressing over the entire salad. Season with salt and pepper and serve immediately.

▶ *Variation:* Replace the portobello mushrooms with cremini mushrooms, button mushrooms, or any other fresh mushrooms. Cut any large mushrooms in half and slice thinly.

▶ *Health Tip:* Use only pasteurized feta or pasteurized goat cheese (see Listeriosis Warning, page 129).

instructions for sautéing tofu

Sautéed tofu, seasoned or plain, adds protein and calcium to many dishes, including salads, chilis, stews, soups, and grain dishes. To sauté tofu, drain it well, then slice it as called for in the recipe or as desired. Arrange it in an even layer on a large plate lined with a double thickness of paper towels. Using a second double thickness of paper towels, blot the tofu to remove as much moisture as possible.

Heat 1 tablespoon canola oil in a large nonstick skillet over medium-high heat. Add the tofu and any seasonings, and sauté for 5 minutes, or until it is heated through and the surface is light golden brown. Remove the tofu from the skillet and drain on paper towels, or add it directly to another dish.

▶ *Complete Meal Ideas:* Serve this salad with:
    Whole wheat roll or bread
    Reduced-fat 2% milk or low-fat yogurt
    Fresh fruit that contains vitamin C

APPROXIMATE NUTRITIONAL INFORMATION: Serving size: one-quarter sautéed tofu and portobello mushroom salad; Calories: 234 cals; Protein: 16 g; Carbohydrates: 11 g; Fat: 24 g; Fiber: 3 g; Sodium: 296 mg; Diabetic Exchange: Bread/Starch 1, Fat 3, Meat (Medium Fat) 2

vegetarian omelet for one

What's in this for baby and me? Protein, calcium, folic acid, and fiber.

HIGH IN PROTEIN, calcium, folic acid, and fiber, and a good source of vitamin A and iron, this power-packed omelet dinner is a winner.

serves 1

2 large eggs
½ teaspoon unsalted butter, or canola oil
    cooking spray
½ cup canned black beans, rinsed, drained,
    and blotted dry with a paper towel

3 tablespoons grated cheddar cheese (or any
    cheese of your choice)
1 tablespoon chopped fresh cilantro (optional)
Salt and freshly ground pepper, to taste
Salsa, for the table

1. Whisk the eggs in a bowl, and set aside.
2. Melt the butter in a medium nonstick skillet over medium-high heat. Add the eggs and swirl to coat the bottom of the pan, then add the black beans, cheddar cheese, and cilantro. Gently tilt the skillet, using a spatula or wooden spoon to pull the cooked egg towards the center of the pan while allowing the raw egg to hit the hot skillet. Season with salt and pepper. Repeat this procedure until the egg is completely cooked. The whole process should take about 2 minutes.
3. Fold the omelet in half and cook about 30 seconds longer, or until the egg is no longer runny (the cheese will be runny), then transfer to a serving plate. Serve immediately, with the salsa.

▶ *Health Tip:* Be sure to cook your eggs thoroughly (both whites and yolks) during your pregnancy (see Eggs and *Salmonella enteritidis*, page 79). If your doctor has restricted your fat intake, use canola oil cooking spray for the skillet instead of butter, and use a reduced-fat grated cheese.

▶ *Serve omelet with:*
    Whole wheat roll or bread
    Tossed salad
    Reduced-fat 2% milk or low-fat yogurt
    Fresh fruit that contains vitamin C

APPROXIMATE NUTRITIONAL INFORMATION: Serving size: one vegetarian omelet; Calories: 366 cals; Protein: 25 g; Carbohydrates: 21 g; Fat: 20 g; Fiber: 7 g; Sodium: 259 mg; Folic Acid: 179 mcg; Calcium: 226 mg; Diabetic Exchange: Bread/Starch 1.5, Fat 1, Meat (Medium Fat) 3

recommendations for optimizing iron and zinc bioavailability in vegetarians[6]

- ▶ Emphasize variety in your diet, especially foods that are nutrient dense.

- ▶ Include plenty of sprouted lentils, chickpeas, and beans.

- ▶ Eat fermented soy foods (such as soy sauce, tempeh, and miso).

- ▶ Choose dried fruits for dessert.

- ▶ Eat plenty of fresh fruits and dark green leafy vegetables.

- ▶ Try not to consume phytate-rich foods and calcium-rich dairy foods in the same meal.

- ▶ Do not consume calcium- and iron-rich foods in the same meal.

- ▶ Drink tea and coffee at times other than mealtime.

- ▶ Try to eat vitamin C–rich foods with iron-rich foods.

- ▶ Evaluate your iron, zinc, calcium, and phytate intake on a regular basis.

- ▶ Use iron- and zinc-fortified foods if recommended by your doctor or nutritionist.

sample menus for optimizing iron and zinc bioavailability[7]

INITIAL MENU	INITIAL MENU MODIFIED TO INCREASE IRON AND ZINC BIOAVAILABILITY
Breakfast	*Breakfast*
Wheat toast	Fortified breakfast cereal with raisins
English muffin	English muffin
Tea with milk	Herbal tea (see Herbal Teas to Avoid, page 70)
Apple	Orange juice
Lunch	*Lunch*
Vegetable salad	Sprouted bean and vegetable salad
Baked potato	Baked potato with low-fat cheese
Whole wheat bread and jelly	Whole wheat bread and peanut butter
Black coffee	Tomato juice
Dinner	*Dinner*
Tomato soup	Black bean soup
Noodles	Brown rice
Stir-fried vegetables	Tempeh with stir-fried vegetables
Strawberry yogurt	Orange-banana juice

lentil, brown rice, and mushroom pilaf

What's in this for baby and me? Protein, folic acid, and fiber.

THIS LENTIL, BROWN rice, and mushroom casserole is an excellent source of protein, folic acid, and fiber, and a good source of iron. For a more intense mushroom flavor, mushroom broth can be used in place of vegetable stock.

serves 4 to 6

2 tablespoons unsalted butter	1 teaspoon dried oregano
1 small onion, finely chopped	¾ cup green lentils, picked over and rinsed
1 garlic clove, minced	½ cup brown rice
8 ounces cremini or button mushrooms, washed, trimmed, and thinly sliced	½ teaspoon salt
1 teaspoon dried thyme	4 cups vegetable stock
	Grated Parmesan cheese, for the table

1. Preheat the oven to 350°F.
2. Melt the butter in a large nonstick skillet over medium-high heat. Add the onion and sauté for 3 minutes. Add the garlic, mushrooms, thyme, and oregano and sauté for 1 minute more. Add the lentils and rice and sauté for 1 minute. Add the salt and stock and bring to a boil.
3. Carefully transfer the contents of the skillet to an 8 x 8 x 2-inch Pyrex baking dish. Bake for 2 hours, or until the rice and lentils in the center of the casserole are soft and the liquid is absorbed. Cover the dish with foil during the last 30 minutes of baking. Serve hot, with Parmesan cheese.

▶ *Variation:* Use long- or medium-grain white rice (not basmati or instant) and reduce the cooking time to about 1 hour.

▶ *Storage Tip:* This pilaf keeps for 5 days refrigerated.

▶ *Complete Meal Ideas:* Serve this pilaf with:
Green or yellow vegetable (you might want to try the Tomato and Mozzarella Salad with Fresh Basil, page 157)
Reduced-fat 2% milk or low-fat yogurt
Fresh fruit that contains vitamin C

APPROXIMATE NUTRITIONAL INFORMATION: Serving size: 1 cup lentil, brown rice, and mushroom pilaf; Calories: 206 cals; Protein: 11 g; Carbohydrates: 30 g; Fat: 5 g; Fiber: 9 g; Sodium: 879 mg; Folic Acid: 110 mcg; Diabetic Exchange: Bread/Starch 2, Fat 1, Meat (Lean Fat) .5

swiss chard or spinach with garlicky soy dressing

~

What's in this for baby and me? Vitamins A and C.

Packed with vitamins A and C, and a good source of iron and folic acid, Swiss chard or spinach with garlicky soy dressing is a tasty side dish for any main course. The soy dressing can also be served with broccoli, asparagus, or eggplant.

serves 2 to 3 (makes about 1 ½ cups)

GARLICKY SOY DRESSING
- 1 tablespoon soy sauce
- ¼ teaspoon minced garlic
- 1 to 2 teaspoons brown sugar, or to taste
- 1 teaspoon canola oil
- A drop or two of toasted sesame oil

- 1 tablespoon canola oil
- 10–12 ounces red or green Swiss chard (see Cooking Tip below) or one 10-ounce package baby spinach leaves, washed, stems trimmed

1. To make the sauce, combine the soy sauce, garlic, and brown sugar in a small bowl. Stir until the sugar dissolves, then add the canola oil and sesame oil, stir, and set aside.
2. Heat the canola oil in a large nonstick skillet over medium-high heat. Add the Swiss chard and sauté just until wilted, about 3 minutes (if it does not fit in the pan all at once, you may need to sauté half of it, then add the rest after it has wilted). Transfer the cooked greens to a serving dish (after draining off any watery juices), add the reserved sauce, and mix gently. Serve hot or at room temperature.

▶ *Advance Preparation: Variation:* The sauce can be made up to 2 days in advance. The greens can be cooked up to 6 hours in advance, covered, and left at room temperature.

▶ *Cooking Tip:* To clean Swiss chard, trim the thick stems, then place the leaves in a large bowl or sink filled with water and gently rub the leaves with your fingers to dislodge any sand. Lift the greens out of the water and place them in a colander to drain. Wash the leaves a second time, or until no more sand remains. Slice the large leaves in half, then roll up a handful of leaves at a time and slice them about ½ inch thick.

▶ *Timesaving Tip:* Use frozen spinach. Cook it according to package directions and drain well.

APPROXIMATE NUTRITIONAL INFORMATION: Serving size: one-third Swiss chard with garlicky soy dressing; Calories: 83 cals; Protein: 2 g; Carbohydrates: 6 g; Fat: 6 g; Fiber: 2 g; Sodium: 477 mg; Vitamin A: 2,966 IU; Vitamin C: 17 mg; Diabetic Exchange: Fat 1, Vegetable 1

APPROXIMATE NUTRITIONAL INFORMATION: Serving size: one-third spinach with garlicky soy dressing: Calories: 87 cals; Protein: 3 g; Carbohydrates: 5 g; Fat: 7 g; Fiber: 2 g; Sodium: 409 mg; Vitamin A: 7,739 IU; Iron: 4 mg; Folic Acid: 139 mcg; Diabetic Exchange: Fat 1.5, Vegetable 1

lima beans with artichoke hearts and dill

What's in this for baby and me? Vitamin C and fiber.

Hɪɢʜ ɪɴ ᴠɪᴛᴀᴍɪɴ C and fiber, and a good source of protein, vitamin A, iron, and folic acid, lima beans and artichokes are among the healthiest vegetables you can eat. If serving to young children, you might want to omit the dill in their portions, and refer to the lima beans as green M&Ms.

serves 5 (makes about 2½ cups)

1 cup fat-free vegetable stock

8 ounces frozen lima beans (about 1¾ cups)

One 14-ounce can artichoke hearts, drained and cut into quarters, or one 8-ounce package frozen sliced artichoke hearts

½ cup half-and-half

1½ tablespoons quick-dissolving flour (such as Wondra), or to desired consistency

¼ cup chopped fresh dill

Salt and freshly ground pepper, to taste

Squeeze of fresh lemon juice, to taste

1. In a large saucepan bring the stock to a boil. Add the lima beans and artichoke hearts and return to a boil. Reduce the heat and simmer, covered, for 5 minutes.
2. Add the half-and-half and return to a simmer, then sprinkle in the flour, stir, and continue to simmer for 2 minutes. Add the dill and season to taste with salt and pepper and lemon juice. Serve warm.

▸ **Storage Tip:** This dish keeps refrigerated for 3 days. Do not freeze.

▸ **Health Tip:** If your doctor has restricted your fat intake, use 1½ cups stock and omit the half-and-half. The dish will be just as tasty but less creamy.

APPROXIMATE NUTRITIONAL INFORMATION: Serving size: ½ cup lima beans with artichoke hearts; Calories: 125 cals; Protein: 6 g; Carbohydrates: 20 g; Fat: 3 g; Fiber: 5 g; Sodium: 265 mg; Vitamin C: 14 mg; Diabetic Exchange: Bread/Starch 1, Fat 1, Vegetable 1

okra and tomatoes

~

What's in this for baby and me? Vitamin C.

OKRA AND TOMATOES are an excellent source of vitamin C, and a good source of vitamin A, calcium, and fiber. This is delicious over rice, couscous, or quinoa, and for ominvores it makes a healthy side dish for grilled meat, broiled chicken, or baked fish.

serves 4 (makes about 3 cups)

1 tablespoon olive oil	**cut into ½-inch slices**
½ cup finely chopped onion	**One 14.5-ounce can diced tomatoes (do not**
1 small garlic clove, minced	**drain)**
1 teaspoon Italian seasoning or dried oregano	**1 teaspoon sugar**
10 ounces okra, washed, ends trimmed, and	**Salt and freshly ground pepper, to taste**

1. Heat the oil in a large saucepan over medium-high heat. Add the onion and sauté for 3 minutes, or until light golden brown. Add the remaining ingredients and bring to a boil, then reduce the heat, cover, and simmer gently for 30 to 35 minutes, or until the okra is tender.
2. Adjust the seasoning and serve.

▶ *Timesaving Tip:* One 10-ounce package sliced frozen okra, defrosted and drained, can be substituted for the fresh okra. Cook the okra according to the time listed on the package.

▶ *Variation:* Add your favorite vegetables, such as cubed zucchini, quartered canned artichoke hearts, or fresh green beans, with the okra.

▶ *Storage Tip:* This dish keeps for 3 days refrigerated, and it can be frozen for up to 1 month.

APPROXIMATE NUTRITIONAL INFORMATION: Serving size: one-quarter okra and tomatoes; Calories: 81 cals; Protein: 2 g; Carbohydrates: 11 g; Fat: 3 g; Fiber: 3 g; Sodium: 346 mg; Vitamin C: 30 mg; Diabetic Exchange: Fat .5, Vegetable 1

classic creamed spinach

What's in this for baby and me? Vitamins A and C, calcium, iron, and fiber.

CLASSIC CREAMED SPINACH is an excellent source of vitamins A and C, calcium, iron, and fiber, and a good source of protein—Popeye would approve!

serves 3 (makes about 1 ½ cups)

One 10-ounce package frozen chopped
    spinach, cooked and drained, or one 10–12
    ounce package fresh baby spinach
1 tablespoon unsalted butter
2 tablespoons finely chopped onion
    (preferably a sweet onion such as Vidalia)

1 tablespoon all-purpose flour
½ cup whole milk
½ cup shredded Monterey Jack cheese
Salt and freshly ground pepper, to taste

1. If using fresh spinach, place about 2 cups of water in a large saucepan, add a pinch of salt, and bring to a boil. Add the spinach and cook for about 3 minutes, or just until wilted. Drain and cool, then squeeze dry, coarsely chop, and set aside.
2. Melt the butter in a large saucepan (you can use the same saucepan used to cook the fresh spinach) over medium-high heat. Add the onion, and sauté for 3 minutes, or until lightly browned. Add the flour and continue to sauté for 30 seconds, then add the milk, stirring constantly, and cook, stirring, until smooth and slightly thickened, about 1 to 3 minutes.
3. Add the spinach and cheese and stir to heat through. Season, and serve immediately.

▶ *Timesaving Tip:* Use a microwaveable 10-ounce bag of baby spinach, available in many grocery stores. Cook according to the directions on the bag.

▶ *Storage Tip:* This dish keeps refrigerated for 3 days. Do not freeze.

▶ *Health Tip:* If your doctor has restricted your fat intake, replace the butter with tub margarine, use reduced-fat 2% milk, and either use a reduced-fat cheese or omit the cheese.

APPROXIMATE NUTRITIONAL INFORMATION: Serving size: ½ cup creamed spinach; Calories: 155 cals; Protein: 9 g; Carbohydrates: 5 g; Fat: 12 g; Fiber: 8 g; Sodium: 260 mg; Vitamin A: 5,395 IU; Vitamin C: 23 mg; Calcium: 259 mg; Iron: 6 mg; Diabetic Exchange: Fat 1, Meat (Medium Fat) 1, Vegetable 1

simple and tasty brussels sprouts

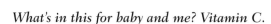

What's in this for baby and me? Vitamin C.

Brussels sprouts are high in vitamin C, and a good source of vitamin A and folic acid. For color and crunch, add toasted sliced almonds and dried cranberries to the sautéed sprouts.

serves 4 (makes about 2 cups)

10–12 ounces Brussels sprouts, washed, bottoms trimmed, loose or damaged outer leaves removed, and cut in half (or quarters, if they are very large)

1½ tablespoons unsalted butter
½ teaspoon sugar
Salt and freshly ground pepper, to taste

1. In a large saucepan, bring ½ cup water to a boil. Add the sprouts and cook for 8 minutes.
2. Drain the sprouts and return to the saucepan. Add the butter and sugar and sauté over high heat for 5 minutes, or until nicely browned. Season, transfer to a serving dish, and serve immediately.

▶ *Timesaving Tip:* Use whole frozen Brussels sprouts and cook according to package directions. Drain and sauté as described above.

APPROXIMATE NUTRITIONAL INFORMATION: Serving size: ¼ cup Brussels sprouts; Calories: 70 cals; Protein: 2 g; Carbohydrates: 7 g; Fat: 5 g; Fiber: 2 g; Sodium: 16 mg; Vitamin C: 44 mg; Diabetic Exchange: Fat 1, Vegetable 1.5

southern-style sweet potato casserole

What's in this for baby and me? Vitamin A and C.

THIS SWEET POTATO casserole, packed with vitamins A and C, and a good source of protein and fiber, is a guaranteed crowd pleaser, particularly during the holidays. Canned sweet potatoes are a fine substitute for fresh, especially if time is scarce. Buy the vacuum-packed variety or those packed in light syrup rather than those in heavy syrup. (See Timesaving Tip for instructions on using canned sweet potatoes.) Adding marshmallows might be a means to get your children to try this vitamin-packed dish.

serves 4 to 6

Canola oil cooking spray or unsalted butter,
    for greasing the baking dish
SWEET POTATO FILLING
    2 pounds (about 3 medium) red sweet
        potatoes, peeled and cut into large
        pieces of equal size
    ½ cup whole milk
    2 tablespoons unsalted butter
    1–2 tablespoons light brown sugar, to taste
        (optional)
    2 tablespoons mild molasses, to taste
        (optional)

1 large egg
½ teaspoon ground cinnamon, cloves, or
    allspice, or a mixture of any of these
    spices
¼ teaspoon salt
NUT CRUMB TOPPING (optional)
    ¼ cup all-purpose flour
    ⅓ cup loosely packed light or dark brown
        sugar
    3 tablespoons unsalted butter
    ½ cup pecans or walnuts, or a mixture

1. Preheat the oven to 375°F. Grease an 8 x 8 x 2-inch baking dish or a 9-inch pie pan with canola oil cooking spray or butter.
2. To make the filling, place the potatoes in a large pot and add just enough water to cover the potatoes. Bring to a boil, then reduce heat and simmer for 20 to 25 minutes, or until the potatoes are soft. Drain.
3. Place the hot potatoes in a large bowl. Beat them with an electric mixer on low speed to break them up, then increase the speed to medium and beat for 1 to 2 minutes, or until fairly smooth. Add the remaining filling ingredients and mix on low speed until well blended and almost smooth, about 1 minute. Transfer the pureed potatoes to the prepared baking dish.
4. To make the optional nut crumb topping, combine the flour and brown sugar in a small bowl. Using a dull knife (such as a table knife) or your fingers, work in the butter until the dough has a crumb-like consistency. Mix in the pecans.

5. Distribute the topping evenly over the sweet potato casserole. Bake for 45 minutes, or until the casserole is heated through and the topping has set. If the topping has not set after 45 minutes, place the casserole under the broiler for a minute or two. Remove from the oven and serve immediately.

▶ *Timesaving Tip:* Substitute 2 pounds vacuum-packed or canned sweet potatoes or yams (in light syrup) for the fresh sweet potatoes. Drain, place the sweet potatoes in a large bowl, and proceed with Step 3. Omit the crumb topping.

▶ *Advance Preparation: Variation:* The filling can be prepared up to 1 day in advance; cover and refrigerate. The nut crumb topping can be made 2 to 5 days in advance; place it on the casserole just before baking.

▶ *Variation:* If you don't need to watch your calorie intake, a marshmallow topping is a decadent treat. To make the topping, cover the top of the baked casserole with mini marshmallows or large ones cut in half. Place the casserole under the broiler for a few seconds. Watch carefully to avoid burning the marshmallows.

▶ *Health Tip:* If your doctor has restricted your fat or calorie intake, use reduced-fat 2% milk and omit the butter, molasses, and sugar; do not use the nut crumb or marshmallow topping.

▶ *Diabetic Tip:* Do not use the nut crumb or marshmallow topping.

APPROXIMATE NUTRITIONAL INFORMATION: Serving size: one-eighth sweet potato casserole (without the marshmallows); Calories: 308 cals; Protein: 6 g; Carbohydrates: 43 g; Fat: 14 g; Fiber: 3 g; Sodium: 109 mg; Vitamin A: 19,707 IU; Vitamin C: 20 mg; Diabetic Exchange: Bread/Starch 3, Fat 3

baked acorn squash with molasses

What's in this for baby and me? Vitamin C and fiber.

HIGH IN VITAMIN C and fiber, and a good source of vitamin A and iron, baked acorn squash makes a sweet and homey dish.

serves 4 (makes about 2 cups)

Canola oil spray for greasing the baking dish

1 large acorn squash (about 2 pounds),
    washed, sliced in half, and seeds removed

1 tablespoon brown sugar, or to taste

1 tablespoon mild molasses, or to taste

½ teaspoon ground cinnamon, cloves, or
    allspice, or a mixture

1 tablespoon unsalted butter

Salt, to taste

1. Preheat the oven to 375°F. Line a baking dish with foil and lightly spray.
2. Place the squash cut-side down in the baking dish and bake for 40 to 50 minutes, or until tender. Check doneness by piercing the squash with the tip of a knife. Let cool slightly.
3. When cool enough to handle, scoop out the squash pulp from the shells with a large spoon and place it in a serving bowl. Add the remaining ingredients and mix gently. Reheat in a microwave oven before serving, if desired.

APPROXIMATE NUTRITIONAL INFORMATION: Serving size: ½ cup acorn squash; Calories: 150 cals; Protein: 2 g; Carbohydrates: 32 g; Fat: 3 g; Fiber: 8 g; Sodium: 10 mg; Vitamin C: 20 mg; Diabetic Exchange: Bread/Starch 2, Fat 1

annie mozer's greens

~

What's in this for baby and me? Calcium, vitamins A and C, and folic acid.

THESE TASTY GREENS will help you get calcium, vitamins A and C, and folic acid into your diet, not to mention iron and fiber.

collard greens with black-eyed peas and tomatoes

serves 4

2 tablespoons canola oil

1 medium onion, chopped

¾ pound fresh greens, washed, tough stems
    trimmed, and sliced into ½-inch strips

Salt, to taste

3 tablespoons red wine vinegar

A couple drops of Tabasco

One 15.5-ounce can black-eyed peas, rinsed
    and drained

2 vine-ripened tomatoes, diced

1. In a large nonstick skillet, heat the canola oil over medium-high heat. Add the onion and sauté for 3 minutes. Reduce the heat to medium, add the collard greens, and continue to sauté until wilted. (Note: You may need to add the collard greens in batches—as one batch wilts, add the next.)
2. Add 1 cup water and the salt and cook, uncovered, for 30 to 50 minutes, or until the collard greens are tender; add more water ¼ cup at a time as needed. Add the vinegar during the last 15 minutes of cooking.
3. Remove from the heat and add the Tabasco sauce, black-eyed peas, and tomatoes. Stir, adjust the seasoning, and serve.

APPROXIMATE NUTRITIONAL INFORMATION: Serving size: one-quarter collard greens with black-eyed peas and tomatoes; Calories: 191 cals; Protein: 8 g; Carbohydrates: 25 g; Fat: 8 g; Fiber: 8 g; Sodium: 343 mg; Vitamin A: 3,059 IU; Vitamin C: 32 mg; Folic Acid: 150 mcg; Diabetic Exchange: Fat 1, Vegetable 5

sautéed kale

serves 4

2 tablespoons canola oil
1 medium onion, chopped
¾ pound kale, washed, tough stems trimmed
and sliced into ½-inch strips
Salt, to taste
3 tablespoons red wine vinegar

1. In a large nonstick skillet, heat the canola oil over medium-high heat. Add the onion and sauté for 3 minutes. Reduce the heat to medium, add the kale and salt, and continue to sauté until wilted. Cook, uncovered, for about 15 minutes, stirring frequently. If the kale sticks to the skillet, add a little water, 2 tablespoons at a time. Add the vinegar during the last 5 minutes of cooking.
2. Adjust the seasoning and serve.

APPROXIMATE NUTRITIONAL INFORMATION: Serving size: one-quarter sautéed kale; Calories: 95 cals; Protein: 2 g; Carbohydrates: 7 g; Fat: 7 g; Fiber: 2 g; Sodium: 20 mg; Vitamin A: 6,294 IU; Vitamin C: 37 mg; Diabetic Exchange: Fat 1, Vegetable 1.5

sautéed mustard greens with dried cranberries

serves 4

2 tablespoons canola oil
1 medium onion, chopped
¾ pound mustard greens, washed, tough stems trimmed, and sliced into ½-inch strips
Salt, to taste
3 tablespoons balsamic vinegar
¼ cup dried cranberries

1. In a large nonstick skillet, heat the canola oil over medium-high heat. Add the onion and sauté for 3 minutes. Reduce the heat to medium, add the mustard greens and salt, and continue to sauté until wilted. Cook, uncovered, for about 15 minutes, stirring frequently. If the mustard greens stick to the skillet, add a little water, 2 tablespoons at a time. Add the balsamic vinegar and dried cranberries during the last 5 minutes of cooking.
2. Adjust the seasoning and serve.

APPROXIMATE NUTRITIONAL INFORMATION: Serving size: one-quarter sautéed mustard greens with dried cranberries; Calories: 124 cals; Protein: 2 g; Carbohydrates: 14 g; Fat: 7 g; Fiber: 3 g; Sodium: 15 mg; Vitamin A: 2,578 IU; Vitamin C: 23 mg; Diabetic Exchange: Fat 1, Vegetable 3

bok choy and arugula with soy sauce

serves 5

1 tablespoon canola oil

2 tablespoons toasted sesame oil

1 medium onion, chopped

2 garlic cloves, minced

2¼ pounds bok choy, washed and cut into
   ½-inch slices (Note: Keep the thicker stem

ends separate from the top leaves, as they
   will be cooked first.)

1 large bunch arugula, washed, and stems
   trimmed (about 3 cups leaves)

2 tablespoons soy sauce, or to taste

Freshly ground pepper, to taste

1. In a large nonstick skillet, combine the canola oil and sesame oil and heat over medium-high heat. Add the onion and sauté for 2 minutes. Add the garlic and sauté for 30 seconds. Reduce the heat to medium, add the white stems of the bok choy, and sauté for 3 minutes. Add the green leaves of the bok choy and the arugula and sauté for 5 minutes. If the skillet seems dry, add 2 tablespoons of water.
2. Add the soy sauce and sauté for 3 more minutes. Adjust the seasoning and serve.

APPROXIMATE NUTRITIONAL INFORMATION: Serving size: one-fifth bok choy and arugula with soy sauce; Calories: 115 cals; Protein: 4 g; Carbohydrates: 7 g; Fat: 9 g; Fiber: 4 g; Sodium: 486 mg; Vitamin A: 5,621 IU; Vitamin C: 57 mg; Folic Acid: 105 mcg; Calcium: 224 mg; Diabetic Exchange: Fat 2, Vegetable 1

twenty-minute tomato sauce

*What's in this for baby and me? Vitamins A and C,
and protein from the whole wheat pasta.*

THIS ASTONISHINGLY SIMPLE tomato sauce, high in vitamins A and C, and a good source of B vitamins, is so easy to make you'll think twice about buying jarred spaghetti sauce again. The thickness of the sauce will depend on the juiciness of the vine-ripened tomatoes. If you would like a thinner sauce, add a bit of water during the last 10 minutes of cooking. Serve it over whole wheat pasta, which offers a good amount of iron.

Makes about 2½ cups

4 tablespoons olive oil

2 garlic cloves, minced

2 pounds (about 7) large, vine-ripened tomatoes, cut into a ½-inch dice (about 4 cups)

1 tablespoon Italian seasoning

1 tablespoon brown sugar

1 teaspoon salt

Freshly ground black pepper, to taste

2 tablespoons tomato puree

⅓ cup chopped fresh basil

1. In a large saucepan, combine 3 tablespoons of the olive oil and the garlic, and sauté over medium heat, stirring frequently, until the garlic turns a light golden brown, about 2 minutes. Be careful not to burn the garlic because it will turn bitter.
2. Add the tomatoes, Italian seasoning, brown sugar, salt, and pepper, and simmer, stirring occasionally, for 10 minutes.
3. Stir in the tomato puree, and continue to simmer for 10 minutes. Stir in the basil and the remaining 1 tablespoon of olive oil, adjust the seasoning, and serve.

▶ ***Storage Tip:*** Cover and refrigerate leftovers or freeze for 1 month.

▶ ***Diabetic Tip:*** Reduce the portion size of cooked spaghetti to ¾ cup per serving. Ideally, use whole wheat pasta.

▶ **Complete Meal Ideas:** Serve this tomato sauce with:

Whole wheat pasta

Green salad or vegetable (you might want to try the Vegetables
with Lemon, Olive Oil, and Fresh Herbs, page 153)

Reduced-fat 2% milk or low-fat yogurt

Fresh fruit

APPROXIMATE NUTRITIONAL INFORMATION: Serving size: ½ cup tomato sauce; Calories: 117 cals; Protein: 2 g; Carbohydrates: 8 g; Fat: 9 g; Fiber: 2 g; Sodium: 398 mg; Vitamin A: 1,409 IU; Vitamin C: 20 mg; Diabetic Exchange: Vegetable 1, Fat 2

APPROXIMATE NUTRITIONAL INFORMATION: Serving size: Whole wheat spaghetti: Serving size: 1 ½ cups cooked spaghetti; Calories: 260 cals; Protein: 11 g; Carbohydrates: 56 g; Fat: 1 g; Fiber: 9 g; Sodium: 6 mg; Diabetic Exchange: Bread/Starch 3

edamame, corn, and bean salad

~

What's in this for baby and me? Vitamin C and folic acid.

Bursting with vitamin C and folic acid, and a good source of protein, iron, and fiber, this colorful salad is a winner with just about any main course. Make variations as you wish, and don't be surprised if your kids take seconds.

Serves 4 (makes about 2½ cups)

DRESSING
- 1 tablespoon vinegar (any kind)
- 1 teaspoon freshly squeezed lemon juice, to taste
- 1 teaspoon Dijon mustard
- 2 tablespoons canola oil
- 1 small garlic clove, crushed (optional)

SALAD
- 1 cup cooked edamame, drained and cooled
- ½ cup cooked fresh, frozen, or canned corn
- ½ cup canned black beans, rinsed and drained
- ¼ cup thinly sliced scallions
- 2 tablespoons chopped fresh cilantro

1. To make the dressing, in a small bowl whisk the vinegar, lemon, and mustard. Add the canola oil and garlic and continue whisking until emulsified; set aside.
2. Combine all of the salad ingredients in a serving bowl, add the reserved dressing, and mix gently. Adjust the seasoning and serve.

▶ **Storage Tip:** This salad keeps refrigerated for 3 days.

▶ **Complete Meal Ideas:** Serve this salad with:
   3 ounces protein (you might want to try the Old Bay
      Tofu Cakes with Cocktail Sauce, page 225)
   Brown rice, whole grains, or noodles
   Reduced-fat 2% milk or low-fat yogurt
   Fresh fruit

APPROXIMATE NUTRITIONAL INFORMATION: Serving size: ½ cup edamame, corn, and bean salad; Calories: 173 cals; Protein: 8 g; Carbohydrates: 15 g; Fat: 10 g; Fiber: 5 g; Sodium: 191 mg; Vitamin C: 12 mg; Folic Acid: 80 mcg; Diabetic Exchange: Bread/Starch 1, Fat 2

brown rice and lentil salad

What's in this for baby and me? Protein, folic acid, and fiber.

POWER PACKED WITH protein, folic acid, and fiber, and decent doses of vitamins C and B and iron—salads don't come much healthier than this. If you like cheese, pasteurized feta cheese adds a nice tang.

Serves 4 (makes about 3 cups)

DRESSING
1 tablespoon vinegar (any kind), to taste
1 teaspoon Dijon mustard
1 small garlic clove, minced
2 tablespoons olive oil
One 15-ounce can lentils, rinsed and drained, or 1½ cups cooked lentils
1½ cups cooked brown rice

⅓ cup finely diced celery
⅓ cup sliced or diced red radishes
1 large vine-ripened tomato, cut into a small dice (about 1 cup), or 12 cherry or grape tomatoes, quartered
2 tablespoons chopped fresh parsley
Salt and freshly ground pepper, to taste

1. To make the dressing, in a small bowl whisk the vinegar, mustard, and garlic. Add the olive oil and continue whisking until emulsified. Set aside.
2. Combine the lentils, brown rice, celery, radishes, tomatoes, and parsley in a serving bowl. Add the reserved dressing, and mix gently. Adjust the seasoning and serve.

▶ *Timesaving Tip:* Pick up as many ingredients as you can from a salad bar.

▶ *Storage Tip:* This salad keeps refrigerated for 3 days.

▶ *Complete Meal Ideas:* Serve this brown rice and lentil salad with:
3 ounces protein (you might want to try the Crispy Fried Tofu with Sesame-Soy Sauce, page 259, or the Quick Broccoli–Red Bell Pepper Frittata, page 253)
Reduced-fat 2% milk or low-fat yogurt or soy yogurt
Fruit that contains vitamin C

APPROXIMATE NUTRITIONAL INFORMATION: Serving size: ¾ cup brown rice and lentil salad: Calories: 239 cals; Protein: 9 g; Carbohydrates: 35 g; Fat: 8 g; Fiber: 8 g; Sodium: 339 mg; Folic Acid: 150 mcg; Diabetic Exchange: Bread/Starch 2, Lean Meat .5, Fat 1

asian-style pickled sesame cabbage

What's in this for baby and me? Vitamin C.

IF YOU ARE craving pickles, this vitamin C–packed cabbage salad might hit the spot.

Makes about 3½ cups

1 pound green cabbage, washed, sliced in
    half, damaged outer leaves and core
    removed
1½ teaspoons salt
¼ cup white vinegar

¼ cup sugar
¼ cup toasted sesame oil
2 tablespoons roasted sesame seeds, for
    garnish (optional)

1. Cut the cabbage into 1½-inch pieces. Place them in a large bowl, and sprinkle with the salt. Toss with your hands, then allow the cabbage to sit for 1½ hours at room temperature.
2. To make the marinade: In a medium bowl, mix the vinegar and sugar until most of the sugar has dissolved. Add the sesame oil, mix again, and set aside.
3. When the cabbage is ready, working in batches, use your hands to pick up some cabbage to gently squeeze most of the juices from it (discard the juices). Places the leaves in the bowl of the reserved marinade and repeat with the remaining cabbage. Mix the cabbage with the marinade until well combined. Cover and refrigerate for 6 hours before serving.
4. At the time of serving, garnish with the sesame seeds. Keep leftovers refrigerated

▶ *Variation:* Substitute half of the cabbage called for in this recipe with thickly sliced carrots.

▶ *Storage Tip:* This pickled cabbage keeps refrigerated for 5 days. It will wilt, but that is not a problem.

▶ *Complete Meal Ideas:* Serve this cabbage with:

    3 ounces protein (you might want to try the Crispy Fried
        Tofu with Sesame-Soy Sauce, page 259)
    Brown rice, whole grains, or noodles
    Reduced-fat 2% milk or low-fat yogurt
    Fresh fruit

APPROXIMATE NUTRITIONAL INFORMATION: Serving size: ½ cup pickled sesame cabbage; Calories: 54 cals; Protein: 1 g; Carbohydrates: 6 g; Fat: 3 g; Fiber: 2 g; Sodium: 344 mg; Vitamin C: 21 mg; Diabetic Exchange: Fat 1, Vegetable 1

tofu with vegetables and coconut milk

What's in this for baby and me? Protein, vitamins A and C.

A LIGHT AND healthy dish that delivers excellent doses of protein and vitamins A and C, and a good dose of folic acid, B vitamins, calcium, and iron.

Serves 4

1 cup green beans, washed, ends trimmed,
   and cut into ½-inch pieces on the diagonal
1 cup sliced red bell peppers
1 tablespoon canola oil
1 cup sliced shitake mushrooms (about 5
   mushrooms)
⅓ cup sliced scallions
7½ ounces firm tofu, drained, cut into ½-inch

cubes, and blotted dry with paper towels
1 cup canned coconut milk
½ cup chopped roasted peanuts
1 tablespoon freshly squeezed lime juice
2 teaspoons brown sugar
2 tablespoons soy sauce, to taste
Pinch of chili flakes (optional)
3 tablespoons chopped fresh cilantro

1. Cook the green beans and red bell peppers in boiling water for 2 minutes, drain, then place them in a serving dish; set aside.
2. In a medium saucepan, heat the canola oil over medium heat. Add the mushrooms and scallions, and sauté for 2 minutes. Add the tofu and the coconut milk, and bring to a boil, then reduce the heat and simmer for 5 minutes.
3. Stir in the peanuts, lime juice, sugar, soy sauce, and chili flakes, if using, and cook for 5 minutes. Pour the tofu mixture over the reserved green beans and red bell peppers, garnish with the cilantro, and serve immediately.

▶ *Variation:* Any vegetables can be used in place of those called for; some good choices are sliced carrots, snow peas, baby corn, or broccoli. Cook the vegetables according to Step 1.

▶ *Health Tip:* If your doctor has restricted your sodium intake, use only 1 tablespoon of low-sodium or light soy sauce.

► **Complete Meal Ideas:** Serve this tofu with:
Brown basmati rice or noodles
Reduced-fat 2% milk or low-fat yogurt
Fresh fruit high in vitamin C

APPROXIMATE NUTRITIONAL INFORMATION: Serving size: one-quarter tofu with vegetables and coconut milk; Calories: 325 cals; Protein: 13 g; Carbohydrates: 16 g; Fat: 16 g; Fiber: 5 g; Sodium: 589 mg; Vitamin A: 2,154 IU; Vitamin C: 66 mg; Diabetic Exchange: Bread/Starch 1, Fat 2, Meat (Medium Fat) 2

quick broccoli–red bell pepper frittata

What's in this for baby and me? Protein and vitamin C.

THIS ELEGANT ITALIAN omelet is similar to a crustless quiche. The fillings are sautéed, then beaten egg is added, and the cooking is finished under the broiler. High in protein and vitamin C, plus a good source of calcium, B vitamins, and folic acid, this hearty frittata might become a staple in your home. Tomatoes on the top add a decorative touch.

Serves 4 to 5

5 large eggs

¼ cup whole milk

½ teaspoon salt

Freshly ground pepper

2 tablespoons olive oil

1 tablespoon unsalted butter

1 small onion, peeled and thinly sliced

½ cup thinly sliced red bell peppers

1 cup very small broccoli florets

2 tablespoons chopped fresh parsley

One small tomato, thinly sliced, with seeds removed from the slices

⅓ cup grated Parmesan cheese

1. Combine the eggs, milk, salt, and pepper in a bowl and mix until well blended; set aside.
2. Heat 1 tablespoon of the olive oil and the butter in a large oven-proof 12-inch skillet over medium heat. Add the onions and red bell peppers, and sauté, stirring for 4 minutes, or until light golden. Smear the oil against the sides of the skillet as you stir to grease the pan. Add the broccoli and 4 tablespoons of water and continue to sauté for about 3 minutes, or until the broccoli is crisp-tender. Stir in the parsley during the last minute of cooking.
3. While the broccoli is cooking preheat the broiler to a high setting.
4. Add the remaining 1 tablespoon of olive oil to the skillet, then evenly scatter the vegetables on the bottom of the pan. Add the reserved beaten egg. Do not stir at this point. Cook for about 1 to 2 minutes, or until the bottom has set. While the frittata is cooking, arrange the tomato slices on top, then sprinkle evenly with the Parmesan cheese.
5. Place the frittata under the broiler for 2 minutes, or until the top has set and the Parmesan cheese is light golden. Serve warm.

▶ *Cooking Tip:* The best way to prepare any frittata is in an oven-proof skillet. If you don't have one, you can complete Steps 1 and 2 in a nonstick skillet, then transfer the broccoli–bell pepper mixture to a greased 9-inch Pyrex pie dish and add the reserved egg mixture. Bake in a preheated 350°F oven for 30 to 35 minutes. The eggs won't be as fluffy if they are cooked in the oven, but the taste will still be good.

▶ **Variation:** You may substitute the broccoli with your favorite cooked vegetables, including zucchini, yellow squash, asparagus, or mushrooms. Artichoke hearts are a tasty (and healthy) addition, but they will turn the eggs slightly gray. Shrimp, diced ham, or sausages also work, and additional cheese does too, of course.

▶ **Calcium Boost:** In a measuring cup combine ⅓ cup pasteurized instant nonfat dry milk with the whole milk. Mix until the milk powder has dissolved, then follow the directions in Step 1.

▶ **Complete Meal Ideas:** Serve this frittata with:
    Green salad (you might want to try mixed greens with a
        French-Style Tarragon Vinaigrette, page 166)
    A slice of whole wheat bread or a whole wheat roll
    Tomato juice or fresh fruit

APPROXIMATE NUTRITIONAL INFORMATION: Serving size: one-quarter of the frittata; Calories: 193 cals; Protein: 10 g; Carbohydrates: 6 g; Fat: 15 g; Fiber: 1 g; Sodium: 398 mg; Vitamin C: 50 mg; Diabetic Exchange: Fat 2, Meat (Medium Fat) 1, Vegetable 1

miso soup with tofu and rice noodles

What's in this for baby and me? Protein, vitamins A and C.

WHEN YOU REALIZE how easy this soup is to make, you'll start keeping a package of miso in your fridge for a quick-fix soup anytime. This dish is an excellent source of protein and vitamins A and C, and it provides a decent dose of B vitamins, folic acid, and fiber.

Serves 2 to 3 (makes about 5 cups)

Handful (about 1 ounce) of rice vermicelli, udon, or soba noodles

2 cups thinly sliced baby bok choy, stems and leaves

2 tablespoons thinly sliced scallions

2 slices peeled fresh ginger

7½ ounces extra-firm tofu, drained, cut into a ½-inch dice (about 1 cup diced tofu)

3 tablespoons miso (any kind), to taste

A few drops of light soy sauce, to taste

1. Bring 3 cups of water to a boil in a medium saucepan. Add the noodles and return to a boil. Add the bok choy, scallions, ginger, and tofu, and simmer for 10 minutes.
2. In a small bowl, combine ½ cup of water with the miso and stir until blended.
3. Add this miso mixture to the soup, stir, then remove the saucepan from the heat. Do not boil the soup after you add the miso. Stir in the soy sauce, adjust the seasoning, and serve immediately.

▶ *Variation:* The baby bok choy can be substituted with your favorite greens, and other vegetables can be added, including diced fresh vine-ripened tomatoes and sautéed mushrooms.

▶ *Cooking Tip:* There are basically three different types of miso: red, yellow, and white. Any of them will work in soup. The amount you add will depend on the strength and saltiness of the miso.

▶ *Health Tip:* If your doctor has restricted your sodium intake, use only a tablespoon of miso.

▶ *Complete Meal Ideas:* Serve this soup with:
    Whole wheat crackers and dip (you might want to try
       the Artichoke-Spinach Dip, page 178)
    Reduced-fat 2% milk or low-fat yogurt
    Fresh fruit

APPROXIMATE NUTRITIONAL INFORMATION: Serving size: 2 cups miso soup with tofu and rice noodles; Calories: 138 cals; Protein: 10 g; Carbohydrates: 17 g; Fat: 4 g; Fiber: 2 g; Sodium: 940 mg; Vitamin A: 4,855 IU; Vitamin C: 30 mg; Diabetic Exchange: Bread/Starch 1, Meat (Lean) 1

tofu with soba noodles, carrots, cucumbers, and sesame sauce

What's in this for baby and me? Protein, iron, and vitamin A.

JAM-PACKED WITH protein, iron, and vitamin A, and a smattering of vitamin C, B vitamins, folic acid, and calcium. Expect rave reviews from adults and kids alike.

Serves 6

Sesame Sauce
- **2 tablespoons toasted sesame oil**
- **1 tablespoon peanut butter**
- **3 tablespoons white vinegar**
- **3 tablespoons soy sauce**
- **1½ teaspoons sugar**
- **1 teaspoon minced garlic**
- **8 ounces Japanese soba or somen noodles**
- **1 tablespoon toasted sesame oil**
- **1 tablespoon rice wine**

- **½ cup grated carrots**
- **1 cup cucumbers cut into matchsticks**
- **1 cup cooked edamame**
- **1 tablespoon canola oil, for sautéing the tofu**
- **15 ounces extra-firm tofu, cut into ½-inch cubes, drained, and dried with paper towels**
- **⅓ cup thinly sliced scallions**
- **2 tablespoons roasted sesame seeds (optional)**

1. To make the sesame sauce, combine all of the ingredients in a small bowl and mix well; set aside.
2. Cook the noodles according to the package directions, rinse with cold water, and drain well. Place the noodles in a serving bowl and mix with the sesame oil and rice wine. Arrange the carrots, cucumbers, and edamame on top of the noodles; set aside.
3. Heat the canola oil in a large nonstick skillet over medium-high heat. Add the tofu and sauté, stirring gently, for 4 minutes, or until light golden on most sides.
4. Arrange the tofu on top of the noodles, evenly spoon the reserved sesame sauce over the dish, and garnish with the scallions and sesame seeds. Serve at room temperature. Refrigerate leftovers.

▶ *Variations:* In place of the tofu, use an equal amount of any other protein, such as cooked chicken, shrimp, or beef. Or you can add more vegetables, including red bell peppers, baby corn, cooked green beans, broccoli, asparagus, or snow peas.

▶ *Health Tip:* If your doctor has restricted your sodium intake, use low-sodium or light soy sauce.

▶ *Advance Preparation:* This noodle dish can be made up to 1 day in advance.

▶ *Complete Meal Ideas:* Serve these noodles with:
Reduced-fat 2% milk or low-fat yogurt
Fresh fruit or sorbet

APPROXIMATE NUTRITIONAL INFORMATION: Serving size: one-quarter tofu with soba noodles; Calories: 379 cals; Protein: 18 g; Carbohydrates: 40 g; Fat: 18 g; Fiber: 5 g; Sodium: 914 mg; Vitamin A: 1,337 IU; Iron: 4 mg; Diabetic Exchange: Bread/Starch 2, Fat 2, Meat (Lean) 2, Vegetable 1

crispy fried tofu with sesame-soy sauce

What's in this for baby and me? Protein.

For those of you who have written off tofu as a mushy, flavorless protein, you must try this version of fried tofu. And yes, this tofu is fried, but it absorbs a minimal amount of oil because it is not breaded. Serve the sauce in small individual bowls for easy dipping.

Serves 4

Sesame-Soy Sauce (makes about ¼ cup)
- 2 tablespoons soy sauce
- 1 tablespoon brown sugar
- ½ teaspoon rice wine
- ½ teaspoon toasted sesame oil
- 1 tablespoon minced garlic

- 1 cup canola oil, for frying the tofu
- 15 ounces (drained weight) firm tofu, drained; cut the block of tofu in half horizontally, then cut each half vertically down the center and diagonally into triangles; dry each triangle

1. To make the sesame-soy sauce: In a small bowl, mix the ingredients with 2 tablespoons of water; set aside.
2. To fry the tofu: Have ready a large plate lined with paper towels. In a medium, high-sided skillet heat the canola oil until hot. Dry off the tofu triangles with paper towels, then carefully add them, one piece at a time, to the hot oil and cook for 3 minutes on each side, or until light golden. Using tongs, transfer the tofu to the paper towel–lined plate. Serve hot with the sesame-soy sauce on the side.

▶ *Advance Preparation:* The sesame-soy sauce can be made a day in advance. Keep refrigerated and bring to room temperature before serving.

▶ *Cooking Tip:* Don't be turned off by the large amount of oil. Only a very small portion of it, less than 1 tablespoon, is absorbed by the tofu. It is important to use this much oil to make sure the tofu gets crispy when it is fried.

▶ *Health Tip:* If your doctor has restricted your sodium intake, use only a smidgen of the sesame-soy sauce, or use a substitute such as salsa.

▶ *Complete Meal Ideas:* Serve this tofu with:

Green salad or vegetable

Brown rice, a whole grain, or noodles (you might want to try the
Very Simple Fried Rice with Vegetables, page 263)

Reduced-fat 2% milk or low-fat yogurt

Fresh fruit

APPROXIMATE NUTRITIONAL INFORMATION: Serving size: one-quarter fried tofu with sesame-soy sauce; Calories: 159 cals; Protein: 11 g; Carbohydrates: 6 g; Fat: 9 g; Fiber: 1 g; Sodium: 516 mg; Diabetic Exchange: Fat 1, Meat (Very Lean) 2, Vegetable 1

veggie burgers

What's in this for baby and me? Protein, vitamin C, and fiber.

Homemade veggie burgers don't get much healthier than these, which are packed with protein, vitamin C, and fiber. They're also a good source of vitamin A, iron, folic acid, and B vitamins. Serve veggie burgers on a bun and dress them up with tomato, lettuce, cheese, and your favorite condiments, or with salsa alongside a salad.

Makes 5 burgers

1½ cups cooked brown rice (from about ½ cup uncooked rice, such as Royal Blend Texmati Brown, Wild, and Red rice)

½ cup canned or frozen corn

¾ cup canned refried beans

2 tablespoons chopped fresh cilantro

2 tablespoons thinly sliced scallions

1 large egg

⅓ cup plain breadcrumbs for the burgers, plus ½ cup for coating

2 tablespoons olive oil

1 cup finely sliced mushrooms (any kind)

½ cup diced red bell peppers

½ teaspoon ground cumin

¼ teaspoon salt, to taste

Freshly ground pepper

4 whole wheat hamburger buns

1. In a large bowl, combine the cooked brown rice, corn, refried beans, cilantro, scallions, egg, and ⅓ cup of the breadcrumbs. Mix gently.
2. Heat 1 tablespoon of the olive oil in a medium nonstick skillet over medium heat. Add the mushrooms and sauté, stirring occasionally, until the mushrooms are golden brown, about 5 minutes. Add the bell peppers and cumin, and cook 1 minute longer. Cool slightly, then add this mixture to the the brown rice mixture and stir until well combined. Allow to cool in the refrigerator for at least 30 minutes or overnight.
3. Place the remaining ½ cup of the breadcrumbs in a pie plate. Using a ½-cup measuring cup, scoop out the burger mixture and form it into 5 patties. Coat each patty with the breadcrumbs and refrigerate until ready to use.
4. Heat the remaining 1 tablespoon of the olive oil in a large nonstick skillet over medium heat. Add the patties and cook for 5 minutes on each side, or until heated through. If they begin browning too fast, lower the heat a bit.
5. Serve immediately on whole wheat buns with your favorite condiments, or with a salad.

▶ *Variation:* Substitute your favorite vegetables for the ones called for in this recipe.

▶ *Complete Meal Ideas:* Serve these veggie burgers with:
> Green salad or vegetable (you might want to try the Spinach Salad
>   with Mandarin Oranges and Toasted Almonds, page 163)
> Reduced-fat 2% milk or low-fat yogurt
> Fresh fruit that contains vitamin C

APPROXIMATE NUTRITIONAL INFORMATION: Serving size: one veggie burger on a whole wheat bun; Calories: 347 cals; Protein: 11 g; Carbohydrates: 53 g; Fat: 11 g; Fiber: 8 g; Sodium: 514 mg; Vitamin C: 43 mg; Diabetic Exchange: Bread/Starch 3, Fat 2, Vegetable 1

very simple fried rice with vegetables

What's in this for baby and me? Vitamins A and C.

Fried rice is a perpetual crowd pleaser, especially among children. This dish is high in vitamins A and C. Protein can be added in the form of tofu or tempeh—or, if you are not a vegetarian, diced ham, cooked shrimp, chicken, or sausages are all tasty (and all very Chinese). Brown or white basmati works best in this stir-fry.

Serves 6

1 cup broccoli florets, cut into small pieces	½ cup shredded carrots
1 cup diced red bell peppers	½ cup canned or frozen corn
1 tablespoon canola oil	½ cup finely sliced scallions
2 tablespoons toasted sesame oil	2 tablespoons soy sauce, to taste
2 tablespoons minced garlic	2 large eggs, beaten
About 4 cups cooked brown basmati rice (from 1½ cups uncooked rice)	Salt and freshly ground pepper, to taste

1. Bring a small pot of water to a boil. Add the broccoli and red bell peppers and cook for 1 minute (the water will not return to a boil). Drain and set aside.
2. In a very large nonstick skillet or wok, heat the canola oil and sesame oil over medium-high heat. Add the garlic and cook for 1 minute, stirring, until golden. Add the cooked rice, break up any large clumps, then, using two wooden spoons, mix the rice in a salad-tossing motion to separate the grains as they cook. This will take about 5 minutes. Add the carrots and continue to mix with the spoons for 1 minute. Add the corn, scallions, soy sauce, and the reserved broccoli and red bell peppers and continue mixing for 2 minutes.
3. Push the rice mixture to the side of the skillet to make room to cook the eggs. Add the eggs to the exposed part of the skillet, and, using one of the spoons, scramble them until cooked. Gently incorporate the cooked egg into the rice mixture. Adjust the seasoning and serve. Refrigerate leftovers.

▶ **Complete Meal Ideas:** Serve this fried rice with:

3 ounces protein (you might want to try the Crispy Fried
    Tofu with Sesame-Soy Sauce, page 259)
Reduced-fat 2% milk or low-fat yogurt
Fresh fruit

APPROXIMATE NUTRITIONAL INFORMATION: Serving size: one-sixth fried rice with vegetables; Calories: 199 cals; Protein: 5 g; Carbohydrates: 26 g; Fat: 9 g; Fiber: 2 g; Sodium: 427 mg; Vitamin A: 2,234 IU; Vitamin C: 64 mg; Diabetic Exchange: Bread/Starch 1, Fat 2, Vegetable 1

spinach risotto

What's in this for baby and me? Vitamin A.

Rich and creamy, risotto is Italian comfort food at its best. Spinach, high in vitamin A and a good source of folic acid and calcium, makes this vegetarian dish nutritious too.

Serves 5 (makes about 4 cups)

1½ cups canned vegetable broth

2 tablespoons olive oil

½ cup finely chopped onion

2 garlic cloves, minced

1 cup Arborio rice

8 ounces fresh baby spinach, washed, stems trimmed, and coarsely chopped, or one

8-ounce package frozen chopped spinach, defrosted, and lightly squeezed

3 tablespoons Parmesan cheese

½ teaspoon grated nutmeg

1 tablespoon unsalted butter

Salt and freshly ground pepper, to taste

1. Dilute the vegetable broth with 1½ cups of water and warm it in a microwave oven or in a saucepan.
2. In a large saucepan, heat the olive oil over medium heat. Add the onion and sauté for 3 minutes, stirring constantly, until light golden. Reduce heat to low, stir in the garlic and rice, and cook for 1 minute. Add 2 cups of the broth and cook over low heat, stirring occasionally, until most of the liquid is absorbed (this will take about 5 minutes). Continue adding the broth, ½ cup at a time, stirring after each addition. The risotto will take about 20 minutes to cook. When done, the rice will be just tender and the mixture slightly creamy. Do not overcook or the rice will become mushy.
3. Stir in the spinach, Parmesan cheese, nutmeg, and butter. Heat just until hot and the spinach leaves wilt. Adjust the seasoning and serve immediately.

▶ *Cooking Tips:* The broth is diluted because most canned stocks have a very intense flavor and tend to overpower milder flavors. Add the spinach at the last minute to retain its bright green color.

▶ *Complete Meal Ideas:* Serve this risotto with:

3 ounces protein (you might want to try the My Big Fat Breek Salad, page 170)

Green salad or vegetable

Reduced-fat 2% milk or low-fat yogurt

Fresh fruit

APPROXIMATE NUTRITIONAL INFORMATION: Serving size: one-fifth spinach risotto; Calories: 173 cals; Protein: 4 g; Carbohydrates: 19 g; Fat: 9 g; Fiber: 2 g; Sodium: 375 mg; Vitamin A: 4,731 IU; Diabetic Exchange: Bread/Starch 1, Fat 1.5, Vegetable 1

roasted new potatoes with garlic and rosemary

~

What's in this for baby and me? Vitamin C.

SMALL POTATOES STAR in this high–vitamin C side-dish, which also offers a good dose of iron, B vitamins, folic acid, and fiber. If available, use rosemary-scented oil or play around with other herbs, such as fresh thyme. The roasting time will vary according to the size of the potatoes. The butter helps brown the potatoes, but it is optional.

Serves 4

1½ pounds red bliss or new potatoes, or other thin-skinned potatoes, scrubbed clean, dried, halved (cut any large potatoes into quarters)

2 tablespoons olive oil

1 tablespoon unsalted butter (optional)

3 garlic cloves, skin on, smashed with the side of a knife

3 fresh rosemary sprigs or 1 tablespoon dried rosemary

1. Preheat the oven to 450°F. Have ready a large baking sheet.
2. Bring a large pot of salted water to a boil. Add the potatoes and cook for 12 minutes. Drain the potatoes well and allow them to air dry for about 2 minutes. Then, spread them out on the baking sheet and drizzle with the olive oil. Add the butter, garlic cloves, and rosemary sprigs, and mix with a large spatula. Season with salt and pepper and mix again.
3. Roast for 15 minutes, then remove the tray from the oven and gently mix the potatoes. The potatoes should be light golden and soft at this point. If they are not, continue to roast. Serve immediately.

APPROXIMATE NUTRITIONAL INFORMATION: Serving size: one-quarter of the roasted new potatoes; Calories: 245 cals; Protein: 4 g; Carbohydrates: 36 g; Fat: 10 g; Fiber: 4 g; Sodium: 308 mg; Vitamin C: 16 mg; Diabetic Exchange: Bread/Starch 2, Fat 2

savory corn cakes with cilantro

What's in this for baby and me? Protein and calcium.

Hᴵɢʜ ɪɴ ᴘʀᴏᴛᴇɪɴ and calcium, and a good source of folic acid, vitamin A, and B vitamins, these corn cakes, topped with a dollop of salsa, are a fantastic accompaniment to grilled meats, poultry, tofu, or vegetables. They also make a tasty snack reheated in a microwave oven.

Makes 12 corn cakes

¾ cup stone-ground yellow cornmeal

½ cup all-purpose flour

1 teaspoon baking soda

1 teaspoon salt

Freshly ground pepper

1 large egg

1 cup low-fat buttermilk

1 cup canned or frozen corn

¼ cup thinly sliced scallions

⅓ cup chopped fresh cilantro

1 cup (about 4 ounces) coarsely grated
     Monterey Jack cheese with or without
     jalapeños

1 tablespoon canola oil

1. In a medium bowl, whisk together the cornmeal, flour, baking soda, salt, and pepper until well combined; set aside.
2. In another medium bowl, combine the egg, buttermilk, corn, scallions, cilantro, and Monterey Jack cheese, and whisk until well combined. Add this mixture to the reserved cornmeal mixture and stir well.
3. Heat the canola oil in a large nonstick skillet over medium heat until hot. Add four or five ¼-cup portions of the corn cake batter to the skillet and spread into 3-inch circles. Cook the corn cakes until the edges are set and the underside is golden brown, about 2 minutes. Flip the corncakes and cook about 2 minutes more. Serve warm. Refrigerate leftovers. Reheat in a microwave oven.

▶ *Complete Meal Ideas:* Serve these corncakes with:
  Green vegetables, salad, or soup (you might want to try
    the Black Bean Soup with Cilantro, page 100)
  Reduced-fat 2% milk or low-fat yogurt
  Fresh fruit

APPROXIMATE NUTRITIONAL INFORMATION: Serving size: 2 corn cakes; Calories: 273 cals; Protein 11 g; Carbohydrates: 41 g; Fat: 10 g; Fiber: 1 g; Sodium: 486 mg; Calcium: 193 mg; Diabetic Exchange: Bread/Starch 2, Fat 1, Milk 1

spinach paneer

~

What's in this for baby and me? Vitamins A and C, folic acid, and calcium.

Spinach paneer is a traditional Indian side dish made with a dry, non-melting farmers' cheese. Many Indians make paneer at home, the old-fashioned way, but a pasteurized version, usually available at whole foods stores, is recommended during pregnancy. This dish is loaded with vitamins A and C, folic acid, and calcium, and provides a good dose of protein and B vitamins. If you can't find paneer, firm tofu cut into small cubes is an excellent substitute. Use chopped frozen spinach to save time. If you have young children, reserve a bit of plain spinach for them as they may not like the spiciness.

Serves 6

2 tablespoons olive oil

1 cup finely chopped onions

1 tablespoon minced fresh ginger

2 garlic cloves, minced

¼ teaspoon tumeric

Dash of chili powder (optional)

7 ounces pasteurized paneer, drained and cut into ½-inch dice

1 cup chopped ripe vine-ripened tomatoes

1½ cups frozen chopped spinach (about 12 ounces), defrosted and drained

Salt and freshly ground pepper, to taste

1. Heat the olive oil in a nonstick saucepan over medium heat. Add the onions and sauté until golden brown, stirring occasionally, about 7 minutes. Add the fresh ginger, garlic, turmeric, and chili powder, if using, and sauté for 30 seconds longer.
2. Add the paneer and tomatoes and cook for 3 minutes, then stir in the spinach and cook until heated through, about 5 minutes. Adjust seasonings and serve immediately. Refrigerate leftovers.

▶ *Cooking Tip:* Twelve ounces of fresh baby spinach can be used instead of frozen spinach. Wash, trim the stems, then coarsely chop the spinach and cook it according to the directions in Step 2.

▶ *Health Tip:* Use only pasteurized paneer (see Listeriosis Warning, page 129).

▶ *Complete Meal Ideas:* Serve this spinach paneer with:

   Brown rice (you might want to try the Lentil, Brown
      Rice, and Mushroom Pilaf, page 232)
   Reduced-fat 2% milk or low-fat yogurt (you might want to try
      the Cucumber-Tomato Yogurt Salad, page 172)
   Fresh fruit or sorbet

APPROXIMATE NUTRITIONAL INFORMATION: Serving size: one-sixth of the spinach paneer (Note: Because paneer is not included in Nutritionist Pro software, 7 ounces of feta cheese was used for the following calculations.); Calories: 156 cals; Protein: 7 g; Carbohydrates: 8 g; Fat: 12 g; Fiber: 2 g; Sodium: 400 mg; Vitamin A: 5,042 IU; Vitamin C: 14 mg; Folic Acid: 86 mcg; Calcium: 232 mg; Diabetic Exchange: Fat 2, Vegetable 2

kshama vyas's traditional indian dal

What's in this for baby and me? Protein, folic acid, vitamin C, iron, and fiber.

THE MAINSTAY OF Indian meals, dal is a stew made from lentils or other split beans, combined with garlic, ginger, and spices. Chock-full of protein, folic acid, vitamin C, iron, and fiber, with some vitamin A and the B vitamins thrown in, this dish provides a whopping amount of nutrients. Please don't be turned off by the long list of spices; many of them are used in recipes throughout this book.

Serves 6 (makes about 4 cups)

1½ cups red lentils, rinsed and drained

2 tablespoons canola oil

½ cup chopped onions

2 tablespoons minced fresh ginger

2 teaspoons minced garlic

1 teaspoon garam masala or curry powder

1 teaspoon ground cumin

1 teaspoon turmeric

1½ cups diced vine-ripened tomatoes (from about 3 large tomatoes)

Salt and freshly ground pepper, to taste

3 tablespoons chopped fresh cilantro leaves, for garnish (optional)

1. Combine the lentils and 4 cups of water in a medium saucepan. Bring to a boil, then reduce the heat and simmer strongly for 15 to 20 minutes, or until the lentils are tender. (It should be the consistency of a very thick pea soup.) Cover and set aside.
2. Heat the canola oil in a medium skillet over medium heat until hot. Add the onions and cook until golden brown, about 7 minutes. Add the ginger, garlic, chili, garam masala or curry powder, cumin, and turmeric, and sauté, stirring constantly, for 1 minute. Stir in the vine-ripened tomatoes and cook for 2 minutes. Remove from heat and stir this onion-spice mixture into the reserved lentils.
3. Adjust the seasonings, garnish with the cilantro, if using, and serve.

▶ *Timesaving Tip:* Use 1 cup canned diced tomatoes, drained.

▶ *Storage Tip:* The dal will keep refrigerated for 5 days, and it can be frozen for up to 1 month.

▶ **Complete Meal Ideas:** Serve this dal with:

Brown rice, a whole wheat pita pocket, or an Indian bread

Green salad or vegetable (you might want to try the Spinach Paneer, page 269)

Reduced-fat 2% milk or low-fat yogurt (you might want to try
the Cucumber-Tomato Yogurt Salad, page 172)

Fresh fruit or sorbet

APPROXIMATE NUTRITIONAL INFORMATION: Serving size: 1¼ cups dal; Calories: 221 cals; Protein: 14 g; Carbohydrates: 32 g; Fat: 5 g; Fiber: 15 g; Sodium: 11 mg; Vitamin C: 17 mg; Folic Acid: 218 mcg; Iron: 5 mg; Diabetic Exchange: Bread/Starch 2, Meat (Lean) 1

uses for tofu

If you are a vegetarian, tofu is most likely a big part of your diet, and you probably consume it in many of the ways listed below. If you are new to tofu, give some of these cooking tips a try.

- ▶ Add marinated firm tofu to stir-fries, curries, fajitas, burritos, tacos, or other Asian, Indian, or Mexican dishes.

- ▶ Use crumbled firm tofu in pasta sauces or to stuff pasta shells.

- ▶ Use grilled firm tofu to make vegetable and tofu sandwiches or roll-ups.

- ▶ Add crumbled or cubed firm tofu to chili, casseroles, and vegetable dishes.

- ▶ Add soft or thinly sliced firm tofu to lasagna layers.

- ▶ Top a green salad with pieces of sautéed or grilled marinated firm tofu.

- ▶ Scramble crumbled tofu instead of eggs and top it with sautéed vegetables.

- ▶ Add cubed firm or soft tofu to miso soup and other soups.

- ▶ Use silken tofu in salad dressings, mayonnaise, tartar sauce, or dips.

- ▶ Use silken tofu in pureed vegetable soups and chowders instead of cream or milk.

- ▶ Use silken tofu in macaroni and cheese instead of cream or milk.

- ▶ Use silken tofu in milk shakes, smoothies, and other blender drinks.

- ▶ Use silken or soft tofu in pie fillings, sorbets, cheesecake, or mousse.

- ▶ Use silken tofu in batters that call for yogurt or sour cream.

marvelous main courses

~

WE ALL LEAD hectic lives. Juggling family and career, or just family alone, is no easy task.

So, what's for dinner?

This is perhaps the most dreaded question of the day. Putting a hot meal on the table at the end of a long day is a true challenge, even for the best home cooks. Menu planning is an art, and, depending on your organizational skills, time constraints, energy level, and general taste preferences, meals can be planned in advance for the week, for the day, or on the spur of the moment in the grocery store. Whatever your method, obstacles such as morning sickness, general fatigue, or the need for bed rest can thwart even the best intentions to plan home-cooked meals. This is where restaurants and stores selling high-quality prepared and semi-prepared foods fit in. Read labels carefully to make the healthiest choices possible. A ready-to-serve well-balanced dinner can be as simple as a store-bought roasted chicken, a salad from the salad bar, V-8 juice, and a glass of milk—all to go.

THINGS TO REMEMBER
WHEN YOU HAVE NO TIME TO COOK

- Healthy meals do not need to be hot, or fancy.
- Keep your freezer well stocked with healthy foods, both homemade and store-bought.
- Vegetable juice or carrot sticks are an adequate substitute for a vegetable.
- Double your favorite recipes to have leftovers for future meals.
- Make meals on the weekends for busy weekdays.
- When grilling chicken, beef, or vegetables, cook extras and use the leftovers in salads, sandwiches, fajitas, or burritos.

- Use easy-to-prepare, fallback recipes that you know your family likes. Don't try a new recipe when you're in a rush: frustration is the most likely outcome.
- Try using a slow cooker to have your meals ready when you get home.
- Cook side dishes, such as grains and vegetables, ahead of time.
- Cook meals in segments whenever you have free time (see How to Make Dinner Ahead, page 281).

EATING OUT

HECTIC WORK SCHEDULES, a heavy social calendar, or a necessary break from the kitchen are some of the reasons we eat out. If you maintain a nutritionally balanced diet when dining out, there is little reason to feel guilty. If, on the other hand, you continually order the greasiest dish on the menu, eat all the bread in the bread basket, and pig out at dessert, you need to reevaluate your eating habits, pregnant or not. Following are some tips to help you make healthy choices when dining out for breakfast, lunch, or dinner.

Tips for Eating in Restaurants

- Inform your waiter of any special dietary needs you have before you order.
- If your dish does not look good or taste good, don't be shy—send it back. After all, you're paying for it!
- Keep in mind your nutritional needs when ordering. Ask yourself: Did I get enough protein today, or should I have the chicken or fish? How am I doing in the fiber department? Vegetables? Calcium? Iron?
- Ask for all meat, poultry, and fish to be cooked well-done.
- Avoid greasy and fatty foods.
- Avoid dishes with lots of sauce or gravy, or ask for it on the side.
- Eat the healthy, whole grain breads and avoid highly salted or greasy breads. Don't add butter to your bread, because most restaurant foods contain more fat than home-cooked meals.
- Stay away from salads made with mayonnaise, especially at salad bars.
- Always survey a salad bar and make sure everything is clean and properly chilled. Choose a light salad dressing without mayonnaise, or, better yet, make your own from the oil and vinegar. Stay away from artificial foods such as bacon bits.
- Avoid high-calorie desserts. Opt for fresh fruit or fruit sorbet for dessert.
- Don't order dairy-based desserts that are served off a dessert cart without refrigeration.
- Avoid buying any food from street vendors, especially hot dogs.

It's a fact of life in our fast-paced society that at least at some time during pregnancy, you will probably eat in a fast food restaurant. It might be at a rest stop along the highway, or you might finally give in to your preschooler begging you for a Happy Meal. Whatever the reason, fast food does not have to put you on a guilt trip as long as you make smart, healthy choices. The three major concerns with fast food are high calories, fat, and sodium.

Tips for Choosing Fast Foods

- Try to select fast food restaurants or chains that offer salad bars, baked potatoes, baked chicken or fish, burritos, or grilled (not fried) meats and poultry.
- Do not order deep-fried foods. Opt for baked, broiled, or grilled items. Batter on chicken, fish, and onion rings acts as a sponge, absorbing large amounts of fat. Deep-fried chicken or fish could end up having three times the amount of fat of a plain grilled hamburger.
- Order your sandwiches without sauces. Add fresh fixings, such as lettuce, tomatoes, onions, and pickles, to them.
- Avoid bacon, sausages, pepperoni, and other processed meats that are high in fat, sodium, nitrites, and nitrates. Opt for a vegetarian pizza or a simple cheese pizza.
- Choose smart toppings for your baked potato. Use a minimal amount of sour cream, margarine, or butter, and opt for vegetable (broccoli or spinach) toppings, salsa, pasteurized cheese, or low-fat cottage cheese.
- Salad bars and packaged salads are excellent low-fat alternatives. However, you can quickly turn your low-fat salad into a high-fat nightmare by piling on the wrong toppings.
- Avoid croissant sandwiches, hot dogs, french fries, onion rings, and deep-fried fruit pies.
- Bean dishes, such as baked beans, chili with beans, and bean salad, are all smart choices because they add protein, iron, and fiber to your diet.
- Avoid fruits in heavy syrup. Opt for fresh fruits if available.
- Do not use fast foods as snack foods or mini meals between your three main meals.
- Be more careful with your food choices for the rest of the day if you have eaten fast food. Try to fit in fresh fruits and vegetables (even V-8 juice) at some point.

Tips for Diabetics Dining Out

Diabetics have unique eating challenges that can be difficult to keep track of, especially when dining out. If you were diabetic before pregnancy or have been diagnosed with gestational diabetes, the following tips should help you make healthy decisions when dining out. Be sure to seek the advice of your doctor, certified diabetes educator, or registered dietitian if you have any questions regarding certain meals or foods, or how they fit into your diabetic meal plan.

- Remember your meal plan. If you have just received your diet plan or are on a new plan, carry a copy of it with you so you can make smart choices from a menu.
- Watch portion sizes. Some restaurants give you more-than-you-could-ever-eat portions, but this does not mean you have to clean your plate. Ask your waiter to modify your portion in accordance with your diet, or modify it yourself when your meal arrives, and take some home. Don't equate the cost of the dish with having to finish it.
- Avoid fats. Choose baked, grilled, or broiled dishes without added fat, gravy, or sauce; or ask that the gravy or sauce be served separately. (This applies to salad dressings as well.)
- Avoid all deep-fried foods, no matter how tempting they sound.
- Trim any visible fat from your meat. If your diet plan has only 1 fat exchange for your meal, use half a portion of butter and half a portion of salad dressing.
- Plan for your starch intake. If you choose the bread as an appetizer, be sure to count it against the starch exchanges in the rest of your meal.
- Always opt for fresh fruit for dessert. Ask your waiter for a piece of fresh fruit, even if it is not on the menu, or plan ahead and carry some fruit with you.
- Order the type of milk that fits your diet pattern.
- Remember your list of "free foods" for simple pleasures.

marvelous main courses

Spaghetti with Meat Sauce

Best-Ever American Meat Loaf

Flank Steak with Salsa Verde

Quick and Easy Chicken Curry

Chicken or Veal Cutlets with Mushroom-Caper Sauce

Mary Mulard's Baked Chicken

Marinated Grilled Chicken or Beef Fajitas

Moroccan-Style Chicken Stew

Chicken with Homemade Barbecue Sauce

Juicy Turkey Burgers

Homemade Chicken Tenders

Spice-Rubbed Pork Chops

Marinated Grilled or Broiled Lamb Chops

Sautéed Shrimp with Pasta

Shrimp and Vegetable Stir-Fry

Crab Cakes with Red Bell Pepper Sauce

Sautéed Salmon on a Bed of Greens with Citrus Vinaigrette

Roasted Salmon with Papaya Salsa

Tilapia Mediterranean Style

Shrimp with Asparagus and Red Bell Peppers

Grilled Arctic Char with Artichoke–Green Olive Tapenade

Sautéed Halibut with Garlic-Herb Butter

Canned Wild Salmon Patties with Dill-Yogurt Sauce

Marinated Grilled Chicken with Cilantro Dipping Sauce

Beef with Broccoli

RECIPE NOTES

SOME NOTES ABOUT the recipes in this chapter:

- Buy the freshest ingredients you can find. Use them promptly to maximize their vitamin and nutrient content. Check all expiration dates.
- Buy high-quality meats and poultry on sale and freeze them. Whenever possible and affordable, choose minimally processed, all-natural meats and poultry that are antibiotic-, hormone-, and preservative-free.
- Fish and shellfish are always best if prepared on the day they are purchased.
- Use an instant-read thermometer to avoid any doubt about whether something is cooked well-done or not. Cook and eat all of your food well-done during pregnancy.
- Avoid cross-contamination from juices of meat, poultry, and seafood. Keep raw meat, poultry, and seafood away from other foods, and after cutting or handling them, wash your hands, the cutting board, knife, and countertops with hot, soapy water, or use an anti-bacterial spray cleanser.
- Marinating food is an extra step, but it greatly improves the taste of any dish.
- Discard all marinades, rubs, or sauces that have come in contact with raw foods, and do not use them to baste foods on the grill or under the broiler.
- Place all cooked foods on clean plates or serving platters.
- Salt to taste, but be cautious when adding salt to dishes that contain high-sodium ingredients, such as olives, anchovies, or canned vegetables or beans.
- All of the sauces, marinades, and rubs in this book can be used with any meat, poultry, seafood, or tofu.
- Allow meat and poultry to rest for 5 minutes after cooking. It will be juicier and more tender if the meat relaxes.
- Slice cooked meats and poultry with a sharp knife against the grain on a slight angle. This particularly applies to flank steak, skirt steak, and chicken breasts.
- Be sure to clean your grill every time you use it. Nothing is worse than a beautiful piece of salmon or steak that tastes like a dirty grill.
- If broiling anything, watch it very carefully. Never leave the broiler unattended.
- Slow cooker instructions are given in some of the recipes.
- Freeze dishes in meal-size portions in zip-lock bags or small plastic containers. Label and date everything.
- Remove the child's portion of a dish before adding spices, fresh herbs, or anything that your child may not like.

protein sources

FOOD	SERVING SIZE	PROTEIN (G)
Cooked chicken	3 ounces	26
Roasted turkey breast	3 ounces	26
Roasted pork loin or chops	3 ounces	24
Cooked beef	3 ounces	23
Cooked shrimp	4 ounces	23
Canned tuna fish	3 ounces	22
Cured ham	3 ounces	19
Cooked salmon	3 ounces	19
Low-fat cottage cheese	½ cup	16
Cooked catfish	3 ounces	15
Tempeh	½ cup	15
Cheddar cheese	1 cup	14
Low-fat yogurt	1 cup	13
Hard-boiled egg	1 egg	13
Cooked edamame	⅓ cup	11
Extra-firm tofu	2 ounces	11
Roasted peanuts	¼ cup	10
Cooked lentils	½ cup	9
Deli ham	2 ounces	9
Peanut butter	2 tablespoons	8
Reduced-fat 2% milk	1 cup	8
Kidney beans	½ cup	7
Cooked chickpeas	½ cup	7
Mozzarella string cheese	1 item	7
Vegetarian baked beans	½ cup	6
Turkey loaf (breast meat)	4 slices	6
Jarlsberg cheese	1 slice	6
Muenster cheese	1 slice	6
Kraft Singles	1 slice	4
Low-fat frozen yogurt	½ cup	4

HOW TO MAKE DINNER AHEAD

- *Spaghetti with Meat Sauce:* Cook the meat sauce ahead; freeze. Cook the pasta ahead. Microwave to reheat.
- *Best-Ever American Meat Loaf:* Form and bake the meat loaf ahead; microwave to reheat.
- *Flank Steak with Salsa Verde:* Marinate the flank steak up to two days in advance. Make the salsa verde ahead; freeze. The flank steak is best just off the grill, but it can be grilled a bit ahead.
- *Quick and Easy Chicken Curry:* Marinate the chicken and vegetables; cook ahead. Make the rice ahead; microwave to reheat.
- *Chicken or Veal Cutlets with Mushroom-Caper Sauce:* Cook ahead. Make the noodles ahead. Microwave to reheat.
- *Mary Mulard's Baked Chicken:* Assemble the casserole up to six hours before baking; refrigerate.
- *Marinated Grilled Chicken or Beef Fajitas:* Marinate the chicken or beef up to two days in advance. Grill, broil, or sauté in advance. Cook the onions and bell peppers up to two days in advance. Microwave to reheat.
- *Moroccan-Style Chicken Stew:* Cook ahead (use a slow cooker); freeze. Microwave to reheat.
- *Chicken with Homemade Barbecue Sauce:* Make the barbecue sauce ahead. Marinate the chicken up to two days ahead. Bake the chicken and grill or broil at the last minute.
- *Juicy Turkey Burgers:* Form the burgers ahead. Cook the burgers ahead. Microwave to reheat.
- *Homemade Chicken Tenders:* Bake the tenders ahead; freeze. Use a conventional oven or microwave to reheat.
- *Spice-Rubbed Pork Chops:* Make the spice rub ahead. Marinate the pork chops ahead. The pork chops are best cooked just before serving, but they can be made ahead and reheated in a microwave or conventional oven.
- *Marinated Grilled or Broiled Lamb Chops:* Make the marinade ahead. Marinate the lamb chops up to two days in advance. The lamb chops are best cooked just before serving, but they can be made ahead and reheated in a microwave or conventional oven.
- *Sautéed Shrimp with Pasta:* Make the shrimp ahead. Make the pasta ahead. Microwave to reheat.
- *Shrimp and Vegetable Stir-Fry:* Prepare all of the vegetables and cook the rice up to one day ahead. Stir-fry at the last minute.
- *Crab Cakes with Red Bell Pepper Sauce:* Make the red bell pepper sauce up to three days ahead. Form the crab cakes ahead; cook ahead. Microwave to reheat.
- *Sautéed Salmon on a Bed of Greens with Citrus Vinaigrette:* Make the vinaigrette up to three days ahead. Sauté the salmon ahead. Mix the salad ahead, but dress it at the last minute.

- *Roasted Salmon with Papaya Salsa:* Make the papaya salsa up to three hours ahead. Cook the salmon ahead. Microwave to reheat.
- *Tilapia Mediterranean Style:* Cook ahead and microwave to reheat. Or, make just the sauce ahead (the herbs will lose their bright green color but this does not affect the taste) and cook the fish just before serving. Make the rice ahead.
- *Shrimp with Asparagus and Red Bell Peppers:* Make the sauce and cook the asparagus and red bell peppers in advance.
- *Grilled Arctic Char with Artichoke–Green Olive Tapenade:* Make the tapenade up to five days ahead. Grill the fish at the last minute.
- *Sautéed Halibut with Garlic-Herb Butter:* Make the garlic-herb butter five days ahead or freeze. Cook the fish at the last minute.
- *Canned Wild Salmon Patties with Dill-Yogurt Sauce:* The dill-yogurt sauce can be made and the salmon patties can be formed one day ahead. Cook the patties ahead. Microwave to reheat.
- *Marinated Grilled Chicken with Cilantro Dipping Sauce:* Marinate the chicken one day ahead. Grill in advance. Microwave to reheat.
- *Beef with Broccoli:* Cook the broccoli one day ahead.

pantry items for marvelous main courses

Fresh Produce
Asparagus
Avocados
Baby greens
Broccoli florets
Carrots: regular and peeled baby carrots
Celery
Cherry tomatoes
Fresh herbs: basil, cilantro, dill, mint, parsley, rosemary, thyme
Garlic
Ginger
Lemons
Limes
Mushrooms: button or cremini
Navel oranges
Onions: sweet (such as Vidalia), yellow, red
Papayas
Red bell peppers
Scallions
Shallots
Snow peas
Zucchini

Meats, Poultry, and Fish
Arctic char
Beef rib eye
Beef skirt steak
Boneless, skinless chicken breasts
Chicken tenders
Flank steak
Ground turkey
Halibut steaks
Jumbo lump crabmeat or back fin crabmeat, or a combination
Lamb chops (about 1½ inches thick)
Lean ground beef

Meat loaf mixture of beef, pork, and veal
Medium shrimp
Pork chops (about 1 inch thick)
Roasted chicken or cooked chicken
Shrimp
Skinless chicken parts (bone-in)
Skinned salmon fillet
Skin-on salmon fillet and steaks
Thin-sliced chicken cutlets
Tilapia
Veal cutlets

Dairy and Soy Products
Grade A large eggs
Half-and-half (preferably ultra-pasteurized)
Heavy cream (preferably ultra-pasteurized)
Parmesan cheese (grated)
Part-skim ricotta cheese
Plain low-fat yogurt
Swiss cheese
Unsalted butter
Whole milk

Canned, Bottled, and Jarred Staples
Anchovy filets or anchovy paste
Artichoke hearts
Canola oil
Canola oil cooking spray
Capers (small or medium)
Chickpeas (7¾-ounce can)
Condensed chicken soup (any kind) (10¾-ounce can)
Dijon mustard
Fat-free low-sodium stock (any kind) (14.5-ounce can)

Fish sauce
Green olives (pitted)
Hoisin sauce
Honey
Kalamata olives or other brine-cured
    black olives (preferably pitted)
Ketchup
Light mayonnaise
Mandarin oranges in light syrup or
    juice (8-ounce can)
Olive oil
Peeled and diced tomatoes
    (14.5-ounce can)
Pineapple juice
Rice vinegar (seasoned)
Rice wine
Sesame oil (toasted)
Soy sauce (regular or light)
Tomato paste
Tomato sauce (15-ounce can)
Wild salmon (red; 14.75-ounce can)
Worcestershire sauce

Dry Staples
Bread crumbs (plain or seasoned)
Cornstarch
Enriched all-purpose flour (preferably
    unbleached)

Enriched linguine and spaghetti (thin
    or regular)
Enriched medium egg noodles
Fajita-size tortillas (6- or 7-inch)
Light or dark raisins
Nuts: cashew nuts, roasted peanuts
Quick-dissolving flour (such as
    Wondra or Pillsbury Shake and
    Blend)
Sugar: brown and white

Herbs and Spices
Chili powder
Dried oregano
Dried tarragon
Garlic powder
Ground allspice, cinnamon, and/or
    cloves
Ground cumin
Ground ginger
Italian seasoning
Mild curry powder
Old Bay seasoning

From the Salad Bar
Diced onions
Broccoli florets
Sliced mushrooms
Sliced red bell peppers

e. coli warning

Escherichia coli O157:H7 is a bacterium, usually found in undercooked contaminated ground beef, that causes food-borne illness. Other known means of infection are drinking unpasteurized milk and juice, swimming in or drinking sewage-contaminated water, and consuming sprouts, lettuce, and salami. The poor hygiene of infected persons (or caretakers of those persons) suffering from diarrhea can also spread the bacteria.

Escherichia coli O157:H7 can be found on a small number of cattle farms and can live in the intestines of healthy cattle. Meat can become contaminated during slaughter, and organisms can be thoroughly mixed into the beef when it is ground. Contaminated meat looks and smells normal. Bacteria present on the cow's udders or on equipment may get into raw milk, causing contamination. The symptoms of infection are usually severe bloody diarrhea and abdominal cramps, but symptoms are not always present. Fever is uncommon, and the illness usually runs its course in five to ten days.

Here are a few tips to prevent infection.[1]

▶ Cook all ground beef and hamburger thoroughly. Because beef can turn brown before disease-causing bacteria are killed, use an instant-read thermometer to check that ground beef has reached the well-done stage of 160°F. Wash the thermometer in between each test of the meat.

▶ Keep raw meat separate from uncooked foods. Wash hands, counters, and utensils with hot, soapy water after touching raw meat.

▶ Never put cooked hamburgers or ground beef back on the plate that held the raw patties.

▶ Drink only pasteurized milk, juice, and cider.

▶ Wash fruits and vegetables thoroughly, especially those that will not be cooked.

▶ Avoid alfalfa sprouts.

▶ Drink municipal water that has been treated with chlorine and other disinfectants, or drink bottled water.

▶ Avoid swallowing lake or pool water while swimming.

▶ Make sure that persons with diarrhea, especially children, wash their hands, to reduce the risk of spreading infection, and that anyone washes his or her hands after changing soiled diapers.

spaghetti with meat sauce

~

What's in this for baby and me? Protein, vitamins A and C, and folic acid.

Hɪɢʜ ɪɴ ᴘʀᴏᴛᴇɪɴ, vitamins A and C, and folic acid, and a good source of iron, this simple and tasty meat sauce is sure to become a dinner staple. Simmering the meat in milk or half-and-half softens it and gives the finished dish a slightly creamy consistency. Feel free to add your favorite sauce ingredients and omit any of the items that your children might not like, such as the mushrooms, red bell peppers, or fresh herbs. One and one-half cups of cooked enriched spaghetti is an excellent source of protein and folic acid, and a good source of iron, B vitamins, and fiber. Top your spaghetti with lots of Parmesan cheese for calcium.

serves 6 to 8 (makes about 8 cups sauce)

2 tablespoons olive oil

1 onion, finely diced

1 garlic clove, minced

2 teaspoons dried oregano

2 teaspoons dried Italian seasoning

1 pound lean ground beef

1 cup whole milk or half-and-half

8 ounces mushrooms (any kind), washed, stems trimmed, and thinly sliced

1 small red bell pepper, washed, cored, seeded, and cut into small dice

One 15-ounce can tomato sauce

One 14.5-ounce can diced tomatoes (do not drain)

Salt and freshly ground pepper, to taste

Enriched spaghetti or your favorite pasta (see headnote), cooked according to package directions

3–4 tablespoons chopped fresh basil, parsley, or dill, for garnish

Grated Parmesan cheese, for the table

1. In a large heavy-based non-reactive saucepan, heat the olive oil over medium-high heat. Add the onion and sauté for 3 minutes. Add the garlic, oregano, and Italian seasoning and sauté for 1 minute longer.
2. Crumble the ground beef into the saucepan and sauté for 5 minutes, stirring and breaking up any large lumps of meat with the back of a wooden spoon. Add the milk (see Cooking Tip below), mushrooms, and bell pepper and simmer gently for 30 minutes, or until most of the liquid has evaporated.
3. Add the tomato sauce and diced tomatoes and simmer for 30 minutes longer, or until the sauce has thickened to the desired consistency. (Cook the pasta while the sauce is simmering.)
4. Adjust the seasoning, add the basil, and serve over the spaghetti. Pass the cheese at the table.

▶ **Cooking Tip:** It is essential to use very fresh milk or half-and-half. You will probably see a little bit of separation as the milk or half-and-half cooks, this is normal.

▶ **Timesaving Tip:** Use jarred pasta sauce.

▶ **Storage Tip:** The meat sauce keeps 3 days refrigerated, and it can be frozen for up to 1 month.

▶ **Diabetic Tip:** Reduce the portion size of cooked spaghetti to ¾ cup per serving.

▶ **Complete Meal Ideas:** Serve this spaghetti with:
   Green salad or a green vegetable (you might want to try a green
      salad with the Caesar Salad Dressing, page 168)
   Reduced-fat 2% milk or low-fat yogurt
   Fresh fruit that contains vitamin C

APPROXIMATE NUTRITIONAL INFORMATION: Meat Sauce: Serving size: 1 cup; Calories: 248 cals; Protein: 19 g; Carbohydrates: 11 g; Fat: 15 g; Fiber: 2 g; Sodium: 627 mg; Vitamin A: 1,489 IU; Vitamin C: 45 mg; Diabetic Exchange: Bread/Starch: .5, Fat 1.5, Meat (Medium Fat) 2

APPROXIMATE NUTRITIONAL INFORMATION: Spaghetti: Serving size: 1 ½ cups cooked spaghetti; Calories: 296 cals; Protein: 10 g; Carbohydrates: 60 g; Fat: 1 g; Fiber: 4 g; Sodium: 2 mg; Folic Acid: 147 mcg; Diabetic Exchange (values per ¾ cup serving): Bread/Starch: 2

best-ever american meat loaf

What's in this for baby and me? Protein.

MEAT LOAF IS to American cuisine what Norman Rockwell is to American art. Both conjure up images of family gatherings and happy times. Make this meat loaf using only beef, or a combination of beef, pork, and veal. If your kids object to green things in their meat loaf, leave out the herbs. You can't beat meat loaf for a powerful dose of protein, and a good dose of iron and vitamin C. Served hot with mashed potatoes or sweet potatoes, or eaten cold in a sandwich with some good mustard and baby pickles, meat loaf is just plain good!

serves 11

Canola oil or canola oil cooking spray for
    greasing the baking pan
GLAZE (optional)
    ¼ cup ketchup
    1 tablespoon molasses
    1 teaspoon seasoned rice vinegar
MEAT LOAF
    2 pounds lean ground beef (preferably
        chuck) or a meat loaf mix of pork, veal,
        and beef
    2 large eggs, lightly beaten

⅔ cup thinly sliced scallions
¼ cup chopped fresh parsley
¼ cup chopped fresh dill
1 teaspoon dried oregano
1 tablespoon Worcestershire sauce
2 teaspoons Dijon mustard
1 cup plain bread crumbs
1½ teaspoons salt
½ teaspoon freshly ground pepper, or a
    couple drops of Tabasco sauce
½ cup plain low-fat yogurt or whole milk

1. Preheat the oven to 350°F. Line a large baking pan with foil and lightly grease it.
2. To make the optional glaze, mix all of the ingredients in a measuring cup or a small bowl; set aside.
3. To make the meat loaf, combine all of the ingredients in a large bowl and mix with a fork or your hands (wet your hands first to reduce sticking) until well blended. (See the Cooking Tip below for checking the seasoning of the meat loaf mixture.) Form the meat loaf mixture into a large ball and transfer it to the baking pan. Using your hands, form it into an oval-shaped loaf approximately 10 inches long and 2½ inches high. Using the back of a spoon, evenly "frost" the meat loaf with the glaze, if using.
4. Bake for 1 hour and 25 to 30 minutes, or until completely cooked: an instant-read thermometer should read 160°F, and the juices should run clear when the center of the loaf is pierced with a knife or skewer. Remove the meat loaf from the oven and allow it to rest for 15 minutes before slicing.

▶ **Cooking Tip:** To check the seasoning before baking, spray a small skillet with canola oil cooking spray and cook about 1 tablespoon of the meat loaf mixture until well-done. Taste the cooked meat, and adjust the seasoning in remaining meat mixture if necessary.

▶ **Advance Preparation:** The meat loaf can be assembled up to 6 hours before baking and refrigerated. The baking time may increase by 10 to 15 minutes.

▶ **Storage Tip:** The meat loaf keeps 3 days refrigerated. It does not freeze well.

▶ **Health Tip:** Be sure to wash your hands thoroughly with warm water and soap for at least 20 seconds after handling the raw meat.

▶ **Complete Meal Ideas:** Serve this meat loaf with:
>   Mashed potatoes, baked potatoes, or sweet potatoes (you might want
>   to try the Southern-Style Sweet Potato Casserole, page 239)
>   Green salad or green vegetable (try one of Annie Mozer's Greens,
>   pages 242, or the Classic Creamed Spinach, page 237)
>   Reduced-fat 2% milk or low-fat yogurt
>   Fresh fruit that contains vitamin C

APPROXIMATE NUTRITIONAL INFORMATION: Serving size: one 4.5-ounce serving (about one-eleventh of the meat loaf); Calories: 300 cals; Protein: 27 g; Carbohydrates: 8 g; Fat: 17 g; Fiber: .5 g; Sodium: 499 mg; Diabetic Exchange: Bread/Starch .5, Meat (Medium Fat) 3.5

flank steak with salsa verde

What's in this for baby and me? Protein and vitamin C.

THE KEY TO a truly great flank steak is marinating it, for as long as possible, before grilling. The salsa verde, an excellent source of vitamin C, is a take on an Argentinean herb-and-garlic sauce called chimichurri that can also be served with poultry or fish, as well as meat. Like pesto, salsa verde can be frozen. The steak provides protein and a good dose of iron.

serves 4

One 1½-pound flank steak

MARINADE

¼ cup soy sauce

1 teaspoon canola oil

2 teaspoons seasoned rice vinegar or freshly squeezed lime juice

1 tablespoon Worcestershire sauce

1 garlic clove, minced

1 tablespoon minced fresh ginger, or 1 teaspoon ground ginger (optional)

1 tablespoon chopped fresh rosemary (optional)

SALSA VERDE (makes ⅓ cup) (optional)

1½ cups packed fresh cilantro leaves

3 anchovy fillets or 1 teaspoon anchovy paste (optional)

1½ tablespoons small or medium capers

1 garlic clove

1½ tablespoons freshly squeezed lemon juice, or to taste

¼ cup olive oil

Freshly ground pepper, to taste

1. Remove any visible fat from the flank steak. Using a fork, pierce the steak all over, then place it in a 1-gallon zip-lock bag or in a shallow pie dish and set aside.
2. To make the marinade, combine all of the ingredients in a small bowl or measuring cup and mix well. Add the marinade to the flank steak, turning to make sure that it is completely covered with the marinade, and refrigerate for at least 1 hour, or up to 48 hours.
3. To make the salsa verde, combine all of the ingredients in the bowl of a food processor and process until pureed and the sauce is slightly emulsified, scraping down the sides of the bowl as needed. Transfer to a serving bowl, cover with plastic wrap, placing it directly against the surface of the sauce (this is to prevent discoloration), and refrigerate.
4. Preheat the grill. Have a serving platter ready for the cooked flank steak. Grill the flank steak for 12 to 15 minutes, or until well-done; an instant-read thermometer should read 160°F. Transfer the meat to the platter and allow it to rest for 5 minutes for the juices to re-distribute and the meat to relax.

5. To serve, using a sharp knife held on a diagonal slant, on a chopping board with gutters to catch juices, slice the flank steak against the grain into ½-inch slices. Place the slices on the serving platter and serve immediately, with the salsa verde.

▶ **Health Tip:** Discard all leftover marinade—do not use it to baste the flank steak on the grill. Place the finished flank steak on a clean serving platter.

▶ **Advance Preparation:** The flank steak should marinate for at least 1 hour, and up to 48 hours.

▶ **Storage Tip:** The cooked flank steak and salsa verde keep 3 days refrigerated. The salsa verde can be frozen for up to 1 month.

▶ **Complete Meal Ideas:** Serve this steak with:
    Baked potatoes, brown rice, pasta salad, or cornbread (you might want to try the Noodles with Spinach, Red Bell Peppers, and Sesame Dressing, page 148, or the Pink Potato Salad, page 155)
    Green vegetable or green salad
    Reduced-fat 2% milk or low-fat yogurt
    Fresh fruit that contains vitamin C (if you are not using the salsa verde)

APPROXIMATE NUTRITIONAL INFORMATION: Flank steak: Serving size: 4 ounces; Calories: 259 cals; Protein: 35 g; Carbohydrates: 0; Fat: 12 g; Fiber: 0; Sodium: 75 mg; Diabetic Exchange: Meat (Lean) 5

APPROXIMATE NUTRITIONAL INFORMATION: Salsa verde: Serving size: 2 tablespoons; Calories: 90 cals; Protein: .9 g; Carbohydrates: 1 g; Fat: 9 g; Fiber: .4g; Sodium: 143 mg; Vitamin C: 15 mg; Diabetic Exchange: Fat 2

quick and easy chicken curry

What's in this for baby and me? Protein and vitamins A and C.

Packed with protein and vitamins A and C, this light curry is flavorful and not too filling.

serves 3

1 pound chicken tenders, cut into ½-inch slices on the diagonal

1 red bell pepper, cored, seeded, quartered, and cut into ¼-inch strips

1 medium sweet onion (such as Vidalia), halved and thinly sliced

1 tablespoon mild curry powder

1 tablespoon sugar

3 tablespoons canola oil

1 tablespoon fish sauce or soy sauce

3 scallions, trimmed and sliced into large pieces

¼ cup chopped fresh cilantro, or to taste

Freshly squeezed lime juice, to taste

Lime wedges for the table

1. Combine the chicken, red bell pepper, onion, curry powder, sugar, 2 tablespoons of the canola oil, and fish sauce in a bowl. Mix until well combined, then allow to marinate, covered and refrigerated, for at least 30 minutes, or overnight.
2. Heat the remaining 1 tablespoon canola oil in a large nonstick skillet over medium-high heat. Add half of the chicken mixture and half of the scallions and sauté for about 5 to 7 minutes, or until the chicken is cooked. (Note: Use a splatter screen to reduce cleanup.) Transfer the cooked chicken to a serving bowl and cover with foil to keep warm. Reheat the skillet, add the remaining chicken mixture and scallions, and repeat the procedure.
3. Garnish with the cilantro and a squeeze of fresh lime juice. Serve immediately, with the lime wedges.

▶ *Variation:* Substitute 1 pound peeled medium or large raw shrimp for the chicken. Allow them to marinate for 20 minutes. The cooking time will be about 5 minutes. You can replace the red bell peppers with broccoli florets, sliced zucchini, or any other vegetable.

▶ *Storage Tip:* This chicken curry keeps 3 days refrigerated, and it can be frozen for up to 1 month.

▶ **Complete Meal Ideas:** Serve this curry with:

Brown rice, rice noodles, quinoa, or soba noodles

Green vegetable or green salad (you might want to try the Vegetables with Lemon, Olive Oil, and Fresh Herbs, page 153)

Reduced-fat 2% milk or low-fat yogurt

Fresh fruit

APPROXIMATE NUTRITIONAL INFORMATION: Serving size: 7 ounces chicken curry dish; Calories: 236 cals; Protein: 25 g; Carbohydrates: 8 g; Fat: 11 g; Fiber: 1 g; Sodium: 397 mg; Vitamin A: 1,824 IU; Vitamin C: 66 mg; Diabetic Exchange: Bread/Starch .5, Meat (Medium Fat) 3

smart choice frozen foods

The frozen foods market is expanding daily to meet the needs of busy people. Many whole foods stores stock their shelves with high-quality frozen foods, ranging from vegetarian lasagna and ravioli to hearty beef stews. Usually these "in-house" prepared frozen foods contain fewer preservatives and less sodium than the big-name brands carried by large-chain grocery stores. When choosing frozen foods, look for foods containing the highest amount of protein (usually about 10 grams) and the least amount of fat per serving. Reduced-fat frozen dinners are good options, and frozen vegetarian dishes tend to be lower in fat. While frozen foods are convenient, they can be expensive—read labels carefully, because a few pennies more might buy you extra protein and less fat. Also, if you are on a reduced-sodium diet, keep in mind that most frozen foods have a high sodium content.

chicken or veal cutlets
with mushroom-caper sauce

What's in this for baby and me? Protein.

Hɪɢʜ ɪɴ ᴘʀᴏᴛᴇɪɴ and a good source of vitamins A and C and iron, this tasty dish is sure to become a favorite. The heavy cream is optional, but it adds a velvety smoothness to the sauce. Do not substitute milk or half-and-half, because they tend to curdle in the sauce. Have your rice or wide egg noodles ready before making the recipe.

serves 4

¼ cup all-purpose flour, for dredging the
    cutlets
½ teaspoon salt
12 to 16 ounces boneless, skinless thin-sliced
    chicken breast cutlets or thin-sliced veal
    cutlets (if cutlets are not available, see
    Cooking Tip below for instructions on
    using boneless, skinless chicken breasts)
1½ tablespoons canola oil
2 tablespoons unsalted butter
8 ounces mushrooms (any kind), washed,
    stems trimmed, and thinly sliced

One 14.5-ounce can fat-free low-sodium stock
2–3 tablespoons drained small or medium
    capers, or to taste
¼ cup heavy cream (optional)
1 tablespoon quick-dissolving flour (such as
    Wondra), to desired consistency
¼ cup chopped fresh parsley or dill or 1
    teaspoon dried tarragon (optional)
1 to 2 tablespoons freshly squeezed lemon
    juice, or to taste
Salt and freshly ground pepper, to taste

1. Have two large plates ready, one for the floured cutlets and the other for the cooked cutlets. Combine the flour and salt in a shallow dish or pie pan. Coat one cutlet at a time with flour, shake off any excess, and place on one of the plates; set aside.
2. Heat 1 tablespoon of the canola oil in a large nonstick skillet over medium-high heat until hot. Add half the chicken cutlets, and cook, turning only once, for about 3 minutes on each side, or until lightly browned and thoroughly cooked. (Note: The cooking time will depend on the thickness of the cutlets.) Transfer the cutlets to the clean plate, and cover loosely with foil. Add the remaining canola oil to the skillet, heat it, and cook the remaining cutlets. Transfer the cutlets to the plate. (Do not rinse the skillet.)
3. Melt the butter in the same skillet over medium-high heat. Add the mushrooms, if using, and sauté for 3 minutes. Add the stock and bring to a boil. Reduce the heat to low, add the capers and the heavy cream, if using, and simmer gently for 2 minutes. Stir in the quick-dissolving flour and simmer for 2 minutes more. Add

the chicken cutlets to the skillet and simmer until they are hot, about 3 to 5 minutes more.

4. Add the chopped parsley and lemon juice, adjust the seasoning, and serve immediately.

▶ *Cooking Tip:* If cutlets are not available, use boneless, skinless chicken breasts. Cut each breast horizontally in half, then pound each piece between two sheets of plastic wrap until 1/8 inch thick.

▶ *Storage Tip:* The cutlets and sauce keep for 3 days refrigerated. They do not freeze well. You may need to add a bit of water or stock to thin the sauce when reheating it.

▶ *Complete Meal Ideas:* Serve these cutlets with:
>   Egg noodles, brown rice, or potatoes (you might want to try the
>   Roasted New Potatoes with Garlic and Rosemary, page 267)
>   Green vegetable or green salad (you might want to try the Spinach
>   Salad with Mandarin Oranges and Toasted Almonds, page 163)
>   Reduced-fat 2% milk or low-fat yogurt
>   Fresh fruit that contains vitamin C

APPROXIMATE NUTRITIONAL INFORMATION: Serving size: one-quarter of the chicken cutlets with mushroom-caper sauce; Calories: 353 cals; Protein: 36 g; Carbohydrates: 5 g; Fat: 20 g; Fiber: 1 g; Sodium: 594 mg; Diabetic Exchange: Meat (Lean) 5

APPROXIMATE NUTRITIONAL INFORMATION: Serving size: one-quarter of the veal cutlets with mushroom-caper sauce; Calories: 483 cals; Protein: 34 g; Carbohydrates: 5 g; Fat: 36 g; Fiber: 1 g; Sodium: 597 mg; Diabetic Exchange: Fat 1, Meat (Medium Fat) 5

mary mulard's baked chicken

~

What's in this for baby and me? Protein and calcium.

FILLED WITH PROTEIN and calcium, and a good source of vitamin A, this baked chicken takes 10 minutes to prepare and about 50 minutes to bake. Serve it with elbow noodles or your kid's favorite pasta, and watch it disappear.

serves 6

1½ pounds (about 4) boneless, skinless
    chicken breasts
8 ounces (about 4 thick slices) Swiss cheese
One 10¾-ounce can condensed chicken soup

¼ cup water
¾ cup herb-seasoned stuffing mix or corn
    bread stuffing, coarsely crushed

1. Preheat the oven to 350°F.
2. Place the chicken breasts in an ungreased 8 x 8 x 2-inch baking dish. Cover them with the cheese slices; set aside.
3. In a small bowl, mix the chicken soup with the water until almost smooth. Pour the soup evenly over the chicken and top with the stuffing mix. Bake for 50 to 60 minutes, or until an instant-read thermometer inserted into the center (through the side) of a chicken breast reads 165°F.

▶ **Storage Tip:** The chicken keeps refrigerated for 3 days. It does not freeze well.

▶ **Complete Meal Ideas:** Serve this chicken with:
    Noodles, brown rice, or couscous
    A salad or vegetable (you might want to try the Asparagus,
        Hearts of Palm, and Tomato Salad, page 159)
    Reduced-fat 2% milk or low-fat yogurt
    Fresh fruit

APPROXIMATE NUTRITIONAL INFORMATION: Serving size: one-sixth baked chicken; Calories: 401 cals; Protein: 48 g; Carbohydrates: 10 g; Fat: 18 g; Fiber: .5 g; Sodium: 634 mg; Calcium: 389 mg; Diabetic Exchange: Bread/Starch .5, Meat (Medium Fat) 6

toxoplasmosis warning

Toxoplasmosis is an infection caused by the parasite *Toxoplasma gondii*, which can be transmitted by eating undercooked infected meat, or by handling soil or cat feces that contain the parasite. Others sources of infection may be raw goat's milk and raw eggs. Insects, such as flies and cockroaches, that have been in contact with cat feces can contaminate food as well.[2]

Swelling of the lymph nodes or flu-like symptoms (fever, fatigue, and sore throat) may be present, although most adults have no symptoms.[3] If a woman contracts toxoplasmosis for the first time during her pregnancy (active infection only occurs once in a lifetime, although the parasite remains in the body indefinitely), there is a 40 percent chance that her unborn child will also become infected. The risk and severity of the baby's infection depend partly on the timing of the mother's infection. Unborn children infected in early pregnancy are the most likely to suffer severe effects, which may include blindness, deafness, hydrocephalus (water on the brain), seizures, and mental retardation. Tests can determine whether an unborn child is infected, and medications can prevent or reduce severity of effects in unborn children. Toxoplasmosis can also result in miscarriage or stillbirth.

Pregnant women should take the following precautions to prevent toxoplasmosis.[4]

- ▶ Don't empty your cat's litter box; have someone else do this.

- ▶ Don't feed your cat raw or undercooked meat.

- ▶ Keep your cat indoors to prevent it from hunting birds or rodents.

- ▶ Don't eat raw or undercooked meat, especially lamb or pork. Meat should be cooked to an internal temperature of 160–165°F throughout.

- ▶ If you handle raw meat, wash your hands immediately with soap. Never touch your eyes, nose, or mouth with potentially contaminated hands.

- ▶ Wash all raw fruits and vegetables before you eat them.

- ▶ Wear gloves when gardening, since soil may contain the parasites from cats. Keep your hands away from your mouth and eyes, and wash your hands thoroughly when finished. Keep gardening gloves away from food products.

- ▶ Avoid children's sandboxes, as cats may use them as a litter box.

marinated grilled chicken or beef fajitas

~

What's in this for baby and me? Protein, iron, and vitamins A and C and folic acid.

GRILLED FAJITAS, AN excellent source of protein, vitamins A and C, and folic acid, and a good source of calcium, iron, fiber, and B vitamins, are always a hit. Some topping ideas include: grated cheese (such as cheddar or Monterey Jack), guacamole (store-bought or homemade) or sliced avocado, diced vine-ripened tomatoes, shredded lettuce, sliced pitted black olives, jalapeño peppers, sprigs of fresh cilantro, salsa, reduced-fat sour cream or plain yogurt, and lime wedges. Any leftover beef, chicken, vegetables, or tofu can be made into delicious sandwiches, quesadillas, or tacos.

serves 4

MARINADE

2 tablespoons canola oil

2 tablespoons seasoned rice vinegar or freshly squeezed lime juice

2 tablespoons Worcestershire sauce

1 large garlic clove, crushed

½ teaspoon ground cumin

1 teaspoon chili powder

1¼ to 1½ pounds beef skirt steak or boneless skinless chicken breasts (cut horizontally in half), or cutlets or a mixture

1 tablespoon canola oil

2 large bell peppers (any color), washed, cored, seeded, and cut into strips

1 sweet onion (such as Vidalia), thinly sliced

Twelve 7-inch flour tortillas

1. For the marinade, combine all of the ingredients in a small bowl, mix well, and set aside. (Note: If you plan to marinate the beef or chicken in a bowl rather than a zip-lock bag, use a large bowl to make the marinade.) Using a fork, pierce the beef (or chicken) all over to allow the marinade to seep in, then place it in a 1 gallon zip-lock bag. Add the marinade, seal (or cover with plastic wrap), and refrigerate for at least 30 minutes, or overnight.

2. Heat the canola oil in a large skillet over medium-high heat. Add the pepper and onion and sauté for 10 minutes. Remove from the heat, cover, and set aside.

3. To grill the beef or chicken, preheat the grill. The chicken will take longer to cook than the beef, so if you are serving both, start the chicken first. Have a clean platter ready for the cooked meat. Grill the chicken for approximately 10 to 12 minutes on each side, or until the juices run clear when the chicken is pierced with the tip of a knife and an instant-read thermometer inserted into the center (through the side) of the chicken breast reads 165°F. Grill the beef for approximately 6 to 8 minutes on each side, or until an instant-read thermometer inserted into the center of the meat reads 160°F. Transfer to the platter.

To broil the beef or chicken, preheat the broiler. Arrange the beef or chicken in a broiler pan lined with foil. Broil the chicken for approximately 12 minutes on each side, the beef for approximately 7 minutes on each side (refer to the well-done temperatures above). Transfer to the platter.

4. While the meat is cooking, heat the tortillas according to package directions. You can also heat them on the grill just before serving by toasting them for a minute or two on each side. Wrap the tortillas in foil to keep them warm.

5. Using a sharp knife and a chopping board with gutters to catch any juices, slice the cooked beef or chicken, against the grain, about ¼ inch thick on the diagonal, and serve immediately. Place all of your chosen toppings, including the pepper-onion mixture, in small bowls on the table.

▶ **Timesaving Tip:** Cut the beef or chicken into ¼-inch strips before marinating. This will cut the marinating time down to about 15 minutes, as the flavor will be more quickly absorbed into the meat. A grill rack might be necessary for the grill, but the strips can also be broiled or sautéed.

▶ **Variation:** You can replace the beef or chicken with peeled fresh large shrimp. Marinate for about 20 minutes, then grill, broil, or sauté for just a couple of minutes on each side—shrimp cook quickly. For vegetarian fajitas, marinate tofu, portobello mushrooms, or your favorite vegetables in the marinade for about 30 minutes, then grill or broil to desired tenderness. Slice into strips before serving.

▶ **Advance Preparation:** The beef or chicken should marinate for at least 30 minutes, and up to 12 hours. The sautéed pepper-onion mixture can be made 2 days in advance, covered, and refrigerated; reheat in a microwave oven.

▶ **Health Tip:** Discard all leftover marinade—do not use it to baste the beef or chicken on the grill or under the broiler. Place the finished beef or chicken on a clean serving platter. If your doctor has restricted your sodium intake, use only 1 tablespoon Worcestershire sauce and don't use olives as a topping. To reduce the fat, use low-fat cheese and low-fat or nonfat sour cream or yogurt as toppings.

▶ **Storage Tip:** The fajitas keep refrigerated for 3 days. They do not freeze well.

▶ **Complete Meal Ideas:** Serve these fajitas with:
  Green salad or vegetable (you might want to try the
    Edamame, Corn, and Bean Salad, page 247)
  Reduced-fat 2% milk or low-fat yogurt
  Fresh fruit that contains vitamin C

APPROXIMATE NUTRITIONAL INFORMATION: Chicken Fajitas: Serving size: one-sixth of the fajitas (including chicken, flour tortilla, and filling); Calories: 402 cals; Protein: 35 g; Carbohydrates: 40 g; Fat: 10 g; Fiber: 3 g; Sodium: 377 mg; Vitamin A: 2,281 IU; Vitamin C: 77 mg; Folic Acid: 95 mcg; Diabetic Exchange: Bread/Starch 2.5, Meat (Lean) 4

APPROXIMATE NUTRITIONAL INFORMATION: Beef Fajitas: Serving size: one-sixth of the fajitas (including beef, flour tortilla, and filling); Calories: 460 cals; Protein: 31 g; Carbohydrates: 40 g; Fat: 19 g; Fiber: 3 g; Sodium: 384 mg; Vitamin A: 2,261 IU; Vitamin C: 77 mg; B Vitamins: Thiamine: .4 mg, Riboflavin: .3 mg, Niacin: 7 mg; Folic Acid: 99 mcg; Iron 5 mg; Diabetic Exchange: Bread/Starch 2.5, Meat (Medium Fat) 3.5

fast food nightmares

The following nutritional contents of fast foods prove that a single meal in the fast food world can consume your entire daily allowance of calories, fats, and cholesterol with very few nutritional benefits.

MCDONALD'S BIG MAC HAMBURGER

600 calories (30% Daily Value of a 2,000-calorie intake)

33 g total fat (51%)

11 g saturated fat (55%)

85 mg cholesterol (28%)

MCDONALD'S LARGE FRENCH FRIES

540 calories (27%)

26 g total fat (40%)

5 g saturated fat (23%)

0 mg cholesterol (0%)

BURGER KING DOUBLE WHOPPER SANDWICH

980 calories (49%)

62 g total fat (95%)

22 g saturated fat (110%)

160 mg cholesterol (53%)

ONE 16-OUNCE COKE

195 calories (10%)

0 fat and cholesterol (0%)

sample smart choice fast food menus

BREAKFAST

English muffin with an egg

¾ cup fortified cereal with skim milk

8 ounces orange juice

8 ounces reduced-fat 2% milk

8 ounces decaf coffee or tea (optional)

LUNCH OR DINNER

Grilled chicken sandwich, plain roast beef sandwich,
or grilled hamburger/cheeseburger (no sauce)

2 cups prepared salad or salad from the salad bar

About 2 tablespoons reduced-fat salad dressing

8 ounces reduced-fat 2% milk

SAMPLE SALAD

2 cups spinach or dark green lettuce

A large spoonful of beans (kidney or chickpeas)

2–4 tablespoons light tuna or chopped egg

1 cup vegetables

¼ cup reduced-fat salad dressing

1 slice whole wheat bread or 2 whole wheat crackers

8 ounces reduced-fat 2% milk

moroccan-style chicken stew

What's in this for baby and me? Protein and vitamins A and C.

THIS FLAVOR-PACKED chicken stew is an excellent source of protein and vitamins A and C, and a good source of iron, folic acid, and fiber. Vegetarians can substitute tofu for the chicken and add more vegetables. Couscous, quinoa, rice, or tiny pasta (such as orzo or acini di pepe) mixed with a pat of butter or olive oil is the perfect side dish and can be cooked while the stew is simmering.

serves 6 to 8

¼ cup canola oil

1 tablespoon ground cumin

1 teaspoon ground ginger

½ teaspoon ground allspice, cinnamon, or
  cloves, or a mixture

2 pounds boneless, skinless chicken breasts
  or chicken tenders, cut into 1-inch cubes

1 medium onion (preferably a sweet onion like
  Vidalia), chopped

4 carrots, peeled and sliced, or 1½ cups sliced
  baby carrots

One 14.5-ounce can diced tomatoes, drained

½ cup fat-free low-sodium stock or water

1 tablespoon tomato paste

1 tablespoon sugar

About 1 cup (one 7¾-ounce can) chickpeas

1 medium zucchini, washed and diced, or one
  8½-ounce can artichoke hearts, drained
  and quartered

1 cup light or dark raisins

1–2 teaspoons quick-dissolving flour (such as
  Wondra), to desired consistency

1 teaspoon salt

Freshly ground pepper, to taste

3 tablespoon chopped fresh parsley or
  cilantro, for garnish

1. Combine the canola oil, cumin, ginger, and allspice in a 6-quart heavy-based non-reactive saucepan or Dutch oven and heat over medium-high heat for 30 seconds, or just until the spices give off their aroma. Add the chicken and sauté for 3 minutes, turning to cook on all sides. Add the onion and sauté for 3 minutes. Add the carrots, diced tomatoes, stock, tomato paste, and sugar and bring to a boil. Reduce the heat and simmer gently, covered, for 20 minutes.

2. Add the chickpeas, zucchini, and raisins, if using, and continue to simmer for 15 minutes, or just until the zucchini is tender. During the last 5 minutes of simmering, add the flour (adjust the amount to desired consistency) and stir gently.

3. Add the salt and pepper, garnish with the parsley, and serve immediately.

▶ *Slow Cooker Instructions:* Use ¼ cup chicken stock instead of ½ cup. Ideally, you should use chicken meat on the bone, such as skinless chicken thighs or breast meat on the bone, as it tends to dry out less than boneless chicken breasts during cooking.

1. Using a large nonstick skillet instead of a saucepan, follow the instructions for Step 1 and cook the onions with the chicken. Transfer the contents of the skillet to a slow cooker, then add the carrots, diced tomatoes, stock, tomato paste, and sugar. Cover and cook on low for 6 to 8 hours, or on high for 4 to 6 hours.

2. Up to 1 hour and at least 30 minutes before turning the slow cooker off, add the chickpeas, zucchini, raisins, and quick-dissolving flour.

3. Once cooked, season with salt and pepper, garnish with parsley, and serve immediately, or bring to room temperature, cover, and refrigerate or freeze.

▶ *Storage Tip:* This stew keeps for 3 days refrigerated, and it can be frozen for up to 1 month. To prevent scorching, reheat over medium heat or in a microwave oven.

▶ *Complete Meal Ideas:* Serve this stew with:
Couscous, quinoa, or brown rice
Green salad or vegetable (if you did not use many vegetables in the stew)
Reduced-fat 2% milk or low-fat yogurt
Fresh fruit that contains vitamin C

APPROXIMATE NUTRITIONAL INFORMATION: Serving size: One-tenth of the Moroccan-style chicken stew; Calories: 288 cals; Protein: 29 g; Carbohydrates: 23 g; Fat: 9 g; Fiber: 3 g; Sodium: 333 mg; Vitamin A: 5,332 IU; Vitamin C: 13 mg; Diabetic Exchange: Bread/Starch: 1.5, Meat (Lean) 3

chicken with homemade barbecue sauce

What's in this for baby and me? Protein.

Aɴʏ ᴄᴜᴛ ᴏꜰ chicken, which is high in protein, can be used with this delicious barbecue sauce. Boneless, skinless breast meat cooks the fastest but it is the least juicy. Skinless thighs or breasts on the bone or drumsticks are good choices. Garnish the chicken with chopped fresh cilantro and lime wedges, if desired.

serves 6

BARBECUE SAUCE
- ½ cup ketchup
- 2 tablespoons molasses
- ⅓ cup soy sauce
- ½ teaspoon ground ginger
- ¼ teaspoon ground cloves, allspice, or cinnamon, or a mixture
- 1 garlic clove, minced
- 2 tablespoons minced fresh ginger
- 2½ pounds skinless chicken parts (see headnote above)

1. To make the barbecue sauce, combine all of the ingredients in a small bowl, mix well, and set aside. (Note: If you plan to marinate the chicken in a bowl rather than a zip-lock bag, make the barbecue sauce in a large bowl.)
2. Remove any visible fat from the chicken pieces. Using a fork, pierce the chicken all over to allow the marinade to seep in. Place the chicken in a 1-gallon zip-lock bag (or in the bowl), add the barbecue sauce, seal (or cover with plastic wrap), and refrigerate for at least 2 hours, or up to 48 hours.
3. To cook the chicken, preheat the oven to 400°F.
4. Transfer the chicken with all of the sauce to a large baking dish. Bake for 30 minutes, or until an instant-read thermometer inserted into the center (through the side) of the breast meat or thigh reads 165°F, and the juices run clear when the chicken is pierced with a knife. Remove from the oven.
5. Before grilling or broiling, have a platter ready for the barbecued chicken. Grill the chicken, turning to cook on all sides, over high heat for about 5 minutes, or until the sauce is caramelized. Or, to broil, remove about half of the sauce from the pan and discard it, then place the chicken under the broiler and cook, turning once, for a couple of minutes on each side.

▶ *Advance Preparation:* Marinate the chicken for at least 2 hours, or up to 48 hours.

▶ *Health Tip:* Discard all leftover marinade—do not use it to baste the chicken on the grill or under the broiler.

▶ *Storage Tip:* The barbecued chicken keeps for 3 days refrigerated. It does not freeze well.

▶ *Complete Meal Ideas:* Serve this chicken with:

> Potato, enriched pasta, or couscous salad (you might want to try
> > the Couscous Salad with Chickpeas and Vegetables, page 149,
> > or the Asian-Style Pasta and Vegetable Salad, page 142)
> Green vegetable or a green salad
> Reduced-fat 2% milk or low-fat yogurt
> Fresh fruit

APPROXIMATE NUTRITIONAL INFORMATION: Serving size: 4 ounces roasted chicken (breast meat); Calories: 187 cals; Protein: 35 g; Carbohydrates: 0 g; Fat: 4 g; Fiber: 0 g; Sodium: 84 mg; Diabetic Exchange: Meat (Very Lean) 5

APPROXIMATE NUTRITIONAL INFORMATION: Serving size: 1 tablespoon homemade barbecue sauce; Calories: 49 cals; Protein: 2 g; Carbohydrates: 11 g; Fat: 0 g; Fiber: .3 g; Sodium: 1,050 mg; Diabetic Exchange: Other Carbohydrate 1

juicy turkey burgers

What's in this for baby and me? Protein.

TURKEY BURGERS DON'T get any better than this! The ricotta cheese keeps the burgers moist and the fresh herbs add a burst of flavor. Serve with or without buns, accompanied by the usual lineup of burger fixin's and condiments. For young children, cut up the burgers and serve them with lots of ketchup. These burgers are an excellent source of protein, and a fine source of calcium and iron.

makes 4 burgers

1 pound ground turkey

½ cup part-skim ricotta cheese

½ teaspoon salt

2 teaspoons Worcestershire sauce

2 teaspoons Dijon mustard

1 tablespoon freshly squeezed lemon juice

2 tablespoons chopped fresh cilantro or parsley

1 tablespoon canola oil, or canola oil cooking spray

1. Combine all of the ingredients except the canola oil in a bowl and mix until well blended. If the mixture is too pasty or sticky, add 1 tablespoon water. (Note: The consistency should be softer than a burger made with ground beef, but firm enough to hold its shape.) Divide the turkey mixture into four portions, form each portion into a patty, and place on a large plate.
2. If panfrying, heat the canola oil in a large nonstick skillet over medium heat. If grilling, before preheating the grill, position a piece of foil over the grill rack and poke holes in it. (This will prevent the burgers from sticking to the grill and falling apart.) Just before cooking the burgers, generously spray the foil with canola oil cooking spray. Add the burgers to the skillet or grill and cook for 6 minutes, or until the underside is dark brown. Flip the burgers and cook on the second side for about 6 minutes, or until the center of the burgers is completely opaque and an instant-read thermometer inserted into the center (through the side of the burger) reads 165°F.
3. Remove from the skillet or grill and serve immediately.

▶ *Advance Preparation:* The burgers can be formed, covered, and refrigerated up to 4 hours in advance.

▶ *Variation:* Substitute ground chicken for the turkey.

► **Storage Tip:** These turkey burgers keep for 3 days refrigerated. They do not freeze well.

► **Complete Meal Ideas:** Serve these burgers with:

Whole wheat bun or enriched pasta or potato salad (you might
   want to try the Best-Ever Tabbouleh Salad, page 151, or the
   Asparagus, Hearts of Palm, and Tomato Salad, page 159)
Green salad or tomato salad
Reduced-fat 2% milk or low-fat yogurt
Fresh fruit

APPROXIMATE NUTRITIONAL INFORMATION: Serving size: one 5-ounce turkey burger; Calories: 316 cals; Protein: 35 g; Carbohydrates: 3 g; Fat: 18 g; Fiber: 0 g; Sodium: 498 mg; Diabetic Exchange: Fat 1, Meat (Lean) 5

salt and high-sodium foods

It is a common misconception that salt intake should be restricted during pregnancy. An adequate sodium intake is essential for maintaining fluid balance and regulating electrolytes (sodium, potassium, and chloride). It is usually advisable to salt to taste unless otherwise advised. Consult your doctor or nurse if you are concerned about your salt intake and its effects on your blood pressure. Look for low-sodium labels on food products if you need to reduce your salt intake.

POPULAR HIGH-SODIUM FOODS

MEATS AND FISH: Bacon; sausage; bologna; salami; ham; corned beef; hot dogs; canned meats; sardines; light tuna fish; smoked meat, chicken, or fish; frozen prepared dinners

SNACK FOODS: Salted chips, pretzels, tortilla chips, and corn chips; salted popcorn; nuts and seeds; salted crackers; rolls or breads with salt toppings; french fries; pickles; olives; fast food

SEASONINGS: Salt, sea salt, "lite" salt; seasoned salt (such as onion and garlic salt); Accent; soy sauce; barbecue sauce; ketchup and mustard; packaged sauces and gravies

OTHER: Canned or packaged soups, broths, and bouillons; processed and prepared foods; canned vegetables; cottage cheese; soft drinks; tomato juice or V-8 juice; pickles

homemade chicken tenders

What's in this for baby and me? Protein, iron and B vitamins.

Aɴʏᴏɴᴇ ᴡɪᴛʜ ᴋɪᴅs knows what a staple chicken tenders are. This homemade version is an excellent source of protein, iron, and B vitamins, and a good source of calcium and folic acid. The tenders can be sautéed or baked and eaten right away, or frozen for later. Grown-ups might like these tenders accompanied by a more sophisticated dipping sauce than ketchup, such as store-bought mango chutney or cocktail sauce.

makes about 20 to 25 chicken tenders

1¼ pounds chicken tenders or boneless
    skinless chicken breasts

½ cup all-purpose flour

1 cup plain or seasoned bread crumbs

⅓ cup finely grated Parmesan cheese

A pinch of Old Bay seasoning, Italian herbs, or
    dried oregano

2 large eggs

Canola oil cooking spray if baking the chicken
    tenders, or 1–3 tablespoons canola oil if
    sautéing the tenders

1. Cut packaged chicken tenders in half. Or, if using boneless breasts, cut one lengthwise into three strips, then cut each strip on the diagonal into 2- to 2¼-inch strips. (Don't worry too much about the size and shape.) Place the tenders in a bowl and set aside.

2. Place the flour in a shallow pie dish or plate with sides; set aside. Combine the bread crumbs, Parmesan cheese, and seasonings in a shallow pie dish or a plate with sides and mix well; set aside. Place the eggs in a bowl and beat; set aside.

3. Set up your work station as follows: chicken tenders, flour, egg, bread crumb mixture, and two large plates. Using your dry hand, place about half of the tenders in the flour, tossing gently to coat all sides. Transfer the tenders in batches to the egg and coat them with egg using your other (wet) hand, then transfer them to the bread crumbs. Using your dry hand, cover the tenders with bread crumbs, pressing gently so they adhere, then place the breaded tenders on the plates. Repeat this procedure with the remaining tenders. (Discard all leftover flour, bread crumbs, and egg.)

4. To bake, preheat the oven to 450°F. Just before baking, preheat a baking sheet for 3 minutes (this helps the tenders brown evenly). Remove it from the oven and spray it generously with canola oil cooking spray. Arrange the tenders on the baking sheet, and lightly spray them with canola oil. Bake for 20 minutes, or until thoroughly cooked, turning once.

To panfry, heat 1 tablespoon canola oil in a large nonstick skillet over medium-high heat. Without crowding, place half of the tenders in the skillet and cook for about 7 to 9 minutes, turning once or twice, until browned and crisp on both sides and fully cooked. Transfer to a clean plate lined with paper towels to drain. Use a big wad of paper towels to wipe out the skillet, then repeat the pan frying procedure with the remaining tenders. (If you use a small skillet, you may need to cook the tenders in three batches.) Serve immediately.

▶ **Storage Tip:** These chicken tenders keep for 3 days refrigerated, and they can be cooked then frozen for up to 1 month.

▶ **Complete Meal Ideas:** Serve these chicken tenders with:
> Potato salad, enriched pasta salad, or rice (you might want to try the Pink
>> Potato Salad, page 155, or the Asian-Style Pasta and Vegetable Salad, page
>> 142, or the Couscous Salad with Chickpeas and Vegetables, page 149)
> Green salad or green vegetable
> Sliced tomatoes or yellow vegetable
> Reduced-fat 2% milk or low-fat yogurt
> Fresh fruit that contains vitamin C

APPROXIMATE NUTRITIONAL INFORMATION: Serving size: about 5 homemade chicken tenders; Calories: 445 cals; Protein: 47 g; Carbohydrates: 26 g; Fat: 16 g; Fiber: .8 g; Sodium: 399 mg; B Vitamins: Thiamine: .3 mg, Riboflavin: .4 mg, Niacin: 19 mg; Iron: 4 mg; Diabetic Exchange: Bread/Starch 1.5, Meat (Lean) 6

spice-rubbed pork chops

What's in this for baby and me? Protein.

THIS SPICE RUB can be used with any type of meat, poultry, or fish. Don't be put off by the number of steps in this recipe—they include instructions for both grilling or broiling the pork chops. Pork is an excellent source of protein and a good source of B vitamins.

makes four 4-ounce chops

SPICE RUB

- 1 teaspoon Italian seasoning
- ½ teaspoon chili powder
- ½ teaspoon garlic powder or 1 small garlic clove, crushed
- ½ teaspoon ground ginger
- ½ teaspoon ground cumin
- 2 teaspoons canola oil
- 1 pound pork chops (about 4 chops)

1. To make the spice rub, combine the ingredients in a small bowl or measuring cup, mix well, and set aside.
2. Trim any visible fat from the pork chops. Smear one side of the pork chops with half of the spice rub. Using a fork, pierce the meat all over to allow the spices to seep in, and repeat on the other side. Place the pork chops in a 1-gallon zip-lock bag, seal, and refrigerate for at least 1 hour, or up to 48 hours.
3. To grill the pork chops, preheat the grill. Have a clean plate ready for the cooked meat. Grease the grill rack. Grill the pork chops for approximately 7 minutes on each side (depending on their thickness), or until an instant-read thermometer inserted into the center of the meat close to the bone reads 160°F.

   To broil the pork chops, preheat the broiler and line a shallow baking pan, or a baking sheet with sides, with foil. Arrange the pork chops in the pan and broil for approximately 5 to 7 minutes on each side (see above for well-done temperature). Watch carefully to prevent burning.

▶ **Advance Preparation:** Rub the spices into the pork chops from 1 to 48 hours in advance; bag and refrigerate.

▶ **Health Tip:** Discard any extra spice rub. Place the finished pork chops on a clean serving platter.

▶ **Storage Tip:** These pork chops keep for 3 days refrigerated. They do not freeze well.

▶ *Complete Meal Ideas:* Serve these pork chops with:

    Baked or boiled potatoes, rice, or enriched pasta (you might want to
        try the Pasta Salad with Basil Pesto, page 146, or the Roasted Beets
        with Goat Cheese, Walnuts and Baby Greens, page 158)
    Green salad or green vegetable
    Sliced tomatoes or yellow vegetable
    Reduced-fat 2% milk or low-fat yogurt
    Fresh fruit

APPROXIMATE NUTRITIONAL INFORMATION: Serving size: one 4-ounce pork chop; Calories: 267 cals; Protein: 32 g; Carbohydrates: 0 g; Fat: 15 g; Fiber: 0 g; Sodium: 64 mg; Diabetic Exchange: Meat (Lean) 4.5

salt substitutes to spice up your food

Here are a few tips to help take the salt out of your diet without sacrificing taste:

▶ **Add fresh or dried leafy herbs (such as basil, parsley, dill, tarragon, and chervil) to salads, vegetables, dips, seafood, and poultry.**

▶ **Rosemary, thyme, basil, oregano, and marjoram (fresh or dried) are wonderful additions to meats, poultry, fish, and vegetables such as carrots and potatoes. These herbs also work well on pizza and in pasta sauces.**

▶ **Use dried spices (such as nutmeg, allspice, and cumin) to enhance flavors. For example, add a dash of nutmeg to creamed spinach or a dash of cumin to a cauliflower gratin.**

▶ **Use curry powder to enhance vegetables, meats, fish, and poultry and to liven up dips, marinades, and mayonnaise.**

▶ **Use freshly squeezed lemon juice to flavor vegetables such as broccoli and asparagus, and on meats such as veal and lamb.**

▶ **Garlic is a great flavor booster for meats, poultry, fish, sauce, marinades, and salad dressings.**

▶ **Fresh ginger is a delicious addition to stir-fried dishes and marinades. Lemongrass adds a strong Asian flavor to curries, soups, and marinades.**

▶ **Use a touch of Parmesan cheese on soups and salads. Parmesan cheese does contain salt; however, it is also high in calcium.**

▶ **Go nuts. Add your favorite unsalted nuts (preferably toasted) to pasta, rice, and vegetable dishes. For example, toasted sliced almonds are wonderful with green beans, and toasted pine nuts combined with fresh herbs transform a bland rice dish into a flavorful creation.**

▶ **Use pepper instead of salt. A dash of Tabasco sauce is another option, if you can handle the heat.**

marinated grilled or broiled lamb chops

What's in this for baby and me? Protein.

Simple and delicious, these lamb chops are an excellent source of protein and a good source of iron. The combination of garlic, lemon, olive oil, and rosemary is a traditional flavoring for many Greek and Italian dishes. These chops require no sauce, but a squeeze of lemon and a sprinkle of chopped fresh parsley add the perfect finishing touch. This marinade and garnish also works beautifully with chicken.

serves 4

1½ pounds lamb chops, about 1½ inches thick

MARINADE

   2 garlic cloves, minced

   3 tablespoons freshly squeezed lemon juice

   1 to 2 tablespoons chopped fresh rosemary, mint, or thyme

1 tablespoon olive oil

Lots of freshly ground pepper

2 tablespoons freshly squeezed lemon juice, for garnish

¼ cup chopped fresh parsley, for garnish

Salt, to taste

1. Trim any visible fat from the lamb chops, then, using a fork, pierce the meat all over to allow the marinade to seep in. Place the lamb chops in a 1-gallon zip-lock bag. Add the garlic, lemon juice, chopped rosemary, olive oil, and pepper to the bag and squish it around to make sure that the chops are completely covered with the marinade. Seal the bag and refrigerate for at least 1 hour, or up to 24 hours.

2. To grill the lamb chops, preheat the grill. Have a clean plate ready for the cooked meat. Grease the grill. Grill the lamb chops approximately 7 minutes on each side (depending on their thickness), or until an instant-read thermometer inserted into the center of the meat close to the bone reads 160°F.

    To broil the lamb chops, preheat the broiler and line a shallow baking pan, or a baking sheet with sides, with foil. Arrange the lamb chops in the pan and broil for approximately 5 to 7 minutes on each side (see above for well-done temperature). Watch carefully to prevent burning.

3. Arrange the cooked lamb chops on the plate and sprinkle with the optional lemon juice, a dash of salt, and chopped parsley.

▶ *Advance Preparation:* Marinate the lamb chops for at least 1 hour, or up to 24 hours.

▶ **Health Tip:** Discard all excess marinade. Place the cooked lamb chops on a clean serving plate.

▶ **Complete Meal Ideas:** Serve these lamb chops with:
  Tabbouleh, couscous, or enriched pasta (you might want to try
    the Best-Ever Tabbouleh Salad, page 151, or the Couscous
    Salad with Chickpeas and Vegetables, page 149)
  Green salad or green vegetable
  Sliced tomatoes or yellow vegetable
  Reduced-fat 2% milk or low-fat yogurt
  Fresh fruit that contains vitamin C

APPROXIMATE NUTRITIONAL INFORMATION: Serving size: one 4-ounce lamb chop; Calories: 245 cals; Protein: 34 g; Carbohydrates: 0 g; Fat: 11 g; Fiber: 0 g; Sodium: 95 mg; Diabetic Exchange: Meat (Lean) 4.5

sautéed shrimp with pasta

What's in this for baby and me? Protein, iron, vitamin C, and folic acid.

THIS SHRIMP-AND-tomato combo—high in protein, iron, vitamin C, and folic acid, and a good source of calcium, fiber, B vitamins, and DHA omega-3—is delicious served over any type of pasta.

serves 4

12 to 16 ounces enriched linguine or thin
   spaghetti

2 tablespoon plus 1 teaspoon olive oil

1 small onion, finely diced

1 garlic clove, minced

1¼ pounds medium-size shrimp, peeled and
   deveined (for cleaning instructions, see
   Cooking Tip below)

One 14.5-ounce can diced tomatoes (do not
   drain)

1 teaspoon grated lemon zest (from about 1
   lemon) (optional)

1 tablespoon freshly squeezed lemon juice, or
   to taste

¼ cup chopped fresh basil, cilantro, dill, or a
   mixture

Salt and freshly ground pepper, to taste

Grated Parmesan cheese, for the table

1. Cook the pasta according to the package directions; drain. Place it back in the hot pot, stir in 1 teaspoon of the olive oil (to prevent sticking), and set aside in a warm place.
2. Heat the remaining 2 tablespoons olive oil in a large nonstick skillet over medium-high heat. Add the onion and sauté for 2 minutes, then add the garlic and sauté for 30 seconds. Add the shrimp and cook for 3 minutes, turning the shrimp once. Gently stir in the diced tomatoes, lemon zest, if using, and lemon juice and sauté for 1 minute longer.
3. Add the herbs, then season with salt and pepper. Serve immediately, over the pasta. Pass the Parmesan cheese at the table.

▶ *Cooking Tip:* To clean shrimp, start by removing the shell from the body of the shrimp by holding the underside of the shrimp with your thumb and pulling the shell off with your other hand in an upward motion. When you reach the tail, carefully pull off the hard shell. (Note: Remove the tail shell gently—if you pull too hard, you could rip the shrimp in half.) To devein the shrimp, make a very shallow incision from the top end to the middle of the outer curve of the shrimp to expose the dark vein. Using your fingers, pull out the vein and discard.

▶ **Complete Meal Ideas:** Serve this shrimp and pasta with:

Green salad or green vegetable (you might want to try the Romaine Lettuce with Olive Oil–Lemon Dressing, page 169, or one of Annie Mozer's Greens, pages 242)

Reduced-fat 2% milk or low-fat yogurt

Fresh fruit that contains vitamin C

APPROXIMATE NUTRITIONAL INFORMATION: Serving size: one-quarter of the shrimp sauce with 1½ cups of enriched pasta; Calories: 474 cals; Protein: 35 g; Carbohydrates: 65 g; Fat: 7 g; Fiber: 5 g; Sodium: 597 mg; Vitamin C: 21 mg; Folic Acid: 156 mcg; Iron: 7 mg; Diabetic Exchange: Bread/Starch 4, Meat (Lean) 3.5

how to buy and cook fish and shellfish[5]

TIPS FOR BUYING FRESH FISH FILETS AND STEAKS

▶ Look for firm, shiny flesh that gives slightly when pressed. Flesh should not be mushy, and it should not separate easily.

▶ If the head is on, the fish's eyes should be clear and should bulge a bit. Avoid dull, cloudy, sunken, or bloody eyes.

▶ The gills should be bright pink or red, not brown or gray.

▶ The fish should have a pleasant ocean-fresh smell, not a fishy or ammonia-like odor.

▶ Scales (if on the fish) should be shinny and should cling tightly to the flesh.

▶ Steaks and filets should be moist, not slimy or dry, and the color should be uniformly bright, not dull.

TIPS FOR BUYING LIVE CRABS, LOBSTERS, AND SHRIMP

▶ The legs of a live lobster should be lively when touched unless the crustacean is soft shelled (such as soft-shell crabs).

▶ The tail of a live lobster should curl under when lifted up. It should not hang limp.

▶ Shellfish should feel weighty, not light or dry.

▶ Raw shrimp should have translucent shells with a grayish green, pinkish-tan, or pink tint. They should be moist and firm, not mealy.

TIPS FOR BUYING LIVE CLAMS, MUSSELS, OYSTERS, SCALLOPS, AND OTHER MOLLUSKS

▶ Shells should be tightly closed. If they are open, they should shut immediately when gently tapped. Discard gaping shells that do not close when tapped.

▶ Shells should be moist and intact, not cracked, dry, or chipped.

▶ Mollusks should have a clean ocean-fresh scent, not a fishy odor.

TIPS FOR BUYING SHUCKED CLAMS, MUSSELS, OYSTERS, SCALLOPS, AND OTHER MOLLUSKS

▶ Meat should be plump, not shriveled, dark, or dry.

▶ Meat should be free of shell and sand particles.

▶ Liquid should be clear, not cloudy or opaque, and it should be less than 10% of the volume.

▶ Mollusks should have a clean ocean-fresh scent, not a fishy odor.

TIPS FOR BUYING FROZEN FISH AND SHELLFISH

▶ Flesh should be frozen solidly.

▶ Fish should be contained in a tight, moisture-proof package.

▶ Fish should not have any freezer burn or ice crystals.

▶ When thawed, fish and shellfish should pass the same tests as outlined above.

▶ Frozen fish should remain frozen until it is thawed for cooking. Do not refreeze fish or shellfish.

TIPS FOR COOKING FRESH FISH

▶ Marinades and dry rubs add tremendous taste to fish. The options are endless—play around to find your favorites.

▶ Keep fish that is marinating in the refrigerator; do not leave it at room temperature.

▶ The healthiest and tastiest ways to cook fish are grilling, broiling, poaching, steaming, pan sautéing, and baking. Try to avoid deep frying.

▶ The 10-Minute-per-Inch Rule for Fish: Measure fish at its thickest point (if stuffed or rolled, measure after stuffing). If baking (at a high temperature), grilling, broiling, poaching, steaming, or sautéing, cook the fish for about 10 minutes per inch of thickness. Add 5 minutes of cooking time to the total cooking time for fish wrapped in foil or covered with a sauce. Double the cooking time for frozen fish that has not been thawed prior to cooking.

▶ Fish is done when the flesh turns from translucent to opaque. It should flake easily with a fork or knife. A thermometer should read 140°F when cooked.

▶ Cook fish skin-side down. The filet or meat will slide off the fish easily when cooked.

shrimp and vegetable stir-fry

What's in this for baby and me? Protein, iron, and vitamins A and C.

THIS STIR-FRY is an excellent source of protein, iron, and vitamins A and C, and a good source of calcium, B vitamins, folic acid, fiber, and DHA omega-3. Use the marinade and sauce as a blueprint for your favorite ingredients.

serves 4 (makes about 8 cups)

MARINADE

2 tablespoons soy sauce

2 tablespoons hoisin sauce

2 tablespoons water

1 garlic clove, minced

1 tablespoon minced fresh ginger

1¼ pounds medium shrimp, peeled and deveined (for cleaning instructions, see Cooking Tip below)

STIR-FRY SAUCE

1 tablespoon hoisin sauce

3 tablespoons water

2 tablespoons soy sauce

1 teaspoon cornstarch

1 teaspoon brown sugar

1 tablespoon canola oil

A few drops of toasted sesame oil (optional)

1 tablespoon minced fresh ginger

1 garlic clove, minced

1 cup sliced or grated carrots

¾ cup fresh snow peas, washed, and ends trimmed

1½ cups fresh broccoli florets, washed and ends trimmed

½ red bell pepper, washed and thinly sliced

1 cup sliced zucchini or yellow squash

3 scallions, trimmed and thinly sliced

⅓ cup cashew nuts, coarsely chopped (optional)

¼ cup chopped fresh cilantro (optional)

Cooked rice or noodles, to serve with the stir-fry

1. To make the marinade, combine all of the ingredients in a medium-size bowl and whisk. Add the shrimp, cover, and refrigerate for at least 15 minutes, or up to 12 hours.

2. To make the stir-fry sauce, combine all of the ingredients in a small bowl and whisk until the cornstarch is completely dissolved; set aside.

3. To cook the stir-fry, heat the canola oil and optional sesame oil in a very large nonstick skillet or large nonstick wok over medium-high heat. Add the ginger and garlic and sauté for 30 seconds. Add the carrots, snow peas, broccoli florets, red bell pepper, and zucchini and cook, stirring occasionally, for 5 minutes, or until crisp-tender. Keep a cover or a piece of foil over the skillet or wok when you are not stirring; if the vegetables stick to the pan, add 1 tablespoon water. Transfer the cooked vegetables to a serving bowl and cover with foil to keep warm. (Do not rinse the skillet.)

4. Reheat the skillet over medium-high heat. Add the shrimp, and its marinade, and the stir-fry sauce, stir, cover, and cook for 3 minutes. Add the scallions and cook 1 minute more. Transfer the contents of the skillet to the serving bowl containing the vegetables, gently mix, and garnish with the cashew nuts and cilantro, if desired. Serve immediately, with the rice.

▶ *Cooking Tip:* To clean shrimp, start by removing the shell from the body of the shrimp by holding the underside of the shrimp with your thumb and pulling the shell off with your other hand in an upward motion. When you reach the tail, carefully pull off the hard shell. (Note: Remove the tail shell gently—if you pull too hard, you could rip the shrimp in half.) To devein the shrimp, make a very shallow incision from the top end to the middle of the outer curve of the shrimp to expose the dark vein. Using your fingers, pull out the vein and discard.

▶ *Advance Preparation:* Marinate the shrimp for 20 minutes. The stir-fry sauce can be made 1 day in advance, covered, and refrigerated, and the vegetables can be prepared up to 3 days in advance and refrigerated.

▶ *Variation:* The shrimp can be replaced with chicken strips, beef strips (use thin-sliced beef rib eye Delmonico steak), scallops, or any other source of protein. For vegetarians, one 15-ounce package (drained weight) extra-firm tofu, cut into ½-inch cubes and blotted dry with paper towels, can be used in place of the shrimp. Use your favorite vegetables, equal to 6 to 7 cups (about 1 to 1¼ pounds). Try to cut all of the vegetables about the same size so they require the same cooking time.

▶ *Timesaving Tip:* Convenient fresh vegetable stir-fry packs are available in some grocery stores. They usually come in 12-ounce packs and can be supplemented with your favorite vegetables—carrots, broccoli, and asparagus are among the healthiest. Avoid fresh bean sprouts (see *E. coli* Warning, page 285). Sixteen-ounce bags of frozen stir-fry vegetables are also available in most grocery stores. Follow the package directions for stir-frying vegetables in oil.

▶ *Health Tip:* If your salt intake has been restricted, use low-sodium soy sauce, use less hoisin sauce, and omit the cashew nuts.

▶ *Complete Meal Ideas:* Serve this stir-fry with:
　　Rice, rice noodles, or quinoa
　　Reduced-fat 2% milk or low-fat yogurt
　　Fresh fruit

APPROXIMATE NUTRITIONAL INFORMATION: Serving size: 2 cups shrimp and vegetable stir-fry; Calories: 301 cals; Protein: 30 g; Carbohydrates: 21 g; Fat: 11 g; Fiber: 3 g; Sodium: 1,377 mg; Vitamin A: 10,807 IU; Vitamin C: 79 g; Diabetic Exchange: Fat .5, Meat (Medium Fat) 2.5

faqs about mercury in fish and shellfish

WHAT ARE MERCURY AND METHYLMERCURY?

Mercury occurs naturally in the environment, and it can also be released into the air through industrial pollution. Mercury falls from the sky, accumulating in streams and oceans, where it turns into methylmercury in the water. Fish absorb methylmercury as they feed. High amounts of methylmercury in certain types of fish can potentially be harmful to the neurological development of an unborn baby and young child.

IS THERE METHYLMERCURY IN ALL FISH AND SHELLFISH?

Nearly all fish and shellfish contain traces of methylmercury. Large fish (shark, swordfish, king mackerel, and tilefish) with long life spans have the highest levels of methylmercury, mainly because they've had more time to accumulate it. These fish pose the greatest risk. Other types of fish should be eaten in amounts recommended by the FDA and EPA.

WHAT ABOUT FISH STICKS AND FAST-FOOD FISH SANDWICHES?

Fish sticks and fast-food sandwiches are usually made from fish that are low in mercury, so they are safe to eat.

WHAT ABOUT TUNA STEAKS?

Because tuna steaks generally contain higher levels of mercury than canned light tuna, you may eat up to 6 ounces (one average meal) of tuna steak per week.

WHAT IF I EAT MORE THAN THE RECOMMENDED AMOUNT OF FISH AND SHELLFISH IN A WEEK?

One week's consumption of fish does not change the level of methylmercury in your body much at all.

I'M TRYING TO CONCEIVE. SHOULD I BE CONCERNED ABOUT METHYLMERCURY?

If you regularly eat fish high in methylmercury, it can accumulate in your bloodstream over time. Methylmercury is excreted from the body naturally, but it may take over a year for high levels to drop significantly. Therefore, it may be present in a woman before she becomes pregnant. For this reason, women who are trying to conceive should also try to avoid eating high-mercury fish, *but they certainly should eat other fish.*

crab cakes with red bell pepper sauce

What's in this for baby and me? Protein and vitamin C.

WHEN YOUR BUDGET allows for a splurge, there is nothing better than these home-made crab cakes laced with fresh herbs and served with a creamy red bell pepper sauce. Crab is an excellent source of protein (and a good source of folic acid and DHA omega-3), and the red bell pepper sauce is high in vitamin C (and a good source of vitamin A). If red bell peppers aren't your thing, other sauces in this book, such as the Salsa Verde (page 290), Papaya Salsa (page 327), or Sun-Dried Tomato and Basil Dressing (page 167), are excellent alternatives—and, of course, store-bought cocktail sauce always works. Any leftover crab cakes can be eaten cold with a salad or made into delectable sandwiches. The recipes for both the sauce and the crab cakes can be cut in half for a smaller yield.

makes 7 crab cakes

RED BELL PEPPER SAUCE (makes about 1 cup)
  1 large red bell pepper, washed, cored, seeded, and coarsely diced
  ¾ cup half-and-half
  Salt and freshly ground pepper, to taste
CRAB CAKES
  8 ounces jumbo lump crabmeat, picked over to remove any shells (see Cooking Tip below)
  8 ounces back fin crabmeat, picked over to remove any shells

  ½ cup plain bread crumbs
  2 tablespoons finely chopped scallions or fresh chives
  ¼ cup chopped fresh dill, cilantro, or basil, or a mixture, or to taste
  2 teaspoons grated lemon zest
  2 teaspoons Dijon mustard
  2 large eggs, lightly beaten
  2 tablespoons light mayonnaise
  2 tablespoons canola oil
  Lemon or lime wedges, for the table

1. To make the sauce, combine the bell pepper and half-and-half in a small non-reactive saucepan. Bring to a boil, reduce the heat, and simmer about 15 minutes, or until the peppers are tender. Cool, then puree in a food processor or blender until smooth. Adjust the seasoning, cover, and set aside.

2. To make the crab cakes, combine all of the crab cake ingredients in a bowl. Mix gently until well incorporated. To form the crab cakes, use a ⅓-cup measuring cup to portion out each crab cake, then form it into a patty and place it on a large plate. Cover and refrigerate until ready to cook.

3. Heat the canola oil in a large nonstick skillet over medium-high heat. Add three crab cakes (avoid overcrowding) and cook on one side for about 3 minutes, or until golden brown. Carefully flip and cook the other side for about 3 minutes, or until golden brown and thoroughly heated. (Note: You may need to adjust the heat if the crab cakes begin browning too quickly.) Transfer the cooked crab cakes to a serving

plate and cover loosely with foil to keep warm. Cook the remaining crab cakes, and serve immediately with the red bell pepper sauce and lemon wedges.

▶ *Cooking Tip:* One pound of jumbo lump or back fin crabmeat (which equals about 2 cups of crabmeat) can be used in place of 8 ounces of each. Generally, back fin crabmeat needs to be picked over more carefully, as it contains more bits of shell.

▶ *Advance Preparation:* The crab cakes can be formed up to 12 hours in advance, covered, and refrigerated. The red bell pepper sauce can be made 1 day in advance, covered, and refrigerated.

▶ *Health Tip:* If your doctor has restricted your fat intake, use light skim evaporated milk instead of half-and-half in the red bell pepper sauce.

▶ *Storage Tip:* The crab cakes and red bell pepper sauce keep for 3 days refrigerated. Neither freezes well.

▶ *Complete Meal Ideas:* Serve these crab cakes with:
Corn on the cob, potato salad, or pasta salad
Green salad or green vegetable (you might want to try some baby
greens with the French-Style Tarragon Vinaigrette, page 166)
Reduced-fat 2% milk or low-fat yogurt
Fresh fruit

APPROXIMATE NUTRITIONAL INFORMATION: Serving size: One crab cake (about 3 ounces); Calories: 163 cals; Protein: 15 g; Carbohydrates: 6 g; Fat: 8 g; Fiber: .2 g; Sodium: 288 mg; Diabetic Exchange: Bread/Starch .5, Fat .5, Meat (Lean) 2

APPROXIMATE NUTRITIONAL INFORMATION: Serving size: 2 tablespoons red bell pepper sauce; Calories: 33 cals; Protein: .7 g; Carbohydrates: 2 g; Fat: 3 g; Fiber: .2 g; Sodium: 10 mg; Vitamin C: 28 mg; Diabetic Exchange: Fat .5

limitations on consumption of certain fish

Fish and shellfish are part of a healthy diet and should *not* be excluded, especially during pregnancy. However, certain types of fish can be contaminated with high levels of mercury that may harm an unborn baby or young child's developing nervous system. The risks from mercury in fish and shellfish depend on the amount of fish and shellfish eaten and the levels of mercury in the fish and shellfish. The U.S. Food and Drug Administration and Environmental Protection Agency are advising women who may become pregnant, pregnant women, nursing mothers, and young children to follow these recommendations.

▶ Do not eat shark, swordfish, king mackerel, or tilefish because they contain high levels of mercury.

▶ Eat up to 12 ounces (two average meals) a week of a variety of fish and shellfish that are lower in mercury. Five of the most commonly eaten fish that are low in mercury are shrimp, canned light tuna, salmon, pollock, and catfish. Albacore (white) tuna has more mercury than canned light tuna; so when choosing your two meals of fish and shellfish, you may eat 6 ounces of albacore tuna per week.

▶ Check local advisories about the safety of fish caught by family and friends in your local lakes, rivers, and coastal areas. If no advice is available, eat up to 6 ounces per week of fish from local waters, but don't consume any other fish during that week.

Pregnant women should also avoid raw fish, especially shellfish (oysters and clams), which can be polluted with raw sewage and can contain harmful microorganisms that can lead to severe gastrointestinal illness. All fish and shellfish should be *thoroughly* cooked. [6]

For further information, visit www.epa.gov/waterscience/fishadvice/advice.html.

sautéed salmon on a bed of greens with citrus vinaigrette

What's in this for baby and me? Protein, vitamins A and C, folic acid, B vitamins, and fiber.

THIS MAIN-COURSE salad is an excellent source of protein, vitamins A and C, folic acid, B vitamins, and fiber, and a good source of iron and DHA omega-3. The leftover dressing is delicious on spinach salad, or any other greens or vegetables. This recipe calls for cutting the salmon into strips before cooking it, but feel free to grill, bake, or broil a whole salmon fillet or steak to serve alongside your salad.

serves 2

Citrus Vinaigrette (makes about ⅔ cup)
- Juice of 1 lemon
- Juice of 1 orange
- 1 tablespoon plus 1 teaspoon honey
- 1 teaspoon finely chopped shallots (optional)
- 1 teaspoon Dijon mustard
- ⅛ teaspoon ground ginger
- A couple drops of toasted sesame oil
- ⅓ cup plus 2 tablespoons canola oil

Salmon
- 12 ounces skinned salmon fillet, cut lengthwise in half, then cut into 1-inch-wide strips
- 1 tablespoon soy sauce
- 1 tablespoon canola oil
- 3–4 cups baby greens, washed and well dried
- 1 avocado, peeled, pitted, and sliced
- 1 cup cherry tomatoes, washed
- 2 tablespoons chopped fresh cilantro (optional)

1. To prepare the citrus vinaigrette, combine the citrus juices (they should equal ⅔ cup, if not add more of either juice) and 1 tablespoon of the honey in a small saucepan and bring to a boil. Reduce the heat and simmer for 10 minutes, or until reduced by half (to ⅓ cup).
2. Transfer the reduced citrus juice to a small bowl or measuring cup and add the remaining honey, the shallots, if using, mustard, and ginger. Mix well, then add the sesame oil and canola oil and whisk until emulsified; set aside.
3. To cook the salmon, combine the salmon with the soy sauce and canola oil in a bowl and mix gently. Have a plate for the cooked salmon ready. Heat a large non-stick skillet over medium-high heat until hot. Add the salmon and cook for 2 minutes on each side, or until cooked through and light golden brown on the outside; use a splatter screen if you have one. (Note: The cooking time will depend on the thickness of the salmon. The flesh should flake easily and the interior should be fully cooked.) Transfer the cooked salmon to the plate; set aside.

4. To assemble the salad, combine the baby greens, and avocado, cherry tomatoes, and cilantro with ¼ cup of the vinaigrette in a bowl and toss gently. Divide the salad between two plates, place the sautéed salmon around the salad, and drizzle with just a bit more citrus vinaigrette. Serve immediately.

▶ *Timesaving Tip:* Use your favorite bottled dressing instead of the citrus vinaigrette and use smoked salmon (about 3 to 4 ounces) instead of cooking fresh salmon.

▶ *Variation:* Use 8 to 12 ounces fresh shrimp, peeled and drained (see Cooking Tip on page 319 for instructions), or scallops in place of the salmon. Adjust the cooking time as needed to thoroughly cook the shellfish.

▶ *Storage Tip:* The salmon keeps for 2 days refrigerated, and the citrus vinaigrette keeps for 5 days refrigerated.

▶ *Complete Meal Ideas:* Serve this salad with:
    Whole wheat roll or bread
    Reduced fat 2% milk or low-fat yogurt
    Fresh fruit that contains vitamin C

APPROXIMATE NUTRITIONAL INFORMATION: Serving size: one-half serving of the sautéed salmon and the salad (about 6 ounces of salmon); Calories: 482 cals; Protein: 34 g; Carbohydrates: 10 g; Fat: 35 g; Fiber: 5 g; Sodium: 480 mg; Vitamin A 1,736 IU; Vitamin C: 29 mg; Folic Acid: 164 mcg; B Vitamins: Thiamine: .6 mg, Riboflavin: .3 mg, Niacin: 13 mg; Diabetic Exchange: Bread/Starch .5, Fat 2, Meat (Medium Fat) 4.5

wild versus farm-raised salmon[7]

There is no doubt that salmon, which is high in DHA and EPA, is excellent for your baby's brain development—and a mother's psychological health too (see Postpartum Depression: How Diet and Exercise Can Help, page 385). There is, however, some debate over the levels of PCBs (polychlorinated biphenyls), antibiotics, and other toxins found in farm-raised salmon, and how much of them is safe to consume during pregnancy and breastfeeding. Here are some answers to common questions about wild versus farm-raised salmon.

What are PCBs and how do they get into the fish? PCBs are pollutants that have been shown to cause cancer in animals, not humans. The toxins come from plastics, waste incinerators, leaky transformers, and insecticide residues. Farmed salmon get concentrated levels of PCBs from their processed food. Wild salmon get PCBs too; however, their natural diet is more varied, so PCB levels are lower. Fortunately, fish food is constantly being improved and tested, so the toxin levels are decreasing.

How do I know if salmon is farm-raised or wild? If this distinction is not labeled in the fish case or on the packaging of the fish (which it should be), ask your fishmonger. Names such as *Atlantic salmon* or *Icelandic salmon* may sound like they refer to wild salmon, but the fish are usually farm-raised. Depending on where you live, the price of salmon can also be an indicator: higher prices usually mean the salmon is wild. Also, wild salmon is generally available fresh on the East coast of the U.S. from May until the end of August. Alaska and the West coast enjoy a year-round supply of wild salmon at a reasonable cost. Canned wild salmon is an excellent and safe choice.

Where do wild salmon come from and are they endangered? Many wild salmon runs are threatened, endangered, or even extinct, but many are also still healthy. As a general rule, wild stocks in Alaska are doing better than those of California and the Pacific Northwest. No harvestable runs of Atlantic salmon remain in the U.S.

How much farm-raised salmon is safe to eat? There are no official guidelines on how much farm-raised salmon is safe for pregnant women, lactating women, or young children to eat. As a matter of common sense, if you tend to consume a lot of salmon, try to buy wild salmon whenever it is available and affordable. If wild salmon is not an option, do *not* completely eliminate farm-raised salmon from your diet. Branch out and cook other fish and shellfish, such as cod, catfish, sardines, scallops, and shrimp.

Can I reduce the levels of PCBs in the farm-raised salmon that I eat? Consumers can reduce their exposure to PCBs by removing the skin and fat from fish before cooking it.

Is canned salmon farm-raised? Almost all of it is wild.

What are some sources for wild salmon? Mail-order sources for wild salmon include SalmonGram.com (www.salmongram.com), SeaBear Smokehouse (www.seabear.com), and Vital Choice Seafood (www.vitalchoice.com).

roasted salmon with papaya salsa

What's in this for baby and me? Protein and vitamins A and C.

REFRESHINGLY LIGHT, COLORFUL, and delicious—this combination of salmon and papaya is heavenly. The roasted salmon is an excellent source of protein and a good source of vitamin C, folic acid, B vitamins, and DHA omega-3. The papaya salsa is rich in vitamins A and C. This recipe can be halved to serve two.

serves 4

1½ pounds salmon filet, skin left on

MARINADE

    2 tablespoons soy sauce

    1 tablespoon canola oil

    Freshly ground pepper, to taste

PAPAYA SALSA (makes about 2½ cups)

    1 small papaya, peeled, seeded, and finely
        diced (about 1 cup diced papaya)

    ⅓ cup finely diced red bell pepper

    ½ cup quartered cherry tomatoes

    ¼ cup finely diced red onion

    2 tablespoons chopped fresh cilantro or mint

    One 8-ounce can mandarin oranges in light
        syrup, drained and sliced

    1 tablespoon freshly squeezed lime juice or
        seasoned rice vinegar, or to taste

1. To marinate the salmon fillet, place it in a 1-gallon zip-lock bag. Add the soy sauce, canola oil, and pepper, swish it around, and seal the bag. Refrigerate for at least 30 minutes, or up to 8 hours.

2. To make the papaya salsa, mix all of the ingredients in a bowl. Cover and refrigerate until ready to serve. (Note: The salsa is best if allowed to sit for 30 minutes before serving, to allow the flavors to develop. It can be made up to 3 hours in advance.)

3. To bake the salmon, preheat the oven to 450°F. Line a baking sheet with sides, or a baking pan, with aluminum foil. (Do not grease the foil; see Cooking Tip below.)

4. Place the salmon on the baking sheet, skin side down, leaving the marinade juices behind. Bake the salmon, uncovered, for 12 to 15 minutes, or until fully cooked. The flesh should flake easily and the interior should be fully cooked. Serve immediately with the papaya salsa.

▶ **Health Tip:** Discard all leftover marinade.

▶ **Cooking Tip:** If you do not grease the foil, the salmon skin will stick to it and the salmon fillets can be separated from the skin easily. You might need to cut the salmon fillet (not the skin) down the center to facilitate removing it.

▶ **Storage Tip:** The salmon keeps for 2 days refrigerated. The papaya salsa becomes a little mushy after 8 hours, but the taste is unaffected.

▶ **Complete Meal Ideas:** Serve this baked salmon with:
Couscous, quinoa, or enriched pasta (you might want to try
    the Quinoa Salad, page 144, or the Noodles with Spinach,
    Red Bell Peppers, and Sesame Dressing, page 148)
Green salad or green vegetable
Reduced-fat 2% milk or low-fat yogurt
Fresh fruit

APPROXIMATE NUTRITIONAL INFORMATION: Serving size: about 6 ounces baked salmon; Calories: 385 cals; Protein: 39 g; Carbohydrates: 0 g; Fat: 24 g; Fiber: 0 g; Sodium: 564 mg; Diabetic Exchange: Meat (Medium Fat) 5

APPROXIMATE NUTRITIONAL INFORMATION: Serving size: ½ cup papaya salsa; Calories: 55 cals; Protein: .8 g; Carbohydrates: 14 g; Fat: .2 g; Fiber: 2 g; Sodium: 7 mg; Vitamin A: 1,276 IU; Vitamin C: 54 mg; Diabetic Exchange: Fruit 1

tilapia mediterranean-style

What's in this for baby and me? Protein and Vitamin C.

A BEAUTIFUL-ON-the-plate Mediterranean dish that works well with just about any kind of fish, including red snapper, sole, or cod. Tilapia is an excellent source of protein (and a good source of DHA omega-3), and the tomato sauce provides vitamin C. This recipe can be cut in half to serve two people. If your kids like olives, they might be willing to give this a try.

serves 4

2 tablespoons olive oil

1 garlic clove, minced

1 cup pitted kalamata olives or other brine-cured black olives, chopped

15 ounces (about 3 cups) cherry tomatoes, halved

⅓ cup chopped fresh parsley

¼ cup chopped fresh basil (optional)

2 tablespoons freshly squeezed lemon juice, or to taste

Salt and freshly ground pepper, to taste

1½ pounds tilapia fillets

1. Heat 1 tablespoon of the olive oil in a large nonstick skillet over medium-high heat. Add the garlic and sauté for 30 seconds. Add the olives, cherry tomatoes, parsley, basil, if using, and lemon juice and cook for 2 minutes, or until the cherry tomatoes are soft and their skin wrinkled. Adjust the seasoning, transfer to a heatproof bowl, cover, and set aside. (Do not rinse the skillet.)
2. Have a serving platter ready. Heat the remaining 1 tablespoon olive oil in the skillet over medium-high heat. Add half the fish, season the fish with salt and pepper, and cook for 3 minutes on each side, turning once, or until cooked through. Transfer the cooked fish to the serving platter and cover with aluminum foil. Repeat this procedure with the remaining fish, making sure to reheat the skillet before adding the second batch of fish.
3. Ladle the reserved sauce over the fish and serve immediately.

▶ **Storage Tip:** This tilapia Mediterranean-style keeps 2 days refrigerated. It does not freeze well.

▶ **Complete Meal Ideas:** Serve this tilapia with:
  Rice, enriched pasta, couscous
  Green salad or green vegetable (you might want to try the Vegetables with Lemon, Olive Oil, and Fresh Herbs, page 153)
  Reduced-fat 2% milk or low-fat yogurt
  Fresh fruit

APPROXIMATE NUTRITIONAL INFORMATION: Serving size: one-fourth tilapia Mediterranean style (about 6 ounces of tilapia); Calories: 110 cals; Protein: 11 g; Carbohydrates: 4 g; Fat: 6 g; Fiber: .9 g; Sodium: 148 mg; Diabetic Exchange: Meat (Medium Fat) 1.5

salmonellosis warning

Salmonellosis is a food-borne illness caused by the bacteria *Salmonella*, which can be acquired from infected animals (usually poultry, swine, and cattle), raw milk and raw milk products, undercooked or raw eggs and egg products (see Eggs and *Salmonella enteritidis*, page 79), and contaminated water. Fecal-oral transmission from person to person, especially in infants, is another cause of *salmonella* poisoning. Certain pets, such as turtles, tortoises, iguanas, chicks, dogs, cats, and rodents, can also carry the bacteria in their intestines.

The symptoms of gastrointestinal infection usually include fever, nausea and vomiting, abdominal cramping, and diarrhea, which may be bloody. Other complications, such as enteric (typhoid) fever or extra-intestinal infections (infections that have spread outside the intestines), may occur. Following are a few tips to help prevent infection:[9]

> ▶ Avoid raw eggs and food that contains raw or partially cooked eggs.

> ▶ Avoid raw (unpasteurized) milk and any food that contains raw milk or raw milk products.

> ▶ Thoroughly cook all poultry and meat (see Well-Done Temperature Guide, page 435). Wash instant-read thermometers in between tests of foods that require further cooking.

> ▶ Keep raw meat separate from uncooked foods. Wash hands, counters, and utensils with hot, soapy water after touching raw meat.

> ▶ Consume only safe drinking water or bottled water, especially when traveling to developing countries.

> ▶ Wash hands thoroughly after touching any of the pets mentioned above.

> ▶ Make sure that persons with diarrhea, especially children, wash their hands to reduce the risk of spreading infection, and that anyone washes his or her hands after changing soiled diapers.

> ▶ Avoid swallowing lake or pool water while swimming.

shrimp with asparagus and red bell peppers

What's in this for baby and me? Protein, vitamins A and C.

To ENSURE SUCCESS with stir-fries, have all of your ingredients ready before you start the actual cooking. This dish is an excellent source of protein and vitamins A and C. It is also a good source of B vitamins, folic acid, and DHA omega-3.

Serves 4

SAUCE

- 1 tablespoon rice wine
- 1 tablespoon toasted sesame oil
- 2 teaspoons cornstarch
- 3 tablespoons soy sauce

½ pound baby asparagus spears, washed, stalk-ends trimmed, and stalks cut into 1-inch pieces (about 2½ cups)

1 small red bell pepper, washed and cut into thin slices

1 pound large shrimp, peeled and deveined (about 15 shrimp)

Dash of salt

1 tablespoon rice wine

1 tablespoon of an egg white from a large egg (this is hard to measure, but it does not have to be exact)

1 tablespoon cornstarch

2 tablespoons toasted sesame oil

½ cup sliced scallions

¼ cup fresh ginger, peeled and thinly sliced

1. To make the sauce, combine all of the ingredients plus ¼ cup water in a small bowl and whisk; set aside.
2. Bring a small pot of water to a boil. Add the asparagus and red peppers and cook for 1 minute (the water will not return to a boil). Drain and rinse the vegetables under cold water; set aside.
3. Place the shrimp in a bowl. Add in the following ingredients in the order listed, and mix well after each addition: salt, rice wine, egg white, and cornstarch.
4. In a large nonstick skillet or wok, heat the sesame oil over medium-high heat. Add the shrimp and cook for 1 minute on each side. Add the scallions and ginger, and sauté for 1 minute.
5. Add the reserved asparagus and red bell peppers and the reserved sauce, and continue to sauté, stirring constantly, for about 2 minutes, or until the sauce thickens. Serve immediately.

▶ *Variation:* Substitute the asparagus with green peas, broccoli florets, or any other small, quick-cooking, thinly sliced vegetable.

▶ **Health Tip:** If your doctor has restricted your salt intake, use low-sodium or light soy sauce and omit the salt.

▶ **Complete Meal Ideas:** Serve this shrimp with:
Brown basmati rice or udon noodles
Green salad
Frozen yogurt or fruit sorbet

APPROXIMATE NUTRITIONAL INFORMATION: Serving size: One-fourth of the shrimp with asparagus and red bell peppers; Calories: 280 cals; Protein: 26 g; Carbohydrates: 16 g; Fat: 12 g; Fiber: 2 g; Sodium: 957 mg; Vitamin A: 1,898 IU; Vitamin C: 78 mg; Diabetic Exchange: Bread/Starch 1, Fat 2, Meat (Very Lean) 3

grilled arctic char
with artichoke–green olive tapenade

What's in this for baby and me? Protein.

While this tapenade is delicious with any type of fish, it is also incredibly good as a dip with whole wheat crackers, crispy pita bread, or melba toasts rounds. (You might want to add ⅓ cup crumbled pasteurized feta cheese if serving this tapenade as a dip.) The arctic char is an excellent source of protein, and a good source of vitamin A, folic acid, B vitamins, and DHA omega-3.

Serves 2

Artichoke–Green Olive Tapenade (makes about
1 cup)
¾ cup artichoke hearts in brine (about 4
   large hearts), drained
15 pitted green olives (about ⅓ cup)
1 to 2 tablespoons freshly squeezed lemon
   juice, to taste
2 tablespoons olive oil

1 small garlic clove
¼ cup chopped fresh dill
Freshly ground pepper
12 ounces Arctic char or salmon steaks, rinsed
   and dried with paper towels, brushed with
   olive oil
Salt and freshly ground pepper, to taste

1. To make the tapenade, combine all of the ingredients except the dill in the bowl of a food processor and process until slightly chunky. Add the dill and pulse a few times. Be careful not to puree. Adjust the seasoning and transfer to a serving bowl. Cover and refrigerate until ready to serve.
2. To grill the Arctic char, preheat the grill. Have a clean plate ready for the cooked fish. Grease the grill rack, season the fish with salt and pepper, then place it on the grill for approximately 5 minutes on each side, or until the fish is cooked through. The cooking time will depend on the heat of the grill and the thicknesses of the fish.
3. Serve immediately with the tapenade on the side.

▶ **Storage Tip:** The artichoke–green olive tapenade keeps refrigerated for 7 days. It does not freeze well.

▶ *Complete Meal Ideas:* Serve this Arctic char and tapenade with:

    Brown rice, whole grains, or potatoes

    A vegetable or salad (you might want to try the Vegetables
       with Lemon, Olive Oil, and Fresh Herbs, page 153)

    Reduced-fat 2% milk or low-fat yogurt

    Fresh fruit

APPROXIMATE NUTRITIONAL INFORMATION: Serving size: 6 ounces salmon (Note: Because Arctic char was not included in Nutritionist Pro software, 6 ounces of salmon was used for the following calculations.); Calories: 292 cals; Protein: 31 g; Carbohydrates: 0 g; Fat: 17 g; Fiber: 0 g; Sodium: 86 mg; Diabetic Exchange: Meat (Medium Fat) 4

APPROXIMATE NUTRITIONAL INFORMATION: Serving size: 2 tablespoons artichoke–green olive tapenade; Calories: 57 cals; Protein: 1 g; Carbohydrates: 4 g; Fat: 4 g; Fiber: 0 g; Sodium: 240 mg; Diabetic Exchange: Fat 1, Vegetable 1

omega-3 sources[8]

Amounts of EPA and DHA in fish and fish oils and the amount of fish consumption required to provide about 1 gram of EPA and DHA per day

FISH SOURCE (3-OUNCE SERVING SIZE)	DHA AND EPA CONTENT IN MG *	DAILY AMOUNT IN OUNCES REQUIRED FOR ABOUT 1 GRAM OF EPA AND DHA**
Tuna, light, canned in water, drained	0.26	12
Tuna, white, canned in water, drained	0.73	4
Sardines	0.98–1.70	2–3
Salmon, chum	0.68	4.5
Salmon, sockeye	0.68	4.5
Salmon, pink	1.09	2.5
Salmon, chinook	1.48	2
Salmon, Atlantic, farmed	1.09–1.83	1.5–2.5
Salmon, Atlantic, wild	0.9–1.56	2–3.5
Mackerel	0.34–1.57	2–8.5
Herring, Pacific	1.81	1.5
Herring, Atlantic	1.71	2
Trout, rainbow, farmed	0.98	3
Trout, rainbow, wild	0.84	3.5
Halibut	0.4–1.0	3–7.5
Cod, Pacific	0.13	23
Cod, Atlantic	0.24	12.5
Haddock	0.2	15
Catfish, farmed	0.15	20
Catfish, wild	0.2	15
Flounder/Sole	0.42	7
Oyster, Pacific	1.17	2.5
Oyster, Eastern	0.47	6.5
Oyster, Farmed	0.37	8
Lobster	0.07–0.41	7.5–42.5
Crab, Alaskan king	0.35	8.5
Shrimp, mixed	0.27	11
Clam	0.24	12.5
Scallop	0.17	17.5
CAPSULES		
Cod liver oil***	0.19	5
Standard fish body oil	0.30	3
Omega-3 fatty acid concentrate	0.50	2

The intakes of fish given above are very rough estimates because oil content can vary markedly (>300%) with species, season, diet, and packaging and cooking methods.

*The EPA and DHA content of fish is per 3-ounce serving (edible portion), and per grams per gram of oil.

**The amount required to provide about 1 gram of EPA and DHA per day is measured in ounces of fish per day, or grams per gram of oil per day.

***This intake of cod liver oil would provide approximately the recommended daily allowance of vitamins A and D.

sautéed halibut
with garlic-herb butter

~

What's in this for baby and me? Protein.

PAIR THIS GARLIC-herb butter with any grilled or sautéed fish, poultry, or meat for delectable results. This recipe makes four tablespoons; you will use only a small portion of it on your fish. The leftovers are fantastic on top of cooked vegetables or baked potatoes, or for making garlic bread. Halibut is an excellent source of protein and a good source of vitamins E and A, B vitamins, calcium, iron, and DHA omega-3.

Serves 2

GARLIC-HERB BUTTER
- 4 tablespoons unsalted butter, at room temperature
- 1 small garlic clove
- ½ cup fresh parsley leaves
- ½ cup fresh dill
- Salt and freshly ground pepper, to taste

- 1 tablespoon olive oil
- 12 ounces halibut steak (1 steak about 1¼-inch thick and 10 to 12 inches long), gently rinsed, dried well with paper towels, with cartilage trimmed at both ends
- Salt and freshly ground pepper, to taste

1. To make the garlic-herb butter, place all of the ingredients in the bowl of a food processor and process until smooth and uniformly green.
2. To sauté the halibut steak, heat the olive oil in a medium nonstick skillet over medium-high heat. Season the fish with salt and pepper, then add it to the skillet. Cook for approximately 3 to 4 minutes on each side, or until completely cooked through. Check by pulling the flesh away from the center bone; it should be opaque and flaky.
3. Serve the halibut with about 1 teaspoon of the garlic-herb butter placed on top of the fish to melt.

▶ *Variations:* Use salmon steaks or any other fish filet or steak instead of halibut.

▶ *Cooking Tip:* Halibut is generally sold three ways: full steaks that have four sections attached to a central bone; belly cut, with two sections; and a boneless steak with one section. A full steak serves two people, depending on the size.

▶ *Storage Tip:* The garlic-herb butter keeps refrigerated for 5 days, and it can be frozen for up to 1 month.

▶ *Complete Meal Ideas:* Serve this halibut with:

Vegetables or green salad (you might want to try Light
and Healthy Vegetable Ragout, page 202)
Whole grains, such as couscous or brown rice, or baked or roasted potatoes
Reduced-fat 2% milk or low-fat yogurt
Fresh fruit or sorbet

APPROXIMATE NUTRITIONAL INFORMATION: Serving size: one halibut steak with 1½ teaspoons garlic-herb butter; Calories: 293 cals; Protein: 45 g; Carbohydrates: 0 g; Fat: 11 g; Fiber: 0 g; Sodium: 119 mg; Diabetic Exchange: Fat 2, Meat (Very Lean) 6

canned wild salmon patties
with dill-yogurt sauce

What's in this for baby and me? Protein and calcium.

LIGHT AND TASTY, these salmon patties are a fabulous source of protein and calcium, and, of course, wild salmon is high in DHA omega-3. But that's not all—the patties contain iron, vitamins D and E, folic acid, and B vitamins. One of the best things about canned wild salmon is that is a lot cheaper than fresh wild salmon. Choose canned red (not pink) wild salmon, such as Bumble Bee Wild Alaska Scotch Red Salmon, for best results. If you don't have time for the sauce, a wedge of lemon or lime will do.

Makes 5 patties

DILL-YOGURT SAUCE (makes about ½ cup)
- 1 tablespoon light mayonnaise
- ¼ cup low-fat plain yogurt
- ½ cup fresh dill
- Salt and freshly ground pepper, to taste

SALMON PATTIES
- One 14.75-ounce can of wild red salmon, drained
- ⅓ cup thinly sliced scallions
- 2 tablespoons chopped fresh cilantro
- ⅓ cup finely diced celery
- Zest of one lemon, about 1 teaspoon zest
- 2 tablespoons light mayonnaise
- 1 cup plain breadcrumbs
- 2 large eggs, beaten
- Freshly ground pepper or a dash of Tabasco sauce, to taste
- 2 tablespoons olive oil

1. To make the sauce, combine all the ingredients in the bowl of a food processor and pulse until well blended (the sauce will be runny). Refrigerate until ready to serve.

2. Carefully flake the salmon into a bowl, discarding any small bones, cartilage, and skin.

3. Add the scallions, cilantro, celery, lemon zest, mayonnaise, ½ cup of the breadcrumbs, and the eggs to the bowl. Mix gently, being careful not to overmix, which would make the salmon mushy.

4. Place the remaining ½ cup of breadcrumbs in a pie plate. Using a ½-cup measuring cup, scoop out the salmon mixture and form it into five patties. Coat each patty with the breadcrumbs and set aside. Refrigerate until ready to cook.

5. Heat the olive oil in a large nonstick skillet over medium-low heat. Add the patties and cook for 5 minutes on each side, or until heated through. If they begin browning too fast, lower the heat a bit. Serve immediately with the dill-yogurt sauce on the side.

▶ *Advance Preparation:* The dill-yogurt sauce and the patty mixture can be made up 1 day in advance; keep both refrigerated.

▶ *Storage Tip:* The cooked salmon patties keep refrigerated for 3 days.

▶ *Complete Meal Ideas:* Serve these salmon patties with:
>   Salad or coleslaw (you might want to try the Lemony
>   Coleslaw with Fresh Dill, page 171)
>   Potato salad, whole grains, or whole wheat noodles
>   Reduced-fat 2% milk or low-fat yogurt
>   Fresh fruit

APPROXIMATE NUTRITIONAL INFORMATION: Serving size: 1 salmon patty; Calories: 351 cals; Protein: 27 g; Carbohydrates: 17 g; Fat: 19 g; Fiber: 1 g; Sodium: 818 mg; Calcium: 284 mg; Diabetic Exchange: Bread/ Starch 1, Fat 1, Meat (Medium Fat) 3

marinated grilled chicken
with cilantro dipping sauce

What's in this for baby and me? Protein.

YOU'LL BE SHARING this high-protein grilled chicken recipe with your friends. Cutting the chicken breasts in half horizontally allows more of the marinade to cover the surface of the poultry. See Cooking Tip for a skewered-chicken option. Add the cilantro to the dipping sauce at the last minute to retain its bright green color. Chicken is also a good source of B vitamins.

Serves 4

MARINADE
- 2 tablespoons minced fresh ginger
- 2 garlic cloves, minced
- 3 tablespoons soy sauce
- ¼ cup canned pineapple juice
- 1 tablespoon brown sugar
- 1 tablespoon canola oil
- ⅓ cup chopped fresh cilantro

1 pound boneless, skinless chicken breasts, each cut in half horizontally

CILANTRO DIPPING SAUCE
- 1 tablespoon white vinegar
- 1 teaspoon sugar
- 1 teaspoon minced garlic
- Chili pepper flakes (optional)
- 2 tablespoons finely chopped fresh cilantro leaves

1. To make the marinade, mix all the ingredients *except* the chicken in a bowl. Add the chicken, mix to cover with the marinade, and refrigerate for at least 2 hours, or up to 24 hours.
2. To make the cilantro dipping sauce, combine all of the ingredients *except* the cilantro in a bowl, add 2 tablespoons of water, stir, and set aside.
3. Preheat the grill. Have a platter ready for the cooked chicken. Grease the grill rack, place the chicken on the grill for approximately 4 to 5 minutes on each side, or until thoroughly cooked. The cooking time will depend on the thickness of the chicken and the heat of the grill.
4. Arrange the cooked chicken on a platter. Add the cilantro to the dipping sauce and serve alongside the chicken.

▶ *Advance Preparation:* Marinate the chicken for at least 2 hours, or up to 24. Keep refrigerated.

► **Cooking Tip:** After marinating, this chicken can also be skewered and grilled. Slice each of the chicken breasts into 1½-inch-wide strips and thread them on 12-inch-long skewers. You will have enough chicken to make about 12 skewers.

► **Health Tip:** Discard all excess marinade. Place the cooked chicken on a clean serving plate.

► **Complete Meal Ideas:** Serve this grilled chicken with:
Brown rice or whole wheat noodles (you might want to try
    Very Simple Fried Rice with Vegetables, page 263)
Green salad or vegetable
Reduced-fat 2% milk or low-fat yogurt
Fresh fruit

APPROXIMATE NUTRITIONAL INFORMATION: Serving size: one-fourth of the marinated grilled chicken; Calories: 198 cals; Protein: 29 g; Carbohydrates: 5 g; Fat: 6 g; Fiber: 0 g; Sodium: 688 mg; Diabetic Exchange: Fat 1, Meat (Very Lean) 4

Note: The sodium and fat numbers are high because they take all of the marinade into account. They do not reflect how much you are consuming, which is much less.

APPROXIMATE NUTRITIONAL INFORMATION: Serving size: 1 teaspoon of the cilantro dipping sauce; Calories: 5 cals; Protein: 0 g; Carbohydrates: 1 g; Fat: 0 g; Fiber: 0 g; Sodium: 1 mg; Diabetic Exchange: FREE

beef with broccoli

What's in this for baby and me? Protein and vitamins A and C.

A STAPLE ON Chinese menus, this dish is surprisingly easy to make at home. Apart from being an excellent source of protein and vitamins A and C, beef with broccoli is a good source of iron, folic acid, and B vitamins. Be sure to use the leanest beef your budget allows, such as rib eye or tenderloin. Have your rice or noodles ready before you start this dish; it will only take 5 minutes to cook.

Serves 6

1 pound beef rib eye, visible fat trimmed, sliced into very thin (about ⅛-inch thick) 1-inch-long strips

5 tablespoons soy sauce

1 pound fresh broccoli florets (about 4 cups florets)

1 tablespoon toasted sesame oil

2 tablespoons rice wine

1 tablespoon hoisin sauce

1 tablespoon brown sugar

1 tablespoon cornstarch

1 tablespoon canola oil

1 tablespoon fresh ginger, peeled and very thinly sliced

½ cup scallions, sliced into ½-inch pieces

1 tablespoon roasted sesame seeds, for garnish (optional)

1. Place the beef in a bowl, add 2 tablespoons of the soy sauce, mix well, cover, and refrigerate for up to 30 minutes.
2. Cook the broccoli in boiling water for 2 minutes, drain, and set aside.
3. In a small bowl combine the remaining 3 tablespoons of the soy sauce and the sesame oil, rice wine, hoisin sauce, brown sugar, 3 tablespoons of water, and the cornstarch. Mix well and set aside.
4. Heat the canola oil and ginger in a large nonstick skillet over high heat for 30 seconds. Add the reserved beef, stirring constantly, and sauté for 2 minutes.
5. Add the reserved soy sauce mixture and the scallions. Cook until the sauce begins to thicken, about 2 minutes. Mix in the reserved broccoli, transfer to a serving dish, sprinkle with sesame seeds, if using, and serve immediately.

▶ *Timesaving Tip:* If you are short on time, skip the marinating process in Step 1. Use 5 tablespoons of soy sauce in Step 3.

▶ *Health Tip:* If your doctor has restricted your sodium intake, use low-sodium or light soy sauce.

▶ *Storage Tip:* This beef with broccoli keeps 3 days refrigerated.

▶ *Complete Meal Ideas:* Serve this beef with:
Brown basmati rice or rice noodles
Reduced-fat 2% milk or low-fat yogurt
Fresh fruit that contains vitamin C

APPROXIMATE NUTRITIONAL INFORMATION: Serving size: one-sixth of the beef with broccoli; Calories: 299 cals; Protein: 16 g; Carbohydrates: 9 g; Fat: 22 g; Fiber: 0 g; Sodium: 976 mg; Vitamin A: 1,503 IU; Vitamin C: 46 mg; Diabetic Exchange: Fat 3, Meat (Medium Fat) 2, Vegetable 2

sweet treats:
desserts and snacks

DESSERTS

ESSERT MAY BE the least essential part of the meal, but for many the most satisfying. If you have a sweet tooth, pregnancy-induced or preexisting, curtailing your sugar intake may be one of your biggest challenges during pregnancy. One thing to keep in mind is that not all sweets are sticky, gooey, high fat, and fabulously rich. A bowl of fresh fruit, a serving of sorbet or frozen yogurt, applesauce, raisins, or a glass of juice can satisfy the urge for something sweet and provide some nutrients at the same time.

It is the empty, high-fat calories (such as pastries, doughnuts, and candy) that a pregnant woman should avoid. One of the best ways to eliminate these nonessential items from your diet is to keep them out of your shopping cart. This is admittedly difficult if you have young children or a husband who also has a sweet tooth, but in the long run, it is better for the entire family to avoid such items.

While homemade desserts and snacks are best (because you can control what goes into them), lack of time, energy, or the desire to bake or cook can keep them off your list of things to do. When buying desserts and snacks, read labels carefully and try to choose those that have the most nutritional value per calorie. Avoid all items with trans fats. Try not to let desserts or snacks take the place of high-nutrient foods, especially if you are diabetic or if you need to watch your calorie intake. We all need to indulge at times, and as long as it is done in moderation, and not on a daily basis, a dessert is a well-deserved treat, pregnant or not!

SNACKS

THE BIGGEST DANGER with snacks is turning them into mini meals. Generally, pregnant women should consume three meals and two or three snacks a day. It is important always to remember portion sizes and to try to choose the most nutrient-dense snacks possible. Incorporating protein into your snack, such as having whole wheat crackers and cheese, satisfies hunger and at the same time helps fulfill your protein requirements.

dairy calcium sources

FOOD	SERVING SIZE	CALCIUM (MG)
Swiss cheese	2 ounces	545
Nonfat plain yogurt	1 cup	488
Low-fat plain yogurt	1 cup	448
Monterey Jack cheese	2 ounces	423
Part-skim low-moisture mozzarella cheese	2 ounces	414
Cheddar cheese	2 ounces	409
Processed cheese	2 ounces	325
Fontina cheese	2 ounces	312
Nonfat milk	8 ounces	301
Reduced-fat 1% milk	8 ounces	300
Reduced-fat 2% milk	8 ounces	298
Whole (3.3%) milk	8 ounces	290
Nonfat dry milk	⅓ cup	283
Pasteurized feta cheese	2 ounces	280
Pasteurized goat cheese	1 ounce	253
Part-skim ricotta cheese	¼ cup	167
Reduced-fat buttermilk	½ cup	142
Parmesan cheese	2 tablespoons	138
Frozen yogurt	½ cup	138
Vanilla ice cream	½ cup	87
Low-fat 2% cottage cheese	½ cup	78

Your biggest snack challenge might be young children who seem to be in constant need of a snack. While you are doling out treats, you might find yourself mindlessly putting handfuls in your mouth too. This goes with the territory of being a tired, overworked, and hungry mom who probably eats lunch standing up and considers her toddler's leftovers part of her own meal. Below is a list of snacks and snack combinations to get you started in the right direction.

Healthy Snacks for 100 to 200 Calories

1 mozzarella cheese stick = 80
1 medium apple = 90
2 tablespoons raisins = 90
5 pieces dried apricots = 90
1 cup grapes = 100
1 medium banana = 105
1 cup fresh strawberries with 2 tablespoons By Nature Sweetened Light Whipped Cream = 105
8 ounces Naked Protein Juice Smoothie = 110
18 dry roasted whole almonds = 120
¼ cup trail mix (1 ounce) = 130
¼ cup hummus with 8 baby carrots = 136
2 tablespoons guacamole with 3 whole wheat crackers = 144
1 slice of whole wheat bread with 1 teaspoon jam = 165
1 brown rice cake with 1 tablespoon almond butter = 171
½ cup fruit salad in light syrup (drained) with ½ cup low-fat vanilla yogurt = 177
½ cup low-fat cottage cheese (2%) with 5 whole wheat crackers = 189
1 celery stalk with 2 tablespoons peanut butter = 199
1 ounce cheddar cheese with 5 whole wheat crackers = 201
1 hard-boiled egg with 1 whole wheat pita = 207
¼ cup dry roasted peanuts = 213
1 cup low-fat fruit yogurt = 257

RECIPE NOTES

SOME DESSERTS ARE associated with seasons, others with holidays, and still others with celebrations. What would summer be without fresh fruit cobblers, or Thanksgiving without pumpkin pie? But don't limit yourself to these dessert stereotypes. Use frozen or canned fruit to create a satisfying soul-warming crisp or cobbler in December, and serve pumpkin pie in the middle of June.

sweet treats: desserts and snacks

~

Peach and Blackberry Cobbler

Apple-Blueberry Granola Crisp

Strawberry Whole Wheat Short Cake

No-Bake Fresh Strawberry-Raspberry Pie

Low-Fat Frozen Raspberry Pie

Reduced-Fat Ricotta Cheese Cake

Pumpkin Pie

Carrot Cake with Cream Cheese Frosting

Angel Food Cake with Lemon Drizzle

Vanilla Flan with Fresh Berries

Orange, Blueberry, and Date Salad with Frozen Yogurt

Patricia Terry's Pumpkin Bread

Fruit-Filled Granola ▼

Rhubarb Sauce ▼

Applesauce with Dried Apricots and Cranberries ▼

Walnut Spice Coffee Cake

Blueberry Buckle

▼ Vegan recipe

Some notes about the recipes in this chapter:

- Avoid the temptation to taste any batter that contains raw egg (see Eggs and *Salmonella enteritidis,* page 79).
- If you are making a custard-type dessert that contains eggs, be sure that the eggs are fully cooked. An instant-read thermometer should read 160°F.
- When measuring dry ingredients, level them off with the back of a knife or another straight edge.
- Use a liquid measure (Pyrex measuring cup) to measure wet ingredients and a dry measure (stainless steel or plastic cups) for dry ingredients.
- Factor in the need for advance planning and cool-down times. Some recipes require chilling or freezing, some need to sit overnight, and others need to cool completely before serving.
- Use your favorite fruits in the cobbler and crisp recipes.
- Use frozen fruit or canned fruit in juice or light syrup in place of fresh fruit if you are in a hurry or if fresh fruit is not in season.
- Buy bags of already chopped walnuts and other nuts to save time and energy.
- All-purpose flour should ideally be enriched and unbleached.
- You can substitute soy beverages and other soy products for dairy products.
- Wherever indicated use trans fat–free 9-ounce graham cracker pie shells "with 2 extra servings" to avoid overspill, or make your own (see Homemade Graham Cracker Crust, page 354).
- To minimize clean up, line the baking sheet with foil before placing pie dishes or other things on it to bake.
- Since all oven temperatures vary, be sure to pay close attention to cooking times and judge the doneness according to your oven's performance, not the exact time given in a recipe.
- Modify the recipes to suit your dietary needs and your family's tastes.
- You will notice that only seven of the recipes in this chapter have ADA diabetic exchange values. We decided to omit the values because diabetics should not consume desserts on a regular basis. Their calories should be used for foods with higher nutrients.

PLANNING AHEAD FOR SWEET TREATS:
DESSERTS AND SNACKS

▶ *Best eaten the day they are made:*

Peach and Blackberry Cobbler

Apple-Blueberry Granola Crisp

Strawberry Whole Wheat Shortcake

No-Bake Fresh Strawberry-Raspberry Pie

Pumpkin Pie

Angel Food Cake with Lemon Drizzle

Orange, Blueberry, and Date Salad with Frozen Yogurt

Blueberry Buckle

▶ *Can be made up to 6 hours ahead or the night before:*

No-Bake Fresh Strawberry-Raspberry Pie

Low-Fat Frozen Raspberry Pie

Reduced-Fat Ricotta Cheesecake

Carrot Cake with Cream Cheese Frosting

Vanilla Flan with Fresh Berries

Orange, Blueberry, and Date Salad with Frozen Yogurt

Applesauce with Dried Apricots and Cranberries

Walnut Spice Coffee Cake

Blueberry Buckle

▶ *Can be made up to 3 days ahead:*

Reduced-Fat Ricotta Cheesecake

Pumpkin Pie

Carrot Cake with Cream Cheese Frosting

Vanilla Flan with Fresh Berries

Patricia Terry's Pumpkin Bread

Rhubarb Sauce

Applesauce with Dried Apricots and Cranberries

▶ *Can be frozen for up to 1 month:*

Carrot Cake with Cream Cheese Frosting (freeze unfrosted)

Patricia Terry's Pumpkin Bread

Walnut Spice Coffee Cake

▶ *Can be kept in an airtight container at room temperature for up to 5 days:*

Fruit-Filled Granola

vitamin a and c fruit and vegetable sources

Vitamin A

VEGETABLES

1 cup broccoli

1 cup Brussels sprouts

⅔ cup cooked spinach, mustard
greens, collard greens, kale,
bok choy, or Swiss chard

1 cup packed sliced romaine
or loose leaf lettuce

½ cup sliced asparagus

8 baby carrots

½ cup chopped or pureed
cooked pumpkin

½ cup chopped or pureed
cooked butternut squash

½ cooked sweet potato

½ large red bell pepper

FRUITS

¾ cup cantaloupe

5 dried apricots

½ mango

2 tangerines

Vitamin C

VEGETABLES

¾ cup cauliflower florets

1 cup Brussels sprouts

1 cup broccoli florets

½ cooked bok choy

½ cup cooked mustard greens

½ cup cooked kale

1 cup raw cabbage

1 baked potato

½ large red bell pepper

½ tomato

FRUITS

½ cup orange or grapefruit juice

½ grapefruit

1 orange or other citrus fruit

1 cup diced cantaloupe

1 cup diced papaya

1 mango

1 cup berries (any kind)

½ cup cooked rhubarb

1 cup pineapple

1 kiwi

pantry items for sweet treats: desserts and snacks

Fresh Produce
Blackberries
Blueberries
Carrots
Granny Smith apples
Lemons
Mint
Navel oranges
Peaches
Raspberries
Rhubarb
Strawberries

Dairy
Reduced-fat or fat-free cream cheese or Neufchâtel
Grade A large eggs
Low-fat buttermilk
Low-fat or nonfat plain yogurt
Part-skim ricotta cheese
Reduced-fat or nonfat dairy sour cream
Unsalted butter
Whole or reduced-fat milk 2%

Dry Staples
9-inch store-bought ready-made pie crusts (preferably whole wheat) and/or frozen pie crusts
9-inch store-bought reduced-fat graham cracker pie crusts
9-ounce capacity store-bought graham-cracker crusts "with 2 extra servings"
Baking powder
Baking soda
Brown sugar
Cake flour

Chopped walnuts and/or pecans
Confectioner's sugar
Cornstarch
Cream of tartar
Dark or light raisins
Dried apricots
Dried banana slices
Dried cherries
Dried cranberries
Dried pitted dates
Enriched all-purpose flour (preferably unbleached)
Granulated sugar
Ground flaxseed
Kellogg's Healthy Choice Low Fat Granola without Raisins
Light or dark brown sugar
Plain or vanilla-flavored meringue cookies (such as Miss Meringue)
Powdered sugar
"Old-fashioned" rolled oats (not quick cooking)
Sliced almonds
Walnuts
Whole wheat flour

Spices and Flavorings
Ground cinnamon
Ground ginger
Ground nutmeg
Pumpkin pie spice mix
Pure vanilla extract

Canned, Bottled, and Jarred Staples
Applesauce
Canola oil
Canola oil cooking spray

Crushed pineapple (8-ounce can)
Honey
Light evaporated skim milk (12-ounce can)
Mandarin orange segments in light syrup or juice (15-ounce can)
Maple syrup
Molasses
Non-fat sweetened condensed milk (14-ounce can)
Solid pack pumpkin (not pumpkin pie mix) (15-ounce can)

Yellow cling peaches in light syrup (29-ounce can)

Frozen Staples
Blackberries
Blueberries
Frozen yogurt or ice cream
Peaches
Raspberries (12-ounce bag)

From the Salad Bar
Grated carrots (not shredded)

reduced-fat ricotta cheesecake

What's in this for baby and me? Protein.

THIS REDUCED-FAT cheesecake is crammed with protein, and it is a good source of calcium. Top with sliced fresh fruit or berries, Diabetic-Friendly Strawberry-Raspberry Syrup (page 59), or Rhubarb Sauce (page 373). A recipe for Homemade Graham Cracker Crust follows.

Makes one 9-inch cheesecake; serves 8

One 9-ounce store-bought graham cracker crust "with 2 extra servings" or one 9-inch store-bought reduced-fat graham cracker crust

One 8-ounce package fat-free or reduced-fat cream cheese or Neufchâtel

1 cup part-skim ricotta cheese

⅓ cup sugar

1 large egg

½ cup nonfat plain yogurt or reduced-fat or nonfat dairy sour cream

1 teaspoon pure vanilla extract

1. Preheat the oven to 350°F. Place the graham cracker crust on a baking sheet lined with foil.
2. Place the cream cheese and ricotta cheese in a large bowl and beat with an electric mixer on medium speed until creamy. Add the sugar and continue to beat for 30 seconds. Add the egg, yogurt, and vanilla extract and beat until well blended.
3. Pour the filling into the graham cracker crust. Bake for 45 minutes, or until the center of the cheesecake is almost firm (it will firm up as it cools). Remove the cheesecake from the oven, and let cool to room temperature, then refrigerate for at least 4 hours before serving. (Refrigerate leftovers.)

APPROXIMATE NUTRITIONAL INFORMATION: Serving size: one-eighth of the reduced-fat ricotta cheesecake with a store-bought crust; Calories: 211 cals; Protein: 10 g; Carbohydrates: 27 g; Fat: 7 g; Fiber: 0 g; Sodium: 299 mg; Diabetic Exchange: Bread/Starch 2, Fat 1

Homemade Graham Cracker Crust

1 cup finely crushed graham cracker crumbs

⅓ cup finely chopped walnuts or pecans

2 tablespoons brown sugar

½ teaspoon ground cinnamon

3 tablespoons unsalted butter, melted

1. Preheat the oven to 350°F.
2. Combine all of the ingredients in a bowl and mix until well blended and the crumbs are moist. Transfer the mixture to a 9-inch pie plate and press it evenly over the bottom and up the sides of the plate. Bake for 9 minutes, or until the crust is slightly firm to the touch. Remove from the oven and let cool before filling.

APPROXIMATE NUTRITIONAL INFORMATION: Serving size: one-eighth of the pie crust; Calories: 126 cals; Protein: 2 g; Carbohydrates: 11 g; Fat: 9 g; Fiber: .6 g; Sodium: 65 mg; Diabetic Exchange: Bread/Starch 1

artificial sweeteners during pregnancy

Are artificial sweeteners, such as saccharin and aspartame (Equal and NutraSweet), safe during pregnancy? Saccharin can cross the placenta to the baby and since the results are unclear, it should be avoided. Aspartame is composed of the amino acids aspartate and phenylalanine. Aspartame seems to be of little concern for pregnant women, because these two amino acids are found in most of the protein we eat. It is unlikely that eating or drinking an average amount (one serving of aspartame-sweetened dessert per day) would be harmful.[1] Consult your doctor for specific recommendations or concerns regarding artificial sweeteners.

peach and blackberry cobbler

What's in this for baby and me? Vitamin C and fiber.

WHEN FRESH PEACHES are in season, by all means use them (see Cooking Tip below for instructions on peeling fresh peaches). Off-season, or if you are short on time, use frozen or canned peaches. The blackberries, or blueberries, can be fresh or frozen. This cobbler is an excellent source of vitamin C and fiber, and a good source of vitamin A, calcium, folic acid, and B vitamins. The cobbler dough can be used to cover any 9-inch baking dish of fruit.

makes one 9-inch cobbler; serves 8

COBBLER DOUGH

- ¾ cup all-purpose flour
- ¾ cup whole wheat flour
- 2 teaspoons baking powder
- ¼ cup sugar
- Pinch of salt
- 6 tablespoons unsalted butter, cut into pieces
- ¾ cup whole or reduced-fat 2% milk
- 1½ teaspoons pure vanilla extract

PEACH AND BLACKBERRY FILLING

- 1½ pounds peaches (about 5) washed, pitted, peeled, and sliced (see variations below)
- 8 ounces (about 2 cups) fresh blackberries or blueberries, washed, or 2 cups frozen berries
- ⅓ cup sugar
- 2 tablespoons all-purpose flour or 1½ tablespoons cornstarch
- ½ teaspoon ground cinnamon

1. Preheat the oven to 425°F. Have a 9-inch baking dish ready.
2. To make the dough, combine the all-purpose and whole wheat flours, baking powder, sugar, and salt in a large bowl and stir to mix. Add the butter, then, using your fingers, rub the mixture until it resembles coarse meal. Stir in the milk and vanilla just until the dough comes together; set aside.
3. To prepare the filling, combine all of the ingredients in a large bowl and mix until well blended. (Note: You do not need to thaw the frozen fruit before baking. If using frozen fruit, your baking time will increase by about 10 to 15 minutes.) Transfer the filling to the baking dish, then drop heaping spoonfuls of the cobbler dough over the fruit, leaving some empty spaces for the fruit to show through.
4. Bake for 12 minutes, then reduce the heat to 400°F and continue to bake for 30 to 35 minutes, or until the peaches are tender when pierced with the tip of a knife and the juices are bubbling. Remove the cobbler from the oven and allow to cool slightly before serving. (Refrigerate leftovers.)

▶ **Cooking Tip:** To peel fresh peaches, bring a pot of water to a rapid boil. Have a bowl filled with ice water ready to stop the cooking process. Add the whole peaches to the boiling water and cook for 30 seconds, then immediately plunge them into the ice water. Cool for about 1 minute, then drain and peel.

▶ **Variations:** An equal amount of all-purpose flour can be substituted for the whole wheat flour. One pound sliced frozen peaches or one 29-ounce can yellow sliced cling peaches in light syrup may be substituted for the fresh peaches. Drain the canned peaches. If you are using canned peaches and have extra space in your baking dish, add a few more blackberries or blueberries.

APPROXIMATE NUTRITIONAL INFORMATION: Serving size: one-eighth peach-blackberry cobbler; Calories: 290 cals; Protein: 4 g; Carbohydrates: 48 g; Fat: 10 g; Fiber: 5 g; Sodium: 114 mg; Vitamin C: 13 mg

apple-blueberry granola crisp

What's in this for baby and me? Folic acid and fiber.

WARM FROM THE oven, topped with a scoop of frozen yogurt, ice cream, or whipped cream, nothing beats this super-crunchy crisp. Rich in folic acid and fiber, the crisp is also a good source of iron and vitamins A, C, and the Bs. The granola topping can be used to cover any 8- or 9-inch baking dish of fruit—peaches or nectarines combined with berries are particularly good.

makes one 9-inch crisp; serves 8

APPLE-BLUEBERRY FILLING

- 4 large Granny Smith apples (about 1¾ pounds), peeled, cored, and cut into ¼-inch slices
- 1 dry pint (2 cups) fresh blueberries, washed and picked over
- ½ cup lightly packed light brown sugar
- 2 teaspoons ground cinnamon (optional)
- 2 tablespoons all-purpose flour or 1½ tablespoons cornstarch

GRANOLA TOPPING

- ½ cup all-purpose flour
- ½ cup lightly packed light brown sugar
- 6 tablespoons cold unsalted butter, cut into pieces
- 1½ cups low-fat granola without raisins

1. Preheat the oven to 375°F. Have an 8- or 9-inch baking dish ready.
2. To make the filling, combine all of the ingredients in a large bowl and mix until well blended. Transfer the filling to the baking dish and set aside.
3. To make the granola topping, combine the flour and brown sugar in a bowl. Add the butter and, using your fingers, rub the mixture until it resembles coarse meal. Add the granola and continue to mix until the granola is incorporated and the topping holds together in small clumps.
4. Distribute the topping evenly over the filling. Bake for about 45 minutes, or until the apples are tender when pierced with the tip of a knife and the juices are bubbling. Remove the crisp from the oven and allow to cool slightly before serving. (Refrigerate leftovers.)

▶ *Timesaving Tip:* Use frozen blueberries instead of fresh.

▶ *Cooking Tip:* Other good baking apple varieties include Stayman, Cortland, Golden Delicious, Winesap, and Rome Beauty.

APPROXIMATE NUTRITIONAL INFORMATION: Serving size: one-eighth apple-blueberry granola crisp; Calories: 366 cals; Protein: 3 g; Carbohydrates: 68 g; Fat: 11 g; Fiber: 5 g; Sodium: 59 mg; Folic Acid: 168 mcg

bed rest

Every woman's dream of an uneventful and pleasant pregnancy doesn't always come true. Some conditions in pregnancy lead to activity restrictions, which can be as simple as elevating your legs or as strict as conservative bed rest with no bathroom privileges. Bed-rest restrictions cause added stress for the entire family, and can make meal planning and food preparation difficult. Often the husband or partner, other family members, and friends will need to help with the cooking, household chores, and care of small children.

TIPS FOR COPING WITH MEALS WHILE ON BED REST

▶ Keep a cooler at your bedside stocked with milk, cheese, fruit, fruit juices, yogurt, and your other favorite foods. Make sure that your cooler is properly chilled (the danger zone is temperatures between 40° and 140°F) and remains cold throughout the day.

▶ If possible, set up a microwave oven or toaster oven at your bedside to reheat precooked, frozen, or semi-prepared meals and to cook vegetables and other simple dishes.

▶ Keep a thermos of soup, pasta, or any other food that can be kept warm for a few hours at your bedside.

▶ Keep cut-up fresh fruits and vegetables, raisins, peanut butter, granola bars, whole grain bread, whole wheat crackers, nuts, individual fruit cups, fruit juices, and other snack items within easy reach.

▶ Keep two to three sport bottles filled with water within reach. Most bed rest situations also mean an increase in fluid requirements.

▶ Keep plastic utensils, napkins, paper cups, and wipes by your bedside.

▶ Discuss your prenatal meal plan with your caretaker (your husband or partner, mother, friend, or hired help) and share recipes with family and friends who may be bringing meals to you.

strawberry whole wheat shortcake

⌒

What's in this for baby and me? Vitamin C.

These shortcakes, high in vitamin C, and a good source of calcium, folic acid, and fiber, are so good you'll have trouble keeping little hands (or big ones) from eating the shortcake before the dessert is assembled. The strawberries should be allowed to sit for at least 2 hours before serving for their juices to release. If you need to speed things up, sauté half of the berries with the sugar, combine with the uncooked berries, and serve.

serves 6

STRAWBERRY FILLING

1½ pounds (about 6 cups) fresh
    strawberries, washed and hulled; half of
    the strawberries cut into quarters, or
    eighths if they are large
⅓ cup sugar, or to taste

SHORTCAKE

½ cup all-purpose flour
½ cup whole wheat flour
1½ teaspoons baking powder
¼ cup sugar
3 tablespoons unsalted butter, cut into
    pieces
½ cup whole milk or reduced-fat 2% milk
Whipped cream, for topping (optional)

1. To make the filling, 2 hours before serving, combine the sliced strawberries and sugar in a bowl, mix and set aside. Place the whole strawberries in the bowl of a food processor and pulse until they are chopped into small pieces; do not puree. Add the chopped strawberries to the sliced strawberries, stir, cover, and refrigerate until ready to serve.
2. Preheat the oven to 450°F. Line a baking sheet with parchment paper or lightly grease with canola oil cooking spray.
3. To make the shortcake dough, combine the all-purpose and whole wheat flour, baking powder, and sugar in a large bowl and mix. Add the butter and, using your fingers, rub the mixture until it resembles coarse meal. Add the milk and stir until just combined; do not overmix.
4. Measure scant ¼-cupfuls of the shortcake dough and arrange on the baking sheet. You should have six shortcakes. Bake for 10 minutes, or until light golden brown. Immediately remove the shortcake biscuits from the baking sheet and cool them on a plate or cooling rack.

5. To serve, slice each shortcake biscuit in half. Put the bottoms of the biscuits on the dessert plates, and cover each with some strawberry filling (and juices). Top with whipped cream if desired, cover with the tops of the biscuits, and serve. (Refrigerate leftovers.)

▶ *Cooking Tip:* An equal amount of all-purpose flour can be substituted for the whole wheat flour.

APPROXIMATE NUTRITIONAL INFORMATION: Serving size: one strawberry shortcake; Calories: 239 cals; Protein: 4 g; Carbohydrates: 42 g; Fat: 7 g; Fiber: 4 g; Sodium: 113 mg; Vitamin C: 65 mg

no-bake fresh strawberry-raspberry pie

What's in this for baby and me? Vitamin C.

THE STRAWBERRIES AND raspberries are an excellent source of vitamin C and a good source of fiber. Don't substitute frozen fruit in this recipe. See page 354 for a Homemade Graham Cracker Crust recipe.

makes one 9-inch pie; serves 8

1 pound fresh strawberries (about 5 cups), washed and hulled, large berries halved or quartered
12 ounces fresh raspberries (about 1½ cups), rinsed quickly
¾ cup sugar
¼ cup cornstarch
½ cup water

2 tablespoons freshly squeezed lemon juice
2 tablespoons unsalted butter
One 9-ounce store-bought graham cracker crust "with 2 extra servings" or one 9-inch store-bought piecrust (preferably whole wheat, prebaked according to the package directions)

1. In a large bowl, combine the strawberries and raspberries. Puree 2 cups of the strawberries and raspberries in a food processor or blender until smooth. (Note: The pureed berries should equal about 1⅓ cups.) Set aside the remaining berries.
2. Combine the strawberry-raspberry puree, sugar, cornstarch, water, lemon juice, and butter in a saucepan, bring to a simmer over medium heat, stirring constantly, and simmer, stirring, for 2 minutes, or until the mixture becomes thick and shiny. Remove from the heat.
3. Place half of the reserved strawberries and raspberries in the pie shell and pour half of the hot berry mixture over them. Add the remaining strawberries and raspberries and top with the remaining hot berry mixture. Using a spoon, gently move the strawberries until all of them are covered with sauce and the sauce touches the sides of the pie crust.
4. Cover tightly with plastic and refrigerate for at least 4 hours, or until the filling is set. Serve chilled. (Refrigerate leftovers.)

▶ *Variation:* A total of about 6 cups of either fresh strawberries or raspberries can be used instead of a mixture of both.

APPROXIMATE NUTRITIONAL INFORMATION: Serving size: one-eighth of the strawberry-raspberry pie; Calories: 232 cals; Protein: 2 g; Carbohydrates: 43 g; Fat: 7 g; Fiber: 3 g; Sodium: 88 mg; Vitamin C: 40 mg

pumpkin pie

What's in this for baby and me? Vitamin A.

Packed with vitamin A and a good source of protein and calcium, pumpkin pie isn't just for Thanksgiving! If you feel like making a crust from scratch, try the Homemade Whole Wheat Pie Crust on page 215 or the Homemade Graham Cracker Crust on page 354.

makes one 9-inch pie; serves 10

One 9-ounce store-bought graham cracker crust "with 2 extra servings" or one 9-inch store-bought piecrust (preferably whole wheat)

One 15-ounce can solid-pack pumpkin (not pumpkin pie mix)

One 12-ounce can light evaporated skim milk

2 large eggs

½ cup light or dark brown sugar

2 tablespoons mild molasses (optional)

½ teaspoon salt

2 teaspoons pumpkin pie spice mix

1. Preheat the oven to 350°F.
2. Place the graham cracker crust on a baking sheet lined with foil and bake for 7 minutes, or until the crust feels crisp. (Prebake any other store-bought crust according to package directions.) Remove from the oven and set aside. (Leave the oven on.)
3. To prepare the filling, combine the remaining ingredients in a large bowl and whisk until well blended.
4. Pour the filling into the prepared crust. Bake for 50 minutes, or until a knife inserted into the center comes out clean. Cool completely before slicing. (Refrigerate leftovers.)

▶ *Calcium Boost:* In a measuring cup, combine the evaporated milk with ⅓ cup pasteurized instant nonfat dry milk. Mix until the powder has dissolved, then proceed as directed in Step 3.

▶ *Cooking Tip:* Two teaspoons mixed ground cinnamon, ginger, and cloves, or just one of these spices, can be substituted for the pumpkin pie spice mix.

APPROXIMATE NUTRITIONAL INFORMATION: Serving size: one-tenth of the pumpkin pie; Calories: 183 cals; Protein: 6 g; Carbohydrates: 25 g; Fat: 6 g; Fiber: 2 g; Sodium: 312 mg; Vitamin A: 11,021 IU; Diabetic Exchange: Bread/Starch 1.5, Fat 1

carrot cake with
cream cheese frosting

What's in this for baby and me? Vitamin A.

Frost this carrot cake for a celebration, or keep it simple for a family dessert or snack. Some grocery stores have salad bars that carry coarsely grated (not shredded) carrots, which makes the cake a cinch to make. Rich in vitamin A and a good source of protein, this carrot cake is a worthy staple.

makes one 13 x 9-inch cake; serves 12

Canola oil cooking spray and flour, for the
   baking pan
¾ cup all-purpose flour
¾ cup whole wheat flour
2 teaspoons baking soda
1½ teaspoons baking powder
2 teaspoons ground cinnamon
½ teaspoon salt
¾ cup canola oil

4 large eggs
1 cup sugar
2 cups grated carrots (about 4 large carrots)
One 8-ounce can crushed pineapple, drained
   (optional)
½ cup chopped walnuts or pecans (optional)
Cream cheese frosting (recipe follows)
   (optional)

1. Preheat the oven to 350°F. Lightly grease and flour a 13 x 9 x 2-inch baking pan.
2. In a large bowl, combine the all-purpose and whole wheat flours, baking soda, baking powder, cinnamon, and salt, stir and set aside.
3. In a large bowl, combine the canola oil and eggs and beat with an electric mixer on medium speed for 3 minutes. Add the sugar and beat for another 3 minutes. Add the dry ingredients in three batches, beating on low speed and scraping the sides of the bowl after each addition. Mix just until the flour is absorbed. With a rubber spatula, fold in the carrots and optional pineapple and walnuts until evenly distributed.
4. Fill the baking pan with the batter and tap gently to release any air bubbles. Bake for about 45 minutes, or until a tester inserted into the center comes out clean. Remove from the oven and let stand for 5 minutes, then invert onto a cooling rack. Cool completely.
5. Frost the cake if desired. Refrigerate leftovers.

▶ *Cooking Tip:* An equal amount of all-purpose flour can be substituted for the whole wheat flour.

APPROXIMATE NUTRITIONAL INFORMATION: Serving size: one-twelfth of the carrot cake; Calories: 308 cals; Protein: 5 g; Carbohydrates: 32 g; Fat: 18 g; Fiber: 2 g; Sodium: 386 mg; Vitamin A: 5,844 IU

cream cheese frosting

makes about 2½ cups

One 8-ounce package reduced-fat cream cheese or Neufchâtel, slightly softened
4 tablespoons unsalted butter, softened
1 tablespoon pure vanilla extract
3 cups confectioners' sugar

Combine the cream cheese and butter in a large bowl and beat with an electric mixer on medium speed for 2 minutes, or until creamy and most of the lumps have disappeared. Add the vanilla and half of the confectioners' sugar and beat for 1 minute, scraping down the sides of the bowl as necessary. Add the remaining sugar and beat until the frosting is smooth. Cover and refrigerate for 1 to 2 hours, or until thickened enough to spread. Use on a completely cooled cake.

APPROXIMATE NUTRITIONAL INFORMATION: Serving size: about 3 tablespoons of the cream cheese frosting; Calories: 178 cals; Protein: 2 g; Carbohydrates: 26 g; Fat: 7 g; Fiber: 0 g; Sodium: 57 mg

leg cramps: a common annoyance

Some pregnant women experience leg cramps, usually during the last three months of pregnancy. These often occur during sleep, but they can hit anytime. Following are some tips for relief:

▶ Stretch your legs (especially your calf muscles) before going to bed.

▶ Avoid pointing your toes while stretching or exercising.

▶ Drink plenty of water.

▶ Try to have three or four servings of calcium-rich food every day.

▶ Massage or apply heat to your calves.

angel food cake with lemon drizzle

～

What's in this for baby and me? A fat-free dessert!

THERE IS NO comparison between package-mix and homemade angel food cake. The key to getting good height on this cake is to bake the cake on the lowest oven rack. Also, it is essential to use cake flour—other flours are too heavy. The optional lemon drizzle adds a nice finish. Fresh berries tossed with a bit of sugar, the Diabetic-Friendly Strawberry-Raspberry Syrup (page 59), or the Rhubarb Sauce (page 373) make wonderful accompaniments.

makes one 9- or 10-inch tube cake; serves 8

1 cup cake flour

1⅓ cups sugar

½ teaspoon salt

1½ cups egg whites (from about 12 large eggs)

1 tablespoon freshly squeezed lemon juice

1 teaspoon cream of tartar

2 teaspoons pure vanilla extract

Lemon drizzle (recipe follows)

1. Adjust an oven rack to the lowest position and preheat the oven to 350°F. Have an ungreased 9- or 10-inch angel food cake tube pan ready.
2. Sift the flour, ⅔ cup of the sugar, and the salt into a medium bowl or onto a piece of parchment or wax paper; set aside.
3. In a large bowl (make sure the bowl is very clean), combine the egg whites, lemon juice, cream of tartar, and vanilla extract. Beat with an electric mixer on low speed for 30 seconds. Increase the speed to medium and beat for about 30 seconds, until frothy bubbles begin to appear. Gradually add the remaining ⅔ cup sugar, increase the speed to high, and continue beating just until soft, glossy peaks form, about 3 minutes.
4. With a rubber spatula, gradually fold in the flour mixture about ¼ cup at a time. Work with a slicing and lifting motion, and make sure to bring up the egg whites from the bottom of the bowl. All of the flour needs to be absorbed, but try not to overmix—that can deflate the whites.
5. Spoon the batter into the tube pan. Bake for 40 minutes, or until the top is golden and springs back when lightly touched.
6. Remove from the oven and allow to cool for 5 minutes. If the pan sides have "feet" to keep them elevated, simply invert the pan onto a cake rack. If not, set the inverted pan on three upside-down mugs or similar objects to keep it suspended.

7. Once cooled, run a long thin knife around the sides of the pan and the center tube and invert the cake onto a serving plate. Cover leftovers with aluminum foil and store in a cool, dry place.
8. Slowly pour the lemon drizzle over the cooled cake.

▶ **Cooking Tip:** Cake flour is a very fine chemically bleached wheat flour. Because its high starch content allows it to support the high proportion of sugar in this recipe, it produces a high-rising cake. Unbleached all-purpose flour is more nutritious, but it produces a cake that will not rise as high. Both flours taste the same.

APPROXIMATE NUTRITIONAL INFORMATION: Serving size: one-eighth of the angel food cake; Calories: 201 cals; Protein: 6 g; Carbohydrates: 43 g; Fat: 0 g; Fiber: .2 g; Sodium: 228 mg; Diabetic Exchange: Bread/ Starch 3

lemon drizzle

makes about ¾ cup

1½ cups confectioners' sugar

1 tablespoon grated lemon zest

3½ tablespoons freshly squeezed lemon juice

1½ teaspoons hot water

Mix all of the ingredients in a bowl until smooth.

▶ **Diabetic Tip:** Omit lemon drizzle.

APPROXIMATE NUTRITIONAL INFORMATION: Serving size: one-eighth of the lemon drizzle; Calories: 75 cals; Protein: 0 g; Carbohydrates: 19 g; Fat: 0 g; Fiber: 0 g; Sodium: 0 mg

vanilla flan with fresh berries

~

What's in this for baby and me? Calcium and vitamin C.

BECAUSE THE CUSTARD needs to sit overnight to absorb as much of the caramel flavor as possible, plan to make this fabulous vanilla flan a day in advance. The flan is an excellent source of calcium and a good source of protein, and the berries are high in vitamin C. A word of advice: because bending is not always easy during pregnancy, have someone help you get this flan (which is baked in a water bath) in and out of the oven.

serves 8

One 14-ounce can nonfat sweetened
   condensed milk
1½ cups whole or reduced-fat 2% milk
2 teaspoon pure vanilla extract
3 large eggs

¾ cup sugar
4 cups fresh raspberries, sliced strawberries,
   blueberries, or a mixture, for garnish
   (optional)

1. Preheat the oven to 325°F. Put a kettle of water on to boil. Have a 2-quart soufflé dish and a baking pan large enough to hold the soufflé dish ready.
2. In a bowl, combine the sweetened condensed milk, regular milk, and eggs, whisk thoroughly, and set aside.
3. Place the sugar in a small nonstick saucepan. Cook, over medium-high heat, stirring with a wooden spoon, until it reaches a rich caramel color. Carefully pour the caramel into the bottom of the soufflé dish, then swirl the soufflé dish to allow some of the caramel to coat 1 inch up the sides of the dish. (Note: The caramel will be extremely hot, so be very careful.) Place the hot saucepan in the sink and immediately fill with water for easier cleanup.
4. Pour the egg mixture through a fine-mesh strainer into the caramel-coated soufflé dish. Add enough boiling water to the baking pan to reach 1½ inches up the sides of the soufflé dish. Bake for 1½ hours: the middle will still be a little jiggly but will harden as it cools. Remove the soufflé dish from the baking pan and let cool to room temperature, then refrigerate for at least 8 hours, or overnight.
5. To serve, fill a baking pan with boiling water. Place the soufflé dish in it for at least 5 minutes to allow the caramel to melt and create a sauce. Loosen the sides of the flan by running a sharp knife around the inside of the soufflé dish. Carefully invert the flan onto a large serving platter with sides to catch the caramel sauce. Serve with fresh berries, if desired. (Refrigerate leftovers.)

APPROXIMATE NUTRITIONAL INFORMATION: Serving size: one-eighth of the vanilla flan; Calories: 285 cals; Protein: 8 g; Carbohydrates: 56 g; Fat: 3 g; Fiber: 2 g; Sodium: 98 mg; Calcium: 202 mg

orange, blueberry, and date salad with frozen yogurt

~

What's in this for baby and me? Vitamin C and fiber.

Tʜɪs ꜰʀᴜɪᴛ sᴀʟᴀᴅ is loaded with vitamin C and fiber, and the frozen yogurt is a good source of protein and calcium. Vary the ingredients to suit your family's taste—raspberries, bananas, and peaches are great additions. Omit the mint leaves, and possibly the cinnamon, for kids.

serves 3 (makes about 2 cups fruit salad)

2 large navel oranges, peeled and cut into segments (see Cooking Tip 1 below)
¾ cup fresh blueberries, washed and picked over
10 pitted dates, thinly sliced

Dash of ground cinnamon
About 12 fresh mint leaves, finely sliced (optional)
1½ cups vanilla frozen yogurt (optional)

Combine all of the ingredients except the frozen yogurt in a bowl. Toss gently. Accompany the fruit salad with the frozen yogurt if desired.

▶ *Timesaving Tip:* Use one 15-ounce can mandarin orange segments, drained, instead of the fresh oranges.

▶ *Cooking Tip 1:* To slice the oranges into segments: Slice the peel and white pith off the top and bottom of each orange. Then stand each orange on a cutting board and, using a sharp thin knife, working from the top of the orange to the base, slice the peel from the orange. (Use the first slice as your guide to know how deep to slice.) Working over a bowl to catch the juices, hold the orange in one hand and slice the orange segments from the membranes, getting the knife as close to the membranes as possible and allowing the segments to drop into the bowl. Once all of the segments have been removed, squeeze the membranes to extract as much juice as possible.

▶ *Cooking Tip 2:* To prevent sticking, oil your knife before slicing the dates.

APPROXIMATE NUTRITIONAL INFORMATION: Serving size: one-third of the fruit salad and ½ cup vanilla frozen yogurt; Calories: 220 cals; Protein: 6 g; Carbohydrates: 52 g; Fat: .3 g; Fiber: 5 g; Sodium: 55 mg; Vitamin C: 52 mg; Diabetic Exchange: Bread/Starch 3.5, Fat 1

fruit-filled granola

~

What's in this for baby and me? Fiber.

IF YOU FEEL a sudden urge to get crunchy during pregnancy, this recipe is for you. Homemade granola goes way beyond the call of duty to get fiber into your diet, and this version is also a good source of protein and iron. Use this surprisingly easy recipe as a blueprint—some other healthy additions include sunflower seeds, unsweetened coconut flakes, unsalted sesame seeds, shelled pumpkin seeds, raisins and other dried fruits, and wheat germ. Freeze-dried fruits are a sweet touch and add a burst of color, not to mention vitamins.

makes about 5 cups

Canola oil or canola oil cooking spray for greasing the baking sheet
½ cup honey, molasses, or maple syrup, or a mixture
¼ cup canola oil

2 cups "old-fashioned" rolled oats (not quick-cooking oats) (see Variation below)
½ cup sliced almonds
⅓ cup dried cherries
⅓ cup chopped dried apricots
⅓ cup dried banana slices

1. Preheat the oven to 250°F. Lightly grease a large baking sheet with sides; set aside.
2. Combine the honey and oil in a small saucepan and heat just until hot (or use the microwave). Place the rolled oats and sliced almonds in a bowl and mix. Add the honey-oil mixture and mix until well combined.
3. Spread the granola mixture evenly on the baking sheet. Bake for about 40 minutes, or until light golden. It will still be soft when it comes out of the oven, but it will harden as it cools. Do not overbake, or the granola will have a bitter, burnt taste. Allow the granola to cool completely.
4. Add the optional dried fruit to the granola and mix well. Store in an airtight container or a zip-lock bag.

▶ *Cooking Tip:* Measure the canola oil first, swirl it around the measuring cup to coat the sides, then measure the honey, which will easily slide out of the measuring cup.

► **Variation:** You can use 2 cups of barley, rye, or wheat flakes in place of the oats, or mix and match all four types.

► **Diabetic Tip:** Reduce serving size to ¼ cup.

APPROXIMATE NUTRITIONAL INFORMATION: Serving size: ½ cup of the fruit-filled granola; Calories: 357 cals; Protein: 7 g; Carbohydrates: 55 g; Fat: 14 g; Fiber: 5 g; Sodium: 2 mg; Diabetic Exchange (values per ¼ cup serving): Bread/Starch 1, Fat 1, Fruit 1

pelvic floor (kegel) exercises

Make pelvis floor exercises, also called Kegel exercises, part of your fitness routine before, during, and after pregnancy. The job of the pelvic floor muscles is to hold your pelvic organs (bladder, uterus, and bowel) in place. These muscles tend to become stretched or weakened during pregnancy, and if they become too weakened, or damaged, they cannot function properly. Ideally, exercises should be done throughout pregnancy to help support the extra weight of the body and to prepare for labor, and continued postpregnancy to re-strengthen the muscles.

How to do Pelvic Floor Exercises: While sitting comfortably on the floor, on a ball, or on a chair, contract your pelvis muscles from the outside area to the inner pelvis. Try to imagine that you are stopping your urine in mid-flow and tightening your anus muscle at the same time. Hold briefly, then release slowly. Keep you stomach relaxed and breathe naturally. Repeat five times. Try to do these exercise five times a day.

patricia terry's pumpkin bread

What's in this for baby and me? Vitamin A.

YOU'LL KEEP COMING back to this recipe for pumpkin bread. Add your favorite ingredients, such as walnuts or mini chocolate chips, to get little ones to try a bite. The pumpkin is a good source of vitamin A.

makes two 8½ x 4½-inch loaves or five 5¾ x 3-inch loaves
(each large loaf serves 12 and each small loaf serves 5)

Canola oil cooking spray for greasing the baking pan	**1 teaspoon ground nutmeg (optional)**
2 cups all-purpose flour	**½ teaspoon ground ginger (optional)**
1½ cups whole wheat flour	**½ cup canola oil**
2½ cups sugar	**½ cup applesauce**
½ teaspoon baking powder	**2 large eggs plus 2 large egg whites**
2 teaspoons baking soda	**⅔ cup water**
½ teaspoon salt	**2 cups solid pack pumpkin (not pumpkin pie mix)**
2 teaspoons ground cinnamon	**1 cup dark or light raisins (optional)**

1. Preheat the oven to 350°F. Spray two 8½ x 4½ x 2½-inch loaf pans or three 5¾ x 3 x 2⅛-inch loaf pans with canola oil cooking spray.
2. In a large bowl, combine the dry ingredients and mix until well blended; set aside.
3. In another large bowl, combine the canola oil, applesauce, eggs, egg whites, and water and whisk to mix. Add this mixture to the dry ingredients and whisk just until combined. Add the pumpkin and raisins, if using, and mix until well blended.
4. Divide the batter among the prepared loaf pans. Bake until a tester inserted into the center of each loaf comes out clean, about 70 minutes for large loaves, about 40 minutes for smaller loaves. Let sit for 5 minutes, then remove from the pans and cool completely before slicing.

▶ *Variation:* An equal amount of all-purpose flour can be substituted for the whole wheat flour.

▶ *Storage Tip:* To freeze, wrap the cooled loaves in aluminum foil and freeze. Wrap leftovers in aluminum foil and store in a cool dry place.

APPROXIMATE NUTRITIONAL INFORMATION: Serving size: one-twelfth of one large loaf of pumpkin bread; Calories: 131 cals; Protein: 2 g; Carbohydrates: 25 g; Fat: 3 g; Fiber: 1 g; Sodium: 104 mg; Vitamin A: 2,718 IU; Diabetic Exchange: Bread/Starch: 1.5, Fat 1

rhubarb sauce

What's in this for baby and me? Vitamin C and calcium.

HIGH IN VITAMIN C and calcium, and a good source of fiber, this sauce is irresistible if you like rhubarb. It's the perfect way to jazz up any snack or dessert, including yogurt, frozen yogurt, or ice cream.

makes about 1 cup

1 pound rhubarb, any leaves trimmed, washed, and cut into ½-inch pieces

½ cup sugar

2 tablespoons water

In a small saucepan, combine all of the ingredients and bring to a boil. Reduce the heat and simmer for 15 to 20 minutes, or until the rhubarb is soft and falling apart. Serve hot or cold. Refrigerate leftovers for up to 3 days. This sauce can also be frozen for up to 1 month.

APPROXIMATE NUTRITIONAL INFORMATION: Serving size: ½ cup rhubarb sauce; Calories: 233 cals; Protein: 2 g; Carbohydrates: 58 g; Fat: .4 g; Fiber: 4 g; Sodium: 10 g; Vitamin C: 18 mg; Calcium: 196 mg

applesauce with
dried apricots and cranberries

What's in this for baby and me? Vitamin A and fiber.

THIS VITAMIN A- and fiber-filled applesauce, with a touch of vitamin C, is the perfect snack or dessert. Feel free to substitute the dried apricots and cranberries with other dried fruit such as cherries or pineapple. For an extra kick, add a cinnamon stick or a dash of ground cinnamon, or a drop of vanilla extract to the finished sauce. See Cooking Tip for apple suggestions.

Makes about 2 cups

1½ pounds apples (about 4), peeled, cored, and cut into eighths
½ cup dried apricots (about 15 pieces)
½ cup dried cranberries
3 tablespoons sugar, to taste

1. Combine the apples, dried apricots, and dried cranberries in a medium saucepan. Add 1¼ cups of water and bring to a boil. Reduce the heat and simmer, stirring occasionally, for 10 to 15 minutes, or until the fruit is soft.
2. Remove saucepan from the heat, stir in the sugar, cool, then puree the apple mixture in a blender or food processor to the desired consistency. (Some people like smooth applesauce, others prefer a chunky consistency. If the sauce is too thick, add 1 tablespoon of water at a time to thin it.) Keep refrigerated.

▶ *Cooking Tip:* The best apples for applesauce include Jonagold, Jonathan, Macoun, Pink Lady, Golden Delicious, Empire, McIntosh, and Rome.

▶ *Storage Tip:* This apple sauce keeps for 1 week refrigerated, and it can be frozen for up to 1 month.

▶ *Diabetic Tip:* Omit the sugar and reduce your portion size to ⅓ cup.

APPROXIMATE NUTRITIONAL INFORMATION: Serving size: ½ cup applesauce with dried apricots and cranberries; Calories: 188 cals; Protein: 1 g; Carbohydrates: 48 g; Fat: 0 g; Fiber: 7 g; Sodium: 2 mg; Vitamin A: 1,432 IU; Diabetic Exchange: Fruit 3

walnut spice coffee cake

~

*What's in this for baby and me? A relatively low-fat cake with a
good dose of vitamins and minerals from the walnuts.*

This MOIST COFFEE cake is packed with walnuts, which offer a good source of ALA
omega-3 and some vitamin and mineral benefits.

Makes one 9-inch round cake, or 12 servings

Canola oil cooking spray, for greasing the
   cake pan
1½ cups chopped walnuts
1 cup all-purpose flour
1 teaspoon baking powder
½ teaspoon baking soda
1 teaspoon ground ginger
2 teaspoons ground cinnamon
½ teaspoon ground nutmeg

¼ teaspoon salt
¾ cup brown sugar
2 large eggs
⅓ cup canola oil
½ cup plus 2 tablespoons reduced-fat sour
   cream
Confectioners' sugar, for dusting the finished
   cake

1. Preheat the oven to 350°F. Grease a 9-inch round cake pan with canola oil cooking
    spray and sprinkle with flour; set aside.
2. Place the walnuts in the bowl of a food processor and process, using the pulse
    button, until finely ground but not to the point of forming a paste.
3. Transfer the ground walnuts to a medium bowl, add the flour, baking powder,
    baking soda, ginger, cinnamon, nutmeg, and salt. Whisk until well combined; set
    aside.
4. In the bowl of an electric mixer, combine the brown sugar and the eggs and beat
    on medium speed for about 4 minutes, or until light and fluffy. Add the canola oil
    and the sour cream and beat 30 seconds more.
5. Using a rubber spatula, fold into the egg mixture using the reserved flour mixture
    until well incorporated. Pour the batter into the prepared cake pan and bake for
    30 minutes, or until a tester inserted in the center of the cake comes out clean.
6. Remove the cake from the oven and let cool for 5 minutes. Run a knife around the
    sides of the pan and invert the cake onto a serving platter. Dust with confectioner's
    sugar before serving.

▶ **_Storage Tip:_** Cover leftovers and store in a cool, dry place. To freeze, wrap the cake in aluminum foil or freezer paper and freeze for up to 1 month.

APPROXIMATE NUTRITIONAL INFORMATION: Serving size: one-twelfth of the walnut spice cake; Calories: 264 cals; Protein: 5 g; Carbohydrates: 23 g; Fat: 18 g; Fiber: 1 g; Sodium: 90 mg

blueberry buckle

What's in this for baby and me? Fiber.

WATCH THE BLUEBERRIES burst and ooze as this luscious dessert bakes. Along with the fiber, this buckle offers a good dose of calcium, iron, folic acid, B vitamins, and protein. Serve with a dollop of thick, low-fat, Greek-style yogurt, a scoop of frozen yogurt, or a bit of whipped cream. A traditional buckle calls for lots of butter, replaced here with canola oil. Since no electric mixer is involved, clean-up is a snap.

Serves 8

CAKE
- Canola oil cooking spray, for greasing the cake pan
- 3 cups fresh blueberries, washed and drained
- ¾ cup plus 1 tablespoon all-purpose flour
- ⅓ cup sugar
- ⅓ cup ground flaxseed
- 2 teaspoons baking powder
- ¼ cup canola oil
- 1 large egg
- ½ cup low-fat buttermilk

CRUMBLE TOPPING
- ¼ cup sugar
- ¼ cup flour
- 1 teaspoon ground cinnamon
- 3 tablespoons unsalted butter
- ½ cup sliced almonds

1. Preheat the oven to 350°F. Grease a 9-inch round cake pan with canola oil cooking spray and set aside.
2. To make the crumble topping, combine all on the ingredients *except the almonds* in a small bowl and quickly mix with your fingers to the consistency of coarse cornmeal. Refrigerate until ready to use.
3. To make the cake, mix the blueberries with 1 tablespoon of the flour and set aside.
4. In a large bowl, whisk the remaining flour, sugar, ground flaxseed, and baking powder; set aside.
5. In a separate bowl, combine the canola oil, egg, and buttermilk, and whisk until well blended. Add this egg mixture to the bowl of dry ingredients and whisk until combined. Using a spatula, gently fold in the reserved blueberries, then transfer the batter to the prepared cake pan.
6. Evenly distribute the crumble topping over the top of the batter. Bake for 45 minutes, or until the top is browned and a tester inserted into the center comes out clean (apart from a bit of blueberry juice). Remove the buckle from the oven and allow to cool slightly before serving. Refrigerate leftovers.

▶ *Variations:* The 3 cups of blueberries may be replaced with other berries or a mix of berries, including raspberries, blackberries, or strawberries. Frozen blueberries may be used; simply thaw, drain, and proceed with Step 3.

APPROXIMATE NUTRITIONAL INFORMATION: Serving size: one-eighth blueberry crumble; Calories: 343 cals; Protein: 7 g; Carbohydrates: 39 g; Fat: 19 g; Fiber: 5 g; Sodium: 151 mg

exercise tips:
fitness for two

Exercise in moderation is a good thing during pregnancy. It promotes general physical health, good muscle tone, and a stronger respiratory system. Exercise helps reduce stress, combat fatigue, relieve backaches, improve posture, combat varicose veins, improve self-image, and keep your digestion on track. Better fitness can also make delivery easier and will probably help with postpartum recovery. Throughout your pregnancy, keep in mind that you are exercising to stay fit, healthy, and relaxed, not to lose weight. Discuss the exercise routine that is appropriate for you at different stages of your pregnancy with your doctor. [2]

WOMEN WHO SHOULD NOT EXERCISE WITHOUT THEIR DOCTOR'S PERMISSION

▶ Women with a history of miscarriage
▶ Women who have experienced preterm labor in this or a previous pregnancy
▶ Women who have obstetrical complications, including an incompetent cervix, ruptured membranes (broken bag of water), or vaginal bleeding
▶ Women with diabetes
▶ Women with preeclampsia or pregnancy-induced high blood pressure
▶ Women whose fetus is not growing as rapidly as it should be
▶ Women carrying multiples
▶ Women with any other pregnancy complication

There are a couple of things to keep in mind while exercising during pregnancy. First, it is more difficult for you to breathe when exercising because oxygen must be supplied to your additional body mass (including your baby) and to your increased volume of red blood cells. Second, as your belly gets bigger, breathing becomes even more difficult, because your uterus increasingly crowds your diaphragm, the large muscle between your chest and abdomen. Third, your increased hormone levels soften your connective tissues, making your joints more susceptible to injury. And fourth, your balance shifts as your abdomen and chest enlarge, which can cause clumsiness and possibly falls.

Two of the best exercises for pregnant women are brisk walking and swimming (but not diving). Swimming is particularly good because it uses many muscle groups while the water supports your extra weight. Another option might be to join a prenatal exercise class. Many prenatal classes offer support group discussions on a range of pregnancy-related topics, including how to stretch your pregnancy wardrobe, how to choose a name for the baby, and tips for breastfeeding.

Following are some exercise guidelines recommended by the American College of Obstetricians and Gynecologists (ACOG).

▶ Regular exercise (three to five days per week) is preferable to occasional activity.

- Swimming, stationary cycling, and brisk walking are highly recommended.
- Exercises that require jumping, jarring motions, or rapid changes in direction should be avoided. These can cause damage to connective tissue.
- Exercises done lying flat on the back or right side should be avoided. These positions can allow a woman's expanding uterus to compress the vein that carries blood to the heart, which could interfere with blood flow to the uterus.
- Exercise sessions should be preceded by a five-minute period of muscle warm-up (for example, slow walking or stationary cycling at low resistance).
- Exercise should be done on a safe surface, such as a wooden floor or a tightly carpeted or outdoor surface, to reduce the risk of injury.
- Strenuous exercise should not be performed in hot, humid weather or during illness accompanied by fever.
- Moderate or intense aerobic activities should be limited to periods of fifteen to twenty minutes. Lower-intensity activities may be conducted continuously over a longer period of time, but should not exceed forty-five minutes.
- Heart rate should be measured at times of peak activity and should not exceed 140 beats per minute.
- A pregnant woman's temperature should not exceed 100.4°F while exercising. She should drink plenty of water before and after exercise to prevent dehydration and hyperthermia and take a break during exercise if more water is needed or she is tired.
- Care should be taken to rise from the floor gradually to avoid an abrupt drop in blood pressure, and to continue some form of activity involving the legs for a brief period.
- Exercise sessions should be followed by a brief cool-down period of gradually declining activity that includes gentle stationary stretching. Stretches should not be taken to the maximum of resistance.
- A pregnant woman should consume enough calories to meet the needs of her pregnancy (300 extra calories per day) as well as her exercise program. Women should not try to lose weight by exercising during pregnancy.

WARNING SIGNS TO STOP EXERCISING

Chest pain

Dizziness

Shortness of breath

Palpitations (pounding, racing, or irregular heartbeat)

Faintness

Tachycardia (rapid heartbeat)

Pubic pain

Uterine contractions

Vaginal bleeding/amniotic fluid leakage

Absence of fetal movement

Muscle weakness

Calf pain or swelling

Headache

SEVEN

nine months later

⌒

Your nine months of pregnancy are finally over, and you just delivered a gorgeous baby. Now the real work of motherhood begins. If this is your first child, enjoy the fact that ignorance is bliss. If it is your second or more, you know exactly how much work is involved in raising children, but you also know that the rewards far outweigh the hardships.

"Nine Months Later" is about you—yes you, mom. At some point you will want to get your life back on track, and we are here to help. If you want to eat optimally while breastfeeding, you've come to the right place. If you need help salvaging your figure, follow the Stay Balanced Diet for Mothers. If you want an exercise plan to shave inches off your waistline, thighs, and buttocks, embrace the Exercise Menu. And, if you think you may have the "baby blues" or postpartum depression, read on.

NUTRITION FOR BREASTFEEDING MOTHERS

Breastfeeding is a natural, economical, and practical way to nourish your baby—and as *all* studies prove, the optimal way too. By consuming the proper nutrients, a nursing mother can produce breast milk that greatly enhances her baby's physical and mental development. In this section, we will focus only on the nutritional side of breastfeeding, not the technicalities.

Basic Guidelines

- Inform your ob-gyn and your child's pediatrician in advance of delivery that you will be breastfeeding. Explain any dietary restrictions or special needs you have.
- Continue taking all of your prenatal vitamins and any supplements prescribed by your doctor as long as recommended. Do *not* self-prescribe vitamins or supple-

ments (synthetic or herbal), because large doses may be toxic. And remember that vitamins and supplements do not replace real food.

- Follow a well-balanced, varied diet that contains nutrient-dense foods. Your baby will taste the foods you consume, so if you eat healthfully, don't be surprised if your baby develops a taste for nourishing peas, carrots, and peaches.
- Consume about 500 extra calories per day (or about 200 calories above your pregnancy caloric intake) for the duration of breastfeeding.
- Do *not* diet while breastfeeding. Most nursing mothers find that even if they consume adequate amounts of food, their weight drops gradually while breast-feeding. Losing one to two pounds per month is normal.
- Avoid all alcohol. It reaches your baby through your breast milk.
- Avoid smoking and secondhand smoke, which present an increased risk for sudden infant death syndrome (SIDS), respiratory infections, and other health problems.
- Do not take any medications, prescription or over-the-counter, without your doctor's approval. Breastfeeding women should not use Retin A or Accutane. Avoid illicit drugs.
- Severely limit or eliminate caffeine, which passes into your breast milk and can agitate your baby. If you need energy, go for a walk or take a few deep breaths.
- Drink 8 fluid ounces of water each time you breastfeed, or at least 6 to 8 cups of water per day. This, along with increased fiber, will help avoid constipation.
- Vegetarians and vegans should be able to meet all of their nutritional needs quite adequately, although certain supplements may be needed.
- If you find that your baby is intolerant of certain foods, work around them. Some common culprits include garlic, onions, cabbage, broccoli, cauliflower, beans, and spicy or acidic foods.
- Contact a lactation consultant or diabetes educator for special situations including:

  - Mothers nursing multiples or tandem nursing (breastfeeding while pregnant)
  - Diabetic nursing mothers
  - Obese or underweight nursing mothers
  - Teenage nursing mothers
  - Mothers nursing babies born with a cleft palate, premature babies, hospitalized babies, or any other babies with special needs
  - Mothers who have had breast surgery

Nutrients for Breastfeeding

Many women are surprised to discover that their daily calorie intake during breastfeeding needs to be higher than it was during pregnancy. The reason for this is that your body works in overdrive to nourish itself and your rapidly growing infant. It takes about 500 extra calories to fuel your body's milk-producing factory, but this number may need to be adjusted based on milk production, rate of weight loss, and any special situations. In general, a minimal food intake for nursing mothers is no less than 1,800 calories per day.

As with pregnancy, the nutritional guidelines for breastfeeding may appear daunting on paper, but rest assured that certain nutrients in breast milk are fairly consistent, regardless of what a mother eats. A mother's body channels her nutrients into her breast milk, even if it means depleting her own stores. Listed below are some of the most important nutrients for breastfeeding and how they help your baby grow.

SOME IMPORTANT NUTRIENTS FOR BREASTFEEDING WOMEN

NUTRIENT	PREGNANCY RDI	LACTATING RDI (AGES 19–50)	HOW IT HELPS YOUR BABY
Protein	71 g	60 g	Building your baby's body
Calcium	1,000 mg	1,000 mg	Bones, muscles, and nerve function
DHA and EPA omega-3s	Not available	Not available	Physical and cognitive development
Zinc	11 mg	12 mg	Organ development, muscles, eyes, skin, and genetic expression
Vitamin B_{12}	2.6 mcg	2.8 mcg	Red blood cells, nerve function, and metabolism
Vitamin B_6	1.9 mg	2.0 mg	Cell formation, nervous and immune system function
Vitamin A	770 mcg	1,300 mcg	Healthy vision, skin, cell development, and immunity
Vitamin D	5 mcg/200 IU	5 mcg/200 IU	Bones
Vitamin E	15 mg	19 mg	Protects cells from damage and boosts immunity
Choline	450 mg	550 mg	Brain development
Iodine	220 mcg	290 mcg	Thyroid functioning and metabolism
Copper	1,000 mcg	1,300 mcg	Iron absorption
Potassium	4,700 mg	5,100 mg	Kidney, cardiac, digestive, and muscular function

Three Important Studies Related to Breastfeeding

▶ *Vitamin D Supplements for Breastfed Babies*

In 2000 and 2001, studies on rickets (a softening of the bones in children caused by a lack of vitamin D) among breastfed infants in North Carolina, Texas, Georgia, and the mid-Atlantic region of the United States prompted researchers to take a closer look at whether all breastfed infants were getting adequate amounts of vitamin D. Based on their findings and other data, in 2003, the American Academy of Pediatrics recommended a daily supplement of 200 IU of vitamin D for all breastfed infants and all non-breastfed babies whose daily intake of vitamin D–fortified formula or milk is less than 500 ml. If you have any concerns, consult your child's pediatrician for guidance.[1]

▶ *Maternal Fish Intake and Developmental Milestones*

A recent study conducted by Harvard Medical School and Statens Serum Institute in Denmark revealed that both higher fish consumption and longer breastfeeding are linked, however independently, to better physical and cognitive development in infants. The study looked at 25,446 children born from 1997 to 2002. Mothers reported child development by a standardized interview, which the researchers used to generate developmental scores at ages 6 months and 18 months. Researchers observed that children whose mothers ate about 60 grams, or 2 ounces, of fish per day on average, had children who were 25 percent more likely to have higher developmental scores at 6 months and almost 30 percent more likely to have higher scores at 18 months. The children of women who ate the least fish did not score as well. The researchers also discussed evidence that DHA omega-3s from fish, in combination with other nutrients, may be more beneficial for nervous system development than DHA from a supplement.[2]

▶ *Challenges of Breastfeeding for Obese Mothers*

Severely overweight and obese mothers often experience increased challenges when it comes to breastfeeding. In fact, studies indicate that they are more likely to experience difficulty with the mechanics of nursing, which may be one reason they are less likely to start breastfeeding in the first place, or more inclined to breastfeed for a short duration. Studies show that obese mothers also tend to take longer to produce sufficient milk, possibly because of a lower prolactin (a milk-producing hormone) response to suckling. If you are overweight and are experiencing any difficulties, please don't give up before seeking support, ideally even before you deliver. In addition to the numerous health benefits your baby receives from mother's milk, another reason to give breastfeeding a try is that some evidence suggests that overweight mothers who breastfeed may reduce their child's likelihood of becoming obese later. This evidence is, however, ambiguous because many factors need to be considered when interpreting the reasons why a child becomes obese or not.[3]

POSTPARTUM DEPRESSION:
HOW DIET AND EXERCISE CAN HELP

YOUR BABY IS healthy, your nursery adorable, your spouse loves you—but there's one big problem: you are painfully depressed, anxious, and angry, and you're not sure why. Even worse, you're scared to share your disturbing feelings and thoughts with anyone, even your partner. If this describes you, please know that you are not alone. Approximately one in seven new mothers worldwide (about 15 percent) suffers from postpartum depression (PPD). PPD usually begins during the first three months, but it may begin anytime during the first year postpartum.

As moms, new and old, we all have bad days, even bad weeks that leave us feeling depressed, frustrated, irritated, or helpless. But our temporary slumps still have a light at the end of the tunnel. With PPD that light goes off. Low self-esteem and a roller-coaster of emotions torture a new mother's head, heart, and soul, leaving her behavior erratic and often self-destructive.

One mother who knows these feeling all too well is Shoshana Bennett, Ph.D. Her journeys through PPD following both of her pregnancies sparked her commitment to helping women all over the world recover from this disorder. She has written three books—*Post Partum Depression for Dummies* (Wiley, 2007), *Beyond the Blues* (Mood-swings Press, 2006, second edition), and *Pregnant on Prozac* (GPP Life, 2009)—and has helped thousands of women. We asked her to share her story and her expertise on the critical role of nutrition and exercise in recovery. For more information, check out her website, ClearSky-Inc.com, or call the Postpartum Depression Stressline at 1–888–678–2669. All of the volunteers are survivors of either prenatal or postpartum depression.

a mother's story

Immediately after I delivered our first baby in 1983, I knew there was something very wrong with me. I became anxious and obsessive—scary thoughts were spinning non-stop in my head about my baby being harmed. I didn't trust myself to be alone with her, thinking I might be the one to hurt her. I was overwhelmed and frightened. I thought my life was over—there was nothing but doom and gloom. I was a mere shell of the person I had been before the birth.

My ob-gyn did what many unfortunately still do, through no fault of their own, since most ob-gyns don't learn about prenatal or postpartum mood disorders in medical school. When I exclaimed, "If life's going to be like this, I don't want to be here anymore," he laughed. He told me that all new mothers feel like that and that I should go home and do something nice for myself, and that feeling would pass. He tried to normalize a serious disorder (postpartum depression) and dismissed it as the baby blues. If this is normal, I thought, then clearly I'm an inadequate mother and I wasn't cut out to do this. I was convinced I was a burden to my family, and my husband and baby would be better off without me. I will say that I'm quite blessed and grateful to still be here—there were a couple of very close calls when I almost took myself out.

When my daughter was two-and-a-half years old, I remember thinking, "maybe I can be a mom." I now realize that my chemistry was starting to return to normal then. My hair started to curl again, I started seeing in color again, instead of in shades of gray, and I began tasting my food again. We decided to have another baby. Everything went well during my pregnancy, just like the first time, until I delivered. I dropped into the same nightmarish state.

One year into my second life-threatening and undiagnosed postpartum depression, I learned that what I had been suffering from had a name and that there may even be help for it! I vowed to myself at that moment that I would do everything in my power to help other families prevent the devastating effects of this illness. It became my mission to educate medical and mental health professionals and the public. Still coming out of the depression, I started pioneering northern California, founded an organization called Postpartum Assistance for Mothers, and became president of California's state organization. More recently I served as president of our international organization, Postpartum Support International. The help I never received but desperately needed is what I've given to over twenty thousand women while helping them recover from postpartum depression. Along with therapy that empowers new mothers to discard the unrealistic expectations of motherhood, a basic plan of action always includes uninterrupted hours of sleep at night, excellent nutrition, exercise, and emotional and physical support that allow them to nurture themselves. With proper help, women recover to 100 percent wellness.

Defining Your Depression

Identifying the symptoms of PPD and distinguishing them from the "baby blues" is an essential first step. A thyroid imbalance, which affects up to 10 percent of postpartum women, can mimic the symptoms of PPD, so it should be ruled out by your doctor as a physiological cause of depression. If you're feeling down, the list below[4] should help you classify your blues.

BABY BLUES	POSTPARTUM DEPRESSION	POSTPARTUM PSYCHOSIS
Symptoms may last only a few days or weeks	PPD may appear to be the "baby blues" at first, but the signs and symptoms are more intense, and they last longer, eventually interfering with your ability to care for your baby and handle other daily tasks	A rare but serious condition that usually develops within the first two weeks after delivery. If you experience any of these symptoms, get help immediately
Mood swings		
Anxiety or restlessness		Thoughts of suicide
Sadness	Sadness and depression	Confusion or disorientation
Irritability	Insomnia	Hallucinations or hearing voices
Crying for no apparent reason	Intense irritability or anger	Delusions
Lack of concentration	Overwhelming fatigue and exhaustion	Paranoia
Trouble sleeping	Loss of interest in sex	Urge to harm your baby
Fatigue	Lack of joy in life	Inability to care for your baby
	Feelings of shame, guilt, or hopelessness	Sleeplessness for more than 48 hours
	Severe mood swings, panic attacks, or chronic worrying	Inability to eat for an extended period of time
	Difficulty bonding with your baby	
	Withdrawal from family and friends	
	Thoughts of harming yourself or your baby	
	Obsessive-compulsive behaviors that cause distress	
	Uncontrollable crying	

Dietary Advice

Dr. Bennett closely follows the extensive research being done on nutrition and other ways of preventing the onset and treating the symptoms of PPD. Following are her words of wisdom on optimal nutrition. If you are interested in trying the simple system she personally uses and recommends to her pregnant and postpartum clients, feel free to contact her directly at http://ClearSky-Inc.com.

- Take a daily multivitamin with minerals to make sure that you are getting all the essential vitamins your body and brain need.
- Do *not* diet if you are suffering from PPD. Depriving your body of nutrients is detrimental to recovery.
- If you've lost your appetite and can't manage to eat three meals a day, nibble foods throughout the day.
- Consume lots of protein, ideally at least 60 grams per day (see Protein Sources, page 280). High-protein foods will help prevent your blood sugar level from rising; keeping it steady is important for balancing your moods.
- Eat complex carbohydrates, such as whole grains, fruits, and vegetables. These slow-releasing sugars are the type your brain likes, especially if it is struggling with depression.
- Avoid refined carbohydrates as much as possible. A box of chocolates may be fleetingly pleasurable, but the sugar high and crash that follow will send your blood sugar levels and emotions into a tailspin. Keep these foods out of the house. If you want a cookie, buy a single, delicious cookie, not a whole bag.
- Ward off sugar cravings with ample chromium, about 45 micrograms per day. It is found in meat, poultry, broccoli, spinach, romaine lettuce, peanuts, potatoes, whole grains, and apples. Chromium helps stabilize serotonin, a neurotransmitter that affects anger, aggression, mood, sleep, and other brain functions. A drop in serotonin can trigger sugar cravings.
- Get adequate iron, at least 9 milligrams per day, to help combat fatigue (see Iron Sources, page 38).
- Get plenty of serotonin-raising DHA and EPA omega-3 fatty acids (3,000 milligrams are usually prescribed) from fish or supplements. (For more information on omega-3 fatty acids and sources, see pages 10–14.) DHA and EPA omega-3s are proven to alleviate all kinds of depression, not just PPD. If you are breastfeeding, they are critical for your baby's brain development too.
- Make sure you are getting sufficient B_{12}, at least 2.8 milligrams per day, which is needed to convert amino acids into serotonin and dopamine, two important neurotransmitters linked to depression and low energy. Animal products, fortified breakfast cereals, and brewer's yeast are good sources.
- Eat foods high in folic acid (see Folic Acid Sources, page 141). Studies show that 15 to 38 percent of adults with depressive disorders have low levels of B vitamins, including folic acid. Raising daily folic acid intake to at least 600 micrograms has

been associated with increased energy and mental clarity. This B vitamin is also believed to enhance the effects of antidepressant medications.

- Consume B₆ from poultry, fish, eggs, whole grains, and nuts, and thiamine from whole grain, brewer's yeast, lean pork, legumes, nuts, and seeds. Among other things, both of these B vitamins help conduct the neurotransmitters responsible for balancing your moods.
- Adequate vitamin D from the sun can help alleviate feelings of depression.
- Stay well hydrated with water—aim for at least 8 glasses a day—particularly when exercising or if you suffer from panic attacks. Dehydration can exacerbate anxiety.
- Try to avoid caffeine; it won't aggravate depression, but may increase anxiety.
- Avoid alcohol, which is a depressant.

Exercise Advice

Exercise is an important part of any PPD recovery plan. One of the best reasons to exercise is that it elevates serotonin and dopamine, and it releases endorphins, or happy hormones. Ironically, during a bout of depression, when you most need those happy chemicals, getting exercise can be extremely difficult. Go easy, and remember your body is still recovering. Dr. Bennett suggests doing whatever you can. If all you can do is walk from the living room to the kitchen on a given day, fine. If you can walk outside only far enough to get your mail, that's okay. It may be hard to imagine being this paralyzed by depression, but some women are. Here are some tips to help you start exercising after your doctor gives you clearance.

- Try to take a walk outside everyday; 10 minutes is a good start.
- Even if you don't exercise, do some body stretches that can help relieve tension and stress.
- If you can't get to a gym or join an exercise group, work out in your home using the Exercise Menu (see page 409) or a video.
- Stay well hydrated.
- Take lots of breaks, and don't push yourself too hard. If a woman is experiencing a panic disorder, she should avoid overly strenuous exercise because it may cause an adrenaline surge, which could spark a panic attack.
- Yoga is an excellent stress reducer, though "hot yoga" is best avoided.
- Oxygen therapy, in the form of deep breathing, is helpful for clearing brain fog. Dr. Bennett suggests checking out Zna's Trade Secret O² Breakthrough Training at www.znatrainer.com, or call 801-651-6115. This system stands out from all the rest, and the research backs it up. It requires only a few minutes a day, and no equipment or traveling to a class.

Catch your ZZZZZZs

Easier said than done, especially if you have a baby who does not sleep through the night. Sleep deprivation can rob mothers of melatonin, a naturally occurring hormone vital to the regulation of circadian rhythms, and it can reduce serotonin. Low levels of either of these brain chemicals may cause depression, anxiety, and other negative feelings. Finding a sleep schedule that works for you and your baby is the best advice. One strategy is to nap when your baby naps. This is wishful thinking for many moms, but explain to family and friends how important sleep is to PPD recovery. Solicit help with child care or chores whenever you can. If you are at the breaking point of requiring medication to sleep (or you want to avoid getting to that point), and want to try a natural option first, Dr. Bennett suggests getting a pair of low blue light glasses at www.lowbluelights.com. In the spectrum of light, blue light suppresses melatonin and keeps you awake. These special lenses are designed to block out 95 percent of blue light. Wearing them two to three hours before bed can start the flow of natural melatonin in the brain.

Remember: you will get well, and you will be happy again. Take the necessary steps to nurture yourself.

STAY BALANCED DIET FOR MOTHERS

ONE DAY, LET'S imagine, you finally devise a baby routine that really works, whether you go to the office or stay at home. You are done with breastfeeding, and you want your prepregnant body back. Those sexy jeans are beckoning you from the closet, but how will you ever squeeze into them? Unless you have a fairy godmother with a magic wand, diet and exercise are the only answers.

Enter Linda Wade, Ph.D., and Elaine B. Trujillo, M.S., R.D.—experts on the psychology and mechanics of successful and sustainable weight loss. According to Dr. Wade, a clinical psychologist in New York, a woman must connect with her inner self before beginning any effective weight loss plan at any stage in her life. She advocates discovering one's complex inner relationships and how they influence the outer controls in our lives, such as food, TV, shopping, and people. Dr. Wade shares some of her wisdom in the answers to our questions below. Elaine Trujillo's detailed weight-loss plan follows.

What are "inner relationships" and "outer controls"?

The therapeutic technique I use most in my practice is based on the Internal Family Systems Model (IFS) developed by Richard C. Schwartz, Ph.D. In a nutshell, IFS is based on the understanding that there are many different parts of our mind that affect our thinking. They are almost like separate individuals subconsciously guiding our thoughts and actions. We must acknowledge our "parts" and possibly even name them.

For instance, one part might be protective and managerial, another might try to keep our vulnerabilities under wraps, and a third might try to keep any emotional pain, past or present, from surfacing, sometimes through unhealthy means such as alcohol abuse, binge eating, or overworking. In addition to our different parts, everyone also has a Self, a curious, compassionate, and nonjudgmental center to their entire being. The goal of this work is to be more and more led by one's Self.

How does this apply to sustainable weight loss?

If one's parts are being heard and understood by one's Self, a person can approach dieting in a calm, confident, and creative way. If one or more parts are not being acknowledged, and food has become an antidote for emotional pain or conflict, trying to diet is going to be tricky and, in the end, could add to a person's emotional distress. The IFS Model is, of course, a lot more intricate than this brief description implies. If you would like to learn more about it, visit www.selfleadership.org. *Introduction to the Internal Family Systems Model* (Trailheads Publications, 2001) is an excellent description of the theory that can be ordered from the website.

How will I know when the time is right to start dieting?

The right time to start dieting depends very much on the individual and can be determined only by you. Don't compare yourself to anyone else. We all carry our own weight, both emotional and physical. Check in with yourself and take inventory of what's going on in your life at the moment. As wonderful as the birth of a child is, there can also be losses associated with it: loss of personal time, loss of your prepregnant body image, and sometimes loss of income due to a change of employment. In general, losses tend to make a woman want to use food for comfort, so begin by understanding how you feel about your new place in life and ask yourself if you are happy there. If you are not, think about why not and how you can adjust. Ideally, try to eliminate as much stress and conflict as possible from your life before you begin dieting. Get support from your partner, family, friends, or a diet group.

What is a reasonable goal I can set for myself?

It is very important to be realistic about what can be accomplished. An initial goal of simply maintaining your weight while you try to reduce your stress and manage your life is an admirable goal. When you get an inner reading that things are calm enough for you to effectively change your food intake and begin exercising, one to two pounds per week is a healthy and realistic goal. Many women have an impatient side that will want to set much higher goals, but this invariably leads to failure, self-judgment, and often to giving up. Dropping a few hundred calories from your day requires a lot of physical and mental work.

How can I make time to exercise and take care of myself when I'm on call 24/7?

Making the time to eat right, exercise, journal, and do other self-care activities is one of the biggest challenges of early motherhood. As tired as you may be, set aside 15 minutes for yourself—maybe before the baby and anyone else in the house wakes up—to make a cup of tea, to read something inspirational, to get quiet within yourself, or to journal. During this time, think through your day with this question in mind: When can I be free to take care of myself? Try to carve out time to exercise, take a walk with your baby, make yourself a nice salad for lunch, or nap if you are exhausted. You will know you are strong and confident enough to make positive changes to your lifestyle when you listen to and connect with yourself.

How can I control my cravings?

There is an old saying—hungry, angry, lonely, and tired, also known as HALT—that reminds us that if we are experiencing one or all of these feelings, we are vulnerable to overeating. Exhaustion is especially difficult—and very common in early motherhood. Again, self-knowledge will serve you well. Don't overcommit yourself to nonessential activities, and ask for assistance with basic chores and shopping. Try to keep only healthy foods and snacks in your home, reach out to friends for advice or support, and share your frustration, anger, or anxieties with your partner. If you can eliminate these four feelings, your cravings and overindulgence will likely subside.

What should I do at special occasions when everyone else is feasting on forbidden foods?

Know yourself—your strengths and weaknesses—and figure out how you can feel satisfied without feeling deprived. Once you find harmony, make a deal with yourself that you will try a small portion of appealing dishes and that you won't take seconds. Eat slowly so you aren't finished before everyone else. Think about the number of calories in the high-sugar desserts and ask yourself if they are really worth the extra hours of exercise that will be necessary to burn them off. The answer is probably no.

What if my weight qualifies me as obese and I see no hope of ever taking off all the pounds I need to. I'm depressed, which makes me eat more. What should I do?

There are two issues here. One is long-term weight loss and the other is depression. While dieting, you need to discover how to live with the knowledge that you are doing the best you can to lose weight, even though from day to day the amount of weight being lost does not seem significant. But think: at the rate of one pound per week you will lose fifty-two pounds in one year! That's a considerable amount. Keep returning to the positive—what you have accomplished so far—and keep moving ahead. If you find that your depression is not lifting with positive self-talk, consulting a professional is the best next step. Psychotherapy and/or medication can be very helpful.

What if my partner or others are not supportive?

While dieting is inner work, it helps to have support from the outside. In fact, the ability to speak up for one's self is an expression of inner work. Letting your friends and partner know that you are following a healthy diet plan to lose weight will help you, particularly if you make decisions in front of them. You might also want to ask them not to take personally any refusal of food they offer you. If your partner wants to have certain foods in the house that are not helpful foods for you, ask him or her to find a special closet or space in the refrigerator for them. Some experts may advise that the partner forgo these foods altogether, but in general, I would not agree with this. Ultimately, we cannot place the control of what we eat on anyone or anything outside ourselves.

What is the best way to start a weight loss plan?

Journaling would be my advice. Getting into the habit of recording your daily thoughts and feelings is important inner work for any life change, including weight loss. You can write in a food journal, or you can use a separate journal for your entries (see Keeping a Journal, page 395). Now, to get started, sit somewhere comfortable with a notebook and a pen. Take a big, deep breath and relax. Then begin to notice your emotional body. What is that? you may ask. Well, it's the part of your body that carries a hunch or feels anxiety or tension. Just notice it. Notice what thoughts are coming. There might be judgment: *I hate this*, or *Why do I have to feel this way?* or *What's wrong with me?* There might be opinions: *I have to go on a diet today*, or *This is impossible, it will never work*. Or just feelings: *I'm feeling kind of down today, I'm happy because the baby finally slept through the night*. Don't judge anything you write, but be curious about your thoughts and feelings. These are some of your parts coming forward. They need space and acknowledgement. After you do this for a while, you will begin to notice your whole self relax. Ultimately, you will be in a better place to take actions, such as making smart food choices and doing exercises, which will serve your entire well-being.

STAY BALANCED DIET FOR MOTHERS

THE ORIGINAL STAY Balanced Diet, created by Elaine Trujillo in *Eating for Lower Cholesterol*, is an eating plan designed to lower cholesterol and prevent heart disease. In this book, she has tailored it to mothers by keeping calcium and fiber high, and calories within a healthy range for dieting. The meal plans will work for *all* family members, not just Mom, although serving sizes and calorie intakes will need to be adjusted for men and children. The ultimate goal is to reduce weight gradually and naturally, so once it's off, it stays off. No food groups have been eliminated, and exercise plays a critical role. There are no gimmicks, no false promises, and no instant results.

Everyone's calorie needs are different. The chart on page 395 outlines calorie guidelines for maintaining weight and for weight loss, depending on your age and how active you are. Generally, when you are in the weight-loss mode, you drop approximately 500 calories from your daily maintenance calories in order to lose one pound per week: one pound equals 3,500 calories (500 calories x 7 days = 3,500 calories).

The guidelines below are just that—guidelines. Your calorie needs may be higher or lower, and might change depending on the results you get. If you find that a suggested calorie level is just too low and you are always hungry, even if you are losing weight, increase your calorie intake a bit. In the end, you are better off losing the weight at a slower pace, while changing your eating habits, than losing pounds quickly and not being able to keep them off. On the other hand, if you are not losing weight at all, and you feel you could cut out a few more calories, go for it.

To determine if you are sedentary, moderately active, or active, in addition to your daily routine (additional activities might include brisk walking, jogging, biking, aerobics, or yard work), think about the amount of moderate or vigorous activity you do on most days of the week. Consider yourself active if you do more than 60 minutes; moderately active, 30–60 minutes; and sedentary, less than 30 minutes.

For example, if you are a 30-year-old female and are moderately active, you require about 2,000–2,200 daily maintenance calories. Therefore, shoot for a 1,500 to 1,700 daily weight-loss calorie intake.

AGE	SEDENTARY MAINTAIN	SEDENTARY WEIGHT LOSS	MODERATELY ACTIVE MAINTAIN	MODERATELY ACTIVE WEIGHT LOSS	ACTIVE MAINTAIN	ACTIVE WEIGHT LOSS
14–18	1,800	1,300	2,000	1,500	2,400	1,900
19–30	2,000	1,500	2,000–2,200	1,500–1,700	2,400	1,900
31–50	1,800	1,300	2,000	1,500	2,200	1,700
51+	1,600	1,200	1,800	1,300	2,000–2,200	1,500–1,700

What does the Stay Balanced Diet for Mothers look like? It is represented by a food pyramid in the shape of a scale. The basic premise is that one should eat a healthy, varied diet, and that daily calories consumed should be burned off with daily exercise. When calories *in* equal calories *out*, the scale is balanced.

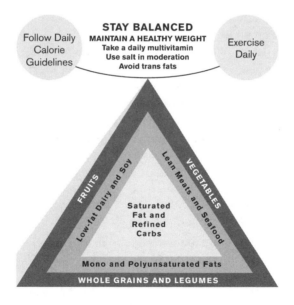

Keeping a Journal

Both Wade and Trujillo strongly advocate journaling your emotions, food intake, and exercise. Results from weight-loss studies indicate that journaling does, in fact, have positive effects on weight reduction. To start a journal, buy a notebook small enough to carry around in your handbag. During the first week, Week 1, track everything you eat and drink—everything—along with your thoughts and feelings. Don't worry about whether you are making good or bad food choices—you will think about that later. Remember that no one is judging you on what you write, except yourself, so be honest and not judgmental with yourself.

What should you record in your journal? A sample entry might contain the following information.

- Date
- Answers to the question, How do I feel today?
- Times of meals and snacks
- Amounts of foods and beverages consumed
- Hunger scale: Rate your hunger at the time of eating on a scale of 1 to 5 (1 = not hungry and 5 = starving)
- Exercise
- Weight, recorded once a week
- Any thoughts associated with eating

Many women find it difficult to initiate dietary changes and to begin exercising at the same time. You do *not* have to do both at the same time. Start with changing your diet while maintaining your current level of activity, whether it is sedentary or very active. Once you have your eating plan under control (which might take a few weeks), then start to add exercise to your daily routine. If you already exercise, by all means continue.

Before you begin, promise yourself *not to get on the scale everyday*. Choose one day a week to weigh yourself when you wake up. Don't be disappointed if the scale does not reflect a decrease right away. Results can sometimes take a few weeks, but they will come. Factors, such as salt intake and your body's fluid status, can alter your weight. Also, if you are toning up and building muscle, the scale may not decrease as much, even though your body is getting leaner. Take out a tape measure or use your old clothes to measure the inches you are losing on your waistline, thighs, and hips.

At the end of Week 1, review your entries. Praise yourself for journaling, and ask yourself how you might make healthier choices the following week. Start Week 2 with a single goal, perhaps to drink more water every day (strive for 8 glasses daily) while cutting out sugar-filled drinks and reducing or eliminating alcohol. Keep in mind that 8 ounces of wine has approximately 200 calories, and 12 ounces of beer has 120.

Journal for a second week, but this time review your entries daily. Patterns will start to emerge, allowing you to pinpoint success areas and trouble spots. You may find yourself eating in response to stress, boredom, or exhaustion. You may notice that you skip breakfast, then binge eat because you're hungry. You may have developed a habit of eating your child's leftovers, or your weekends look like an I-made-it-through-the-week gorge. Think about ways of overcoming snags, and begin implementing some of your ideas.

Week 3: Choose another goal, such as eating complex carbohydrates instead of simple ones. In other words, aim for whole grain everything, from cereal to pasta, with whole wheat crackers in between. Whole grains fill you up faster, and they are infinitely healthier. Evaluate your entries everyday. Make written notes to yourself to avoid junk foods, fast foods, greasy foods, sugar, trans fats, and saturated fats. Remind yourself to eat lots of fresh fruits and vegetables, filled with nutrients and fiber.

Week 4: The real work begins. Now that you are in the habit of writing things down, take it one step further and *really* think about what you are eating. To find your ideal calorie intake, refer to the Daily Maintenance and Weight-Loss Calorie Guidelines for Women table. Let's assume it is 1,500, down from 2,000 calories. Locate 1,500 on the Food Group Servings per Day Based on Calorie Level chart (below), then use a front page of your journal to record the amount of servings you should be eating from each of the six food groups daily. Refer to the Sample Serving Sizes chart (below) to design meals and snacks within your calorie range.

The bottom line is this: Aim for a healthy, balanced diet within your calorie limits and shun all unhealthy foods. Don't get hung up on exact calorie counts or food groups— menu planning is not an exact science. Just do your best. Once your extra weight is gone, which it will be, try your best to maintain your reduced-calorie level. You can increase it slightly on special occasions, but ideally, keep your calories to a minimum and exercise daily to sustain your new weight. Record how you feel in order to stay connected with yourself and your goals. Nine months up, nine months down. Be patient.

FOOD GROUP AND DAILY SERVINGS BASED ON CALORIE LEVELS

DAILY CALORIES	FRUITS	VEGETABLES	WHOLE GRAINS AND LEGUMES	DAIRY	MEATS, SEAFOOD, AND SOY	FATS
1,200	2	4	3	3	5	4
1,300	3	4	4	3	5	4
1,400	3	4	4	3	6	5
1,500	3	4	5	3	6	5
1,600	3	5	5	3	7	5
1,700	4	5	5	3	8	5
1,800	4	5	6	3	8	5
1,900	4	5	6	3	9	6
2,000	5	5	7	3	9	6
2,100	5	5	7	3	10	6
2,200	5	5	8	3	11	6

SAMPLES SERVING SIZES

FOOD GROUP	RECOMMENDED SERVING	SAMPLE SINGLE-SERVING SIZE
Fruits	1–2½ cups daily, or 2–5 servings	▸ 1 medium fruit ▸ ½ cup fresh, frozen, or canned fruit ▸ ½ cup fruit juice ▸ ¼ cup dried fruit
Vegetables	1–4 cups daily, or 4–5 servings	▸ 1 cup raw leafy vegetable ▸ ½ cup cut-up raw or cooked vegetable ▸ ½ cup vegetable juice
Whole Grains and Legumes	3–8 servings daily	▸ 1 slice bread ▸ 1 cup dry fortified cereal ▸ ½ cup cooked rice, pasta, cereal ▸ ½ cup cooked dry beans ▸ ½ baked potato ▸ ½ medium pita ▸ 5 whole wheat crackers
Nonfat or Low-Fat Dairy	3 cups daily, or 3 servings	▸ 1 cup reduced-fat or fat-free milk or yogurt ▸ 1 cup soy milk or soy yogurt ▸ 1½ ounces low-fat or fat-free cheese
Lean Meats, Seafood, and Soy	5–11 ounces daily	▸ 1 ounce of cooked lean meat, poultry, or fish ▸ ¼ cup cooked tofu ▸ 1 egg or egg substitute
Mono- and Polyunsaturated Fats (Good Fats from Vegetable Oils, Nuts, and Seeds)	4–6 servings daily	▸ 1 tsp vegetable oil ▸ 1 tsp soft margarine ▸ 1 tbsp regular salad dressing or 2 tbsp reduced-fat salad dressing ▸ 1 tbsp low-fat mayonnaise ▸ 2 tbsp or 1 ounce avocado ▸ 8 large black or 10 large green olives ▸ 1 tbsp peanut butter ▸ ½ ounce nuts or seeds ▸ 1½ tbsp reduced-fat cream cheese ▸ 1 tbsp pesto sauce

Seven Days of 1,500-Calorie Menus

The following seven menus were created to give you an idea of what a 1,500-calorie day looks like on paper. They are broken down by food groups, and the nutritional values are calculated for the entire day. You do not need to follow them exactly; substitute by using the Sample Serving Sizes chart. Needless to say, make the most of your calorie allowance by choosing nutrient-dense foods high in protein, vitamins, minerals, and fiber. As much as possible, eat home-cooked meals, and choose low-fat frozen or prepared foods, whole grains, good fats, fish, and low-fat dairy and protein sources. Be sure to read labels carefully. Eat mindfully and slowly. It takes about 15 to 20 minutes for your brain to realize that your stomach is full—you can do a lot of unnecessary damage in 15 minutes. Go back and reread Dr. Wade's advice from time to time.

Day One

Breakfast
1 scrambled egg (1 meat)
1 slice whole wheat toast with 1½ teaspoons soft margarine
(1 grain, 1.5 fat)
1 tablespoon jam
½ cup calcium-fortified orange juice (1 fruit)

Lunch
3 slices lean deli ham (2 ounces) with mustard (2 meat)
2 cups romaine lettuce with ½ tomato (2 vegetable)
2 tablespoons reduced-fat Italian dressing (1 fat)
1 whole wheat pita (2 grain)
1 banana (1 fruit)

Snack
1 reduced-fat Colby-Jack cheese stick (1 dairy)
2 large, fat-free, whole wheat crackers (such as Wasa crackers) (1 grain)
1 medium apple (1 fruit)

Dinner
1 cup shrimp stir-fry (see Shrimp and Vegetable Stir Fry, page 318)
(3 meat, 1 vegetable, 1 fat)
1 cup brown rice (2 grain)
½ cup broccoli with 1½ teaspoons soft margarine (1 vegetable, 1.5 fat)
1 cup fat-free chocolate frozen yogurt (2 dairy)

Nutrition Information for Day One
Calories: 1,504 cals   Fat: 38 g
Carbohydrates: 245 g   Protein: 58 g
Fiber: 25 g   Iron: 8 mg
Calcium: 899 mg
Total Food Groups: Fruits: 3; Vegetables: 4;
Grains: 6; Dairy: 3; Meats: 6; Fats: 5

Day Two

Breakfast
1 cup instant oatmeal made with water (1 grain)
½ cup fresh blueberries (1 fruit)
½ cup calcium-fortified orange juice (1 fruit)

Lunch
2 ounces smoked salmon lox with a squeeze of lemon (2 meat)
1 whole wheat pita (2 grain)
1½ ounces low-fat cheddar cheese (1 dairy)
2 cups mixed greens, 5 cherry tomatoes, 6 baby carrots (2 vegetable)
2 tablespoons Italian dressing (2 fat)

Snack
1 cup fruit-flavored nonfat yogurt (1 dairy)
1 banana (1 fruit)

Dinner
4 ounces roasted pork loin with 2 tablespoons gravy (4 meat, 1 fat)
1 medium baked potato with 2 tablespoons fat-free sour cream
(2 grain, 1 fat)
1 cup green beans with 1 teaspoon olive oil (2 vegetable, 1 fat)
½ cup low-fat frozen yogurt (1 dairy)

Nutrition Information for Day Two
Calories: 1,515 cals
Fat: 33 g
Carbohydrates: 219 g
Protein: 95 g
Fiber: 28 g
Iron: 12 mg
Calcium: 1,132 mg
Total Food Groups: Fruits: 3; Vegetables: 4;
Grains: 5; Dairy: 3; Meats: 6; Fats: 5

Day Three

Breakfast
1 cup fortified whole grain cereal (1 grain)
½ cup raspberries (1 fruit)
1 cup reduced-fat 1% milk (1 dairy)

Lunch
1⅓ cups lentil soup (see Lentil Soup with Brown Rice and Spinach, page 102) (2 grain, 1 meat, 2 vegetable)
1½ ounces low-fat cheddar cheese (1 dairy)
1 orange (1 fruit)
½ cup low-sodium tomato or V-8 juice (1 vegetable)
2 large, fat-free, whole wheat crackers (such as Wasa crackers) (1 grain)

Snack
1 cup fruit-flavored nonfat yogurt (1 dairy)
2 tablespoons roasted almonds (2 fat)
2 tablespoons granola (½ grain)

Dinner
5 ounces cod or tilapia, sautéed, or roasted (5 meat)
1 cup spinach salad with 2 tablespoons walnuts and 1 tablespoon vinaigrette (1 grain, 2 fat, 1 vegetable)
½ cup mango sorbet (1 fruit)
1 small whole wheat dinner roll with 1 teaspoon soft margarine (1 grain, 1 fat)

Nutrition Information for Day Three
Calories: 1,490 cals   Fat: 43g
Carbohydrates: 191 g   Protein: 91 g
Fiber: 30 g   Iron: 35 mg
Calcium: 2,453 mg
Total Food Groups: Fruits: 3; Vegetables: 4;
Grains: 6.5; Dairy: 3; Meats: 6; Fats: 4

Day Four

Breakfast
1 cup fortified whole grain cereal (1 grain)
1 cup low-fat 1% milk (1 dairy)
1 banana (1 fruit)
½ cup calcium-fortified orange juice (1 fruit)

Lunch
1 cup romaine lettuce, ½ tomato, 5 cucumber slices (2 vegetable)
2 tablespoons low-fat Thousand Island dressing (1 fat)
1 cheese stick (1 dairy)
2 large, fat-free, whole wheat crackers (such as Wasa crackers) (1 grain)

Snack
1 cup nonfat plain yogurt (1 dairy)
4 tablespoons granola (1 grain, 1 fat)

Dinner
5 ounces store-bought roasted or grilled chicken breast (5 meat)
1 cup brown rice with 1½ teaspoons soft margarine (2 grain, 1.5 fat)
1 cup broccoli with 1½ teaspoons soft margarine (2 vegetable, 1.5 fat)
½ cup unsweetened apple sauce (see Applesauce with Dried Apricots and
Cranberries, page 374) (1 fruit)

Nutrition Information for Day Four
Calories: 1,533 cals
Fat: 44 g
Carbohydrates: 194 g
Protein: 93 g
Fiber: 19 g
Iron: 31 mg
Calcium: 2,636 mg
Total Food Groups: Fruits: 3; Vegetables: 4;
Grains: 5; Dairy: 3; Meats: 5; Fats: 5

Day Five

Breakfast
1 slice whole wheat bread (1 grain)
1 tablespoon low-fat cream cheese (1 fat)
1 hard-boiled egg (1 meat)
1 cup low-fat 1% milk (1 dairy)
½ cup grapefruit slices (1 fruit)

Lunch
1 bean and cheese burrito (1 grain, 2 meat)
2 tablespoons salsa
1 cup romaine lettuce, 6 baby carrots (2 vegetable)
2 tablespoons reduced-fat Italian dressing (1 fat)

Snack
4 tablespoons roasted peanuts (2 fat)
¼ cup raisins (1 fruit)

Dinner
1½ cups vegetarian lasagna with 1 ounce tofu (see Best-Ever Vegetarian
Lasagna, page 208) (2 grain, 1 vegetable, 1 dairy, 2 meat)
1 cup broccoli with 1 teaspoon soft margarine (2 vegetable, 1 fat)
1 cup fat-free plain yogurt with 1 teaspoon honey (1 dairy)
½ cup blueberries (1 fruit)

Nutrition Information for Day Five
Calories: 1,500
Fat: 58 g
Carbohydrates: 186 g
Protein: 74 g
Fiber: 24 g
Iron: 10 mg
Calcium: 1,386 mg
Total Food Groups: Fruits: 3; Vegetables: 5;
Grains: 4; Dairy: 3; Meats: 5; Fats: 5

Day Six

Breakfast
1 cup smoothie (see Super Fruit Smoothies, page 76) (1 fruit, 1 dairy)
1 cup fortified whole grain cereal (1 grain)
1 cup low-fat 1% milk (1 dairy)

Lunch
2 cups baby spinach salad with 1 hard-boiled egg (2 vegetable, 1 meat)
2 tablespoons reduced-fat blue cheese dressing (1 fat)
1 whole wheat pita (2 grain)

Snack
¼ cup (about 5) dried apricots (1 fruit)
3 tablespoons pumpkin seeds (2 fat)
1 part-skim mozzarella cheese stick (1 dairy)

Dinner
4 ounces meat loaf with 2 tablespoons gravy (see Best-Ever American
Meat Loaf, page 288) (4 meat, 1 fat)
¾ cup brown rice (2 grain)
1 cup green beans with 1 teaspoon soft margarine (2 vegetable, 1 fat)
1 peach (fresh or canned in natural juices) (1 fruit)

Nutrition Information for Day Six
Calories: 1,523 cals
Fat: 46 g
Carbohydrates: 226 g
Protein: 63 g
Fiber: 31 g
Iron: 38 mg
Calcium: 2,088 mg
Total Food Groups: Fruits: 3; Vegetables: 4;
Grains: 5; Dairy: 3; Meats: 5; Fats: 5

Day Seven

Breakfast
1 cup oatmeal prepared with water (2 grain)
1 cup reduced-fat 1% milk (1 dairy)
½ cup blueberries (1 fruit)

Lunch
2 ounces turkey slices or leftover meat loaf (2 meat)
5 low-fat whole wheat crackers (1 grain)
1 dill pickle
8 baby carrots and celery sticks (3 vegetable)
2 tablespoons fat-free ranch dressing for dipping (1 fat)
1 banana (1 fruit)

Snack
1 reduced-fat Colby-Jack cheese stick (1 dairy)
4 tablespoons roasted, salted peanuts (2 fat)
1 cup low-sodium tomato juice or V-8 (1 vegetable)

Dinner
4 ounces salmon, grilled, roasted, or broiled (4 meat)
1 tablespoon basil pesto (1 fat)
1 cup tabbouleh with tomatoes and parsley (see Best-Ever Tabbouleh
Salad, page 151) (2 grain, 1 fat)
½ cup fat-free frozen yogurt (1 dairy)
½ cup strawberries (1 fruit)

Nutrition Information for Day Seven
Calories: 1,537   Fat: 60
Carbohydrates: 182   Protein: 76 g
Fiber: 25 g   Iron: 8 mg
Calcium: 886 mg
Total Food Groups: Fruits: 3; Vegetables: 4;
Grains: 5; Dairy: 3; Meats: 6; Fats: 5

GET IN SHAPE AFTER BABY
. . . OR BEFORE IF YOU NEED TO

Exercise is one of the greatest gifts you can give your body at any stage of your life. By exercising, you are preventing illnesses (such as cancer and cardiovascular disease), strengthening your bones to evade osteoporosis, and increasing your blood circulation to nourish your organs and work your heart. Most noticeably, you are also creating a healthier, stronger, and happier you.

If exercise has always been a part of your life, you are extremely fortunate. Keep it that way. When you are ready to shed your pregnancy weight, first and foremost get medical clearance, then gradually resume your old routines. If you don't have an old routine, and exercise is new to you, don't worry. It's never too late to start.

Even with the best intentions, finding the time, energy, and motivation to exercise is not easy, and a demanding new baby makes it even more difficult. Start with 15 minutes a day and gradually work your way up. Keep reminding yourself that exercise is not an all-or-nothing proposition. A 10-minute walk has benefits. Get as much support as you can, and share your goals with your partner.

Getting Started

- Medical clearance from your doctor or health care provider is *essential*. Explain your exercise plan and ask if there are any exercises you should avoid. Inform your doctor if you are breastfeeding.
- Complications during pregnancy or a C-section will prolong postdelivery healing time, and abdominal exercises may need to be delayed. Check with your doctor to make sure.
- Stomach muscle separation requires special attention. Ask about exercises that are safe and beneficial to your healing process.
- Back pain can often be relieved with stretching and exercise, but start slowly, don't push yourself, and be aware of any warning signals. Stop immediately if something does not feel right.
- Nursing mothers should not burn off an excessive amount of calories, which could compromise their optimal milk output.

good heart rates

Check your heart rate periodically to make sure you are exercising within your limits. These limits are prescribed by the American College of Obstetrics and Gynecologists.

FORMULA FOR FINDING YOUR MAXIMUM HEART RATE: 220 – YOUR AGE

AGE	TARGET HEART RATE (BEATS PER MINUTE)	MAXIMUM HEART RATE (BEATS PER MINUTE)
20	120–160	200
25	117–156	195
30	114–152	190
35	111–148	185
40	108–144	180
45	105–140	175

Before and During Each Routine

- Get well hydrated before exercising. Drink a glass or two of water (even if you don't feel thirsty) about an hour *before* you begin your routine. Sip water during your routine if you need to.
- Change into comfortable clothes. Wear a sports bra with strong support.
- Factor your warm-up time and after-exercise stretches into your routine. It is vital to warm up your body before you exercise to prevent injuries, muscle sprains, and strains.
- If advised by your doctor or health practitioner, check your pulse before, during, and after exercise (see Heart Rates During Exercise, above).
- Be aware of your body as you workout. Know when to stop. Warning signals include pain, dizziness, feeling faint, shortness of breath, palpitations (irregular heartbeats), back pain, pelvic pain, and bleeding.

After Your Routine

- Stretch to prevent muscle cramping.
- If you have the time, lie on the floor on your back with your arms and legs relaxed for five minutes of total relaxation. This is called the "corpse pose" in yoga; it is designed to relax your body and clear your mind.

- Your muscles may feel sore, which is okay, but they should not feel painful. Take a minute to distinguish between feeling sore and being in pain. If pain is what you feel, refrain from exercising for a day or two. If the pain is severe, consult your doctor immediately.
- Stand tall for the rest of the day. Suck in your tummy, straighten your back, and distribute your weight evenly on both feet.

THE EXERCISE MENU

WELCOME TO THE Exercise Menu! Because every woman's body and trouble spots are unique, work-out routines will vary. There are, however, some standard guidelines. Ideally, cardio workouts (lasting 20 to 30 minutes) should be done three to five times a week, and muscle-toning exercises at least twice. Abdominal routines can be done everyday.

Read through all of the exercises and practice them slowly the first few times. When you feel the proper muscles working, increase your speed. If possible, have your partner read out the directions to you as you do them the first few sessions. The numbers of repetitions for each exercise are listed as guidelines. Do as many as you can, and gradually work your way up. Do not work your muscles to the point of exhaustion.

NOTE: Please note that the exercises in this section are NOT intended for pregnancy. They are pre- or postpregnancy workouts.

Warm-Up Routines

All exercise *must* begin with a warm-up to protect your muscles and increase your blood flow. Five minutes is adequate; ideally do ten. A good warm-up should leave you a bit sweaty and warm. This can be accomplished with a 10-minute

- jog or brisk walk,
- stationary bike ride or another cardio-machine workout,
- jump rope session, or
- series of squats, lunges, and jumping jacks.

Squats: Stand with your feet a bit farther than shoulder-width apart. Cross your arms in front of you and raise them to shoulder height (they should form a rectangle). Stick out your buttocks; then, keeping your back straight, bend your knees into a squatting position. Go as far down into a sitting position as possible, then rise and straighten your legs, but do not lock your knees. **Repeat 10 times, then take a 10-second break.**

Lunges: Stand with your feet together and your hands on your hips. Take a big step forward with your right foot, find your balance, then bend your right knee. Drop your left knee toward the floor, keeping it about 6 inches above the ground. Pivot off your right foot to return to starting position. Work one leg, then switch to the other. **Repeat 10 times (on each leg), then take a 10-second break.**

Jumping Jacks: Stand with your feet together and your arms at your sides. Jump your feet apart, moving your legs about 3 feet apart, while simultaneously lifting both arms over your head. Jump back into starting position. This movement should be fluid, and your knees should always be bent. **Repeat 10 times, then take a 10-second break.**

exercise mantras

I will do what I can, when I can, without feeling guilty.

I won't compare myself to others.

I won't give up.

Sample Workouts from the Exercise Menu

TWENTY-MINUTE SAMPLE WORKOUT

▸ **Warm-Up**

▸ **2 Arm Routines (2 sets each)**   Bicep Curls and Front Arm Raises

▸ **2 Stomach Routines (1 set each)**   Traditional Abdominal Crunches and Double Crunches

▸ **1 Leg Routine (1 set)**   Lying-Down Leg Lifts

▸ **1 Buttocks Routine (1 set)**   Buttocks Crunches

▸ **After-Exercise Stretches**   After-Exercise Stretches

FORTY-MINUTE SAMPLE WORKOUT

▸ **Warm-Up**

▸ **3 Arm Routines (3 sets each)**   Overhead Shoulder Press, Bicep Curls, and Overhead Tricep Extensions

▸ **3 Stomach Routines (2 sets each)**   Abdominal Crunches on the Ball, Side Crunches, and Bicycle Crunches

▸ **2 Leg Routines (2 sets each)**   Lying-Down Leg Lifts and Deep Squats

▸ **2 Buttocks Routines (2 sets each)**   Buttocks Crunches and Fire Hydrant Leg Lifts

▸ **After-Exercise Stretches**   After-Exercise Stretches

SIXTY-MINUTE SAMPLE WORKOUT

▸ **Warm-Up**

▸ **4 Arm Routines (3 sets each)**   Overhead Shoulder Press, Bicep Curls, Front Arm Raises, and Hand weight Flies on the Ball

▸ **4 Stomach Routines (3 sets each)**   Traditional Abdominal Crunches, Side Crunches, Double Crunches, and Bicycle Crunches

▸ **2 Leg Routines (3 sets each)**   Lying-Down Leg Lifts and Deep Squats

▸ **2 Buttocks Routines (3 sets each)**   Buttocks Crunches and Fire Hydrant Leg Lifts

▸ **After-Exercise Stretches**   After-Exercise Stretches

RECOMMENDED EQUIPMENT

Exercise ball

3- and 5-pound hand weights

Floor mat

NOTE: All breathing should be done through your nose at a natural rate. Start with 3-pound hand weights and work up to 5-pound hand weights. If you are in shape, you can use ankle or wrist weights for more resistance.

ARM ROUTINES

Bicep Curls

Stand with your feet hip-width apart. Hold a 3-pound hand weight in each hand with your palms facing the sides of your thighs. This is your starting position. Keeping your abdominal muscles engaged and your chest lifted, simultaneously raise the hand weights toward your chest, bending only your elbows; your palms will face your chest at the top of the motion. Hold for a second, then slowly lower your arms to starting position. **Repeat 8 times for 2 or 3 sets with a 10-second rest between sets. Work up to 5-pound hand weights.**

Where should I feel it? Biceps and forearms as you raise the hand weights.

Remember: Keep your abdominal muscles engaged, do not lock your elbows, and breathe naturally.

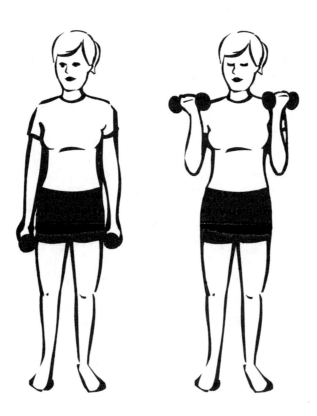

Overhead Shoulder Press

Sit on the ball with your feet hip-width apart and flat on the floor. Find your balance. Hold a 3-pound weight in each hand on either side of your body and raise both of your arms to shoulder height. Bend your elbows to form 90-degree angles. Your palms should be facing forward. Your arms will look like goal posts. This is your starting position. Keeping your abdominal muscles engaged and your chest lifted, raise and almost straighten your arms above your head, so the ends of the hand weights almost touch. Keep your elbows slightly bent. Hold for a second, then slowly lower your arms to your goal-post starting position. **Repeat 8 times for 2 or 3 sets with a 10-second rest between sets. Work up to 5-pound hand weights.**

Where should I feel it? Shoulder area and biceps.

Remember: Keep your abdominal muscles engaged, do not lock your elbows, and breathe naturally.

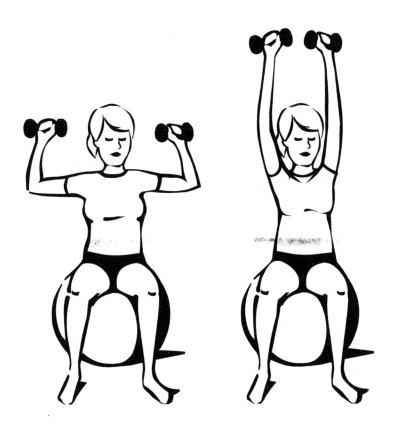

Front Arm Raises

Stand with your feet hip-width apart, knees slightly bent. Hold a 3-pound weight in each hand with your palms facing the sides of your thighs. This is your starting position. Keeping your abdominal muscles engaged and your chest lifted, simultaneously raise the hand weights straight out in front of you to shoulder height. Hold for a second, then slowly lower your arms to starting position without bending them. **Repeat 8 times for 2 or 3 sets with a 10-second rest between sets. Work up to 5-pound hand weights.**

Where should I feel it? Front shoulders and biceps.

Remember: Keep your abdominal muscles engaged, do not lock your elbows, and breathe naturally.

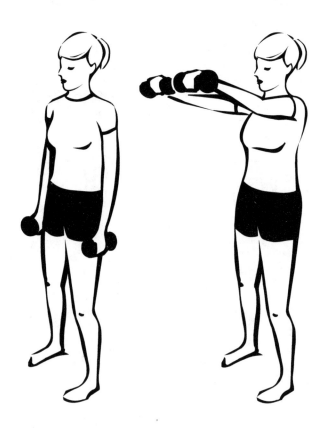

Side Arm Raises

Stand with your feet hip-width apart, knees slightly bent. Hold a 3-pound weight in each hand with your palms facing the sides of your thighs. This is your starting position. Keeping your abdominal muscles engaged and your chest lifted, simultaneously raise the hand weights from your sides to shoulder height. Your body will look like a T. Hold for a second, then slowly lower your arms to starting position. **Repeat 8 times for 2 or 3 sets with a 10-second rest between sets. Work up to 5-pound hand weights.**

Where should I feel it? Front shoulders and biceps.

*Remember: Keep your abdominal muscles engaged, do
not lock your elbows, and breathe naturally.*

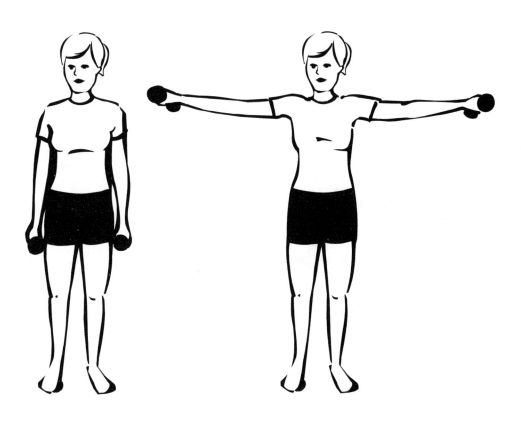

Overhead Tricep Extensions

Sit on the ball with your feet wide enough apart to give you good balance. Hold a 3-pound weight in your right hand. Keep your abdominal muscles engaged and your chest lifted. Raise your right arm above your head with the round ends of the hand weight facing forward and backward. Bend your left arm, rest it on the top of your head, and place your left hand in the hinge of your right elbow. This will support your right arm. Your arms will look like a lowercase H. This is your starting position. Bend your right elbow behind your head, lowering the hand weight toward your shoulders. Stop when your right elbow is at a 90-degree angle. Hold for a second, then straighten your arm to starting position. Repeat 8 times, then work the left arm. **Repeat 8 times for 2 or 3 sets with a 10-second rest between sets. Work up to 5-pound hand weights.**

Where should I feel it? Triceps.

Remember: Keep your abdominal muscles engaged, relax your neck, and breathe naturally.

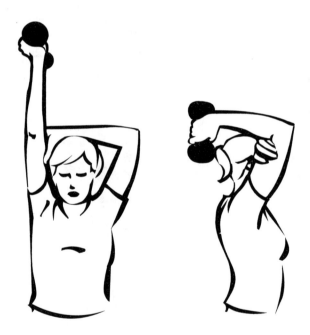

Hand Weight Flies on the Ball

Holding a 3-pound weight in each hand, lie on the ball with your back, neck, and head flush with the surface of the ball. Keep your abdominal muscles engaged, and raise your pelvis to be in a straight line with your abdomen. Engage your thigh and buttocks muscles to support your body and to stabilize the ball. Raise your arms straight up so your palms holding the hand weights face each other. This is your starting position. Slowly lower your arms, twisting the hand weights so your palms face forward, until your elbows are bent to 90-degree angles at your sides. Hold for a second then raise your arms to starting position. **Repeat 8 times for 2 or 3 sets with a 10-second rest between sets. Work up to 5-pound hand weights.**

Where should I feel it? Chest and all arm muscles.

Remember: Keep your abdominal muscles engaged, your pelvis raised and in line with your stomach, and your thighs and buttocks tight. Relax your neck and breathe naturally.

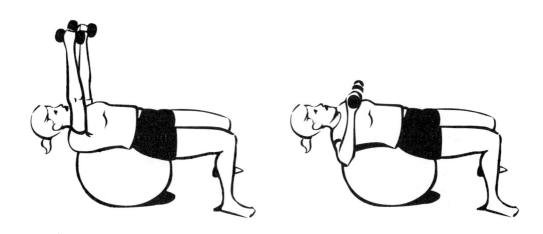

Tricep Kickbacks

Place the ball in front of you. Hold a 3-pound weight in your right hand. Stand behind the ball with your left foot about 9 inches in front of your right foot, as if you are taking a step forward. Place your left hand on top of the ball, but put only a small portion of your body weight on it. It is for balance, not support. Engage your abdominal muscles, bend your front knee slightly, stick out your buttocks, and keep your back straight and at an upward angle. Your head should be in line with your back, and your eyes should be looking forward. Lift your upper right arm to be parallel to your torso and keep your elbow bent down at a 90 degree angle. This is your starting position. While keeping your upper arm immobilized, raise the lower part of your arm to shoulder height. Your right arm will be fully extended behind your back. Hold for a second, then lower your right arm to starting position. **Repeat 8 times for 2 or 3 sets on each arm with a 10-second rest between sets. Work up to 5-pound hand weights.**

Where should I feel it? Triceps.

Remember: Keep your abdominal muscles engaged and your knees bent, relax your neck, keep your gaze forward, and breathe naturally. You should not feel any strain on your back. If you do, adjust your leg and/or back positions.

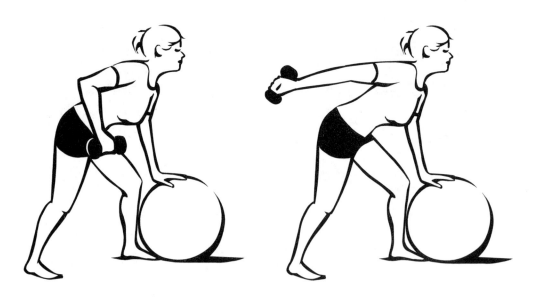

STOMACH ROUTINES

Traditional Abdominal Crunches

Lie on your mat with your back flat. Bend your knees, positioning your feet about hip-width apart. Place your hands behind your neck. Your hands will be used to support your neck, not to pull it up. Relax your neck and curl your chest forward, hold for two counts, and then slowly lower your chest. Keep your stomach muscles continuously engaged, and do not touch the back of your head to the floor. Count like this: Lift-one-two, two-one-two, three-one-two, and so on. When finished with each set, bring your knees to your chest and hold them for 10 seconds. Slowly release.

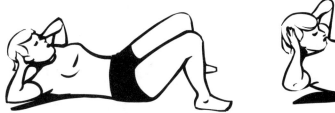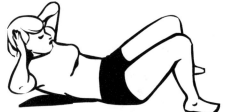

Ball Variation

Place your back and shoulders on the ball. Place your hands behind your neck. Your hands will be used to support your neck, not to pull it up. Relax your neck, and raise your pelvis to be in a straight line with your abdomen. Engage your thigh and buttocks muscles to support your body and to stabilize the ball. Curl your chest forward, hold for two counts, and then slowly lower your chest. Do not let your head go lower than your shoulders; this would strain your neck. Count like this: Lift-one-two, two-one-two, three-one-two, and so on. When finished with each set, bring your knees to your chest and hold them for 10 seconds. Slowly release. **Repeat 15 to 20 times for 1 to 3 sets with a 10-second rest between sets.**

Where should I feel it? Abdominal muscles.

Remember: Relax your neck and breathe naturally. If you are on the ball, keep your pelvis raised and in line with your stomach, and keep your thighs and buttocks tight.

Side Crunches

Lie on your mat with your back flat on the floor. Bend your knees, positioning your feet about hip-width apart. Cross your left leg on top of your right knee. Place your right hand behind your neck. Your hand will be used to support your neck, not to pull it up. Position your left arm on the floor by your side. Relax your neck and curl your chest forward so your right elbow almost touches your left knee. Count like this: Lift-one-two, two-one-two, three-one-two, and so on. Repeat with the other leg and elbow. When finished with each set, bring your knees to your chest and hold them for 10 seconds. Slowly release. **Repeat 10 times on each side for 1 to 3 sets with a 10-second rest between sets.**

Where should I feel it? Upper abdominal muscles.

Remember: Relax your neck and breathe naturally.

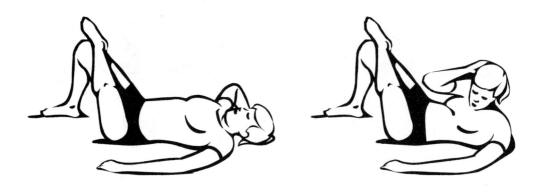

Double Crunches

Lie on your mat with your back flat on the floor. Bend your knees, positioning your feet about hip-width apart. Place your hands behind your neck. Your hands will be used to support your neck, not to pull it up. Lift your chest and both of your legs simultaneously, keeping your knees bent. Your face will be about 3 inches from your knees. Release by moving your legs out, away from your body but not down, and lowering your chest slightly, but not to the floor. When finished with each set, bring your knees to your chest and hold them for 10 seconds. Slowly release. **Repeat 15 to 20 times for 1 to 3 sets with a 10-second rest between sets.**

Where should I feel it? Upper abdominal muscles.

Remember: Relax your neck and breathe naturally. Keep your stomach muscles continuously engaged.

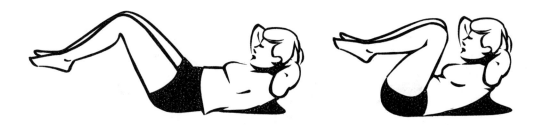

Bicycle Abs

Lie on your mat with your back flat on the floor. Bend your knees, positioning your feet about hip-width apart. Place your hands behind your neck. Your hands will be used to support your neck, not to pull it up. Relax your neck. Move your legs as if you are riding a bike while lying on your back. Now, curl your chest forward, and bring your left elbow to the outside of your bent right knee. Then switch, and bring your right elbow to the outside of your left bent knee. When finished with each set, bring your knees to your chest and hold them for 30 seconds. Slowly release. **Repeat 15 to 20 times for 1 to 3 sets with a 10-second rest between sets.**

Where should I feel it? Lower and side abdominals. When crunching your right arm to your left knee, you should feel it on your right abs, and vice versa.

Remember: Relax your neck and breathe naturally.

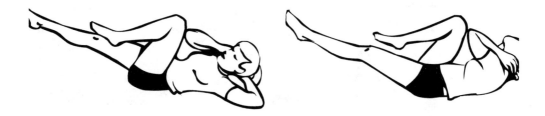

Double Leg Lifts

Note: This exercise puts a lot of strain on your lower abdomen. Women who have had a C-section or abdominal muscle separation should be fully healed before they try it.

Lie on the mat with your back flat on the floor. Bend your knees, positioning your feet flat on the floor about hip-width apart. Place your hands under your buttocks, palms down, with the tips of your thumbs about 2 inches apart. Keeping your legs together, and your knees slightly bent, raise your legs about 60 degrees, then slowly lower them to about 3 inches off the ground. Do not let your heels touch the ground. Raise your legs again, and repeat. When finished with each set, bring your knees to your chest and hold them for 10 seconds. Slowly release. **Repeat 10 to 15 times for 1 to 3 sets with a 10-second rest between sets.**

Where should I feel it? Lower abdominal muscles.

Remember: Relax your upper body, and don't let your heels touch the ground. Breathe naturally.

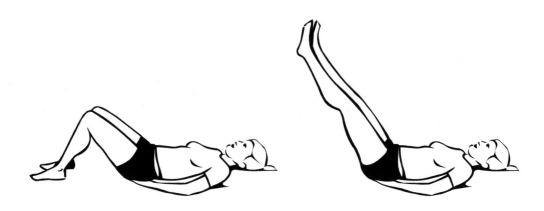

LEG ROUTINES

Lying-Down Leg Lifts

Lie on your mat on your right side. Bend your right arm and cradle your head in your right hand. Bend your right leg along the floor for extra support. Keeping your left leg straight and your ankle at a 90-degree angle, raise your left leg about 60 degrees and hold for two counts. Count like this: Lift-one-two, two-one-two, and so on. Slowly lower your leg. You can stretch your thigh by holding your foot and pulling it back slightly. **Repeat 10 to 15 times on each leg for 1 to 3 sets with a 10-second rest between sets.**

Where should I feel it? Thigh muscles and buttocks.

Remember: Relax your upper body and breathe naturally.

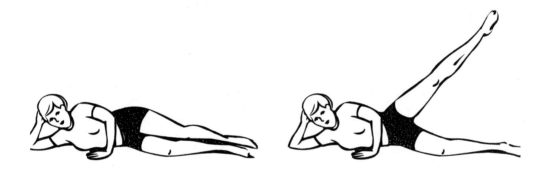

Wide-Legged Squat

Stand with your feet a bit farther than shoulder-width apart. Place your hands on your hips, and stick out your buttocks. Keeping your back straight, bend your knees into a squatting position. Go as far down into a sitting position as possible, then rise and straighten your legs, but do not lock your knees. **Repeat 15 times for 1 to 3 sets with a 10-second rest between sets.**

Where should I feel it? Thighs and buttocks.

Remember: Keep your legs far enough apart so you don't put any strain on your knees. Breathe naturally.

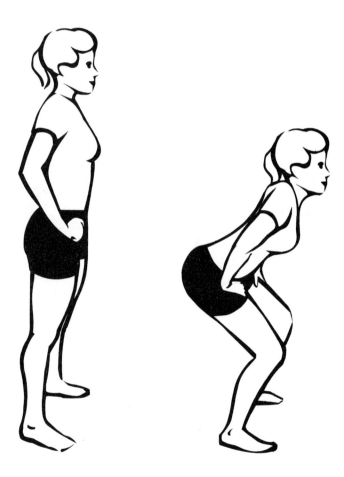

BUTTOCKS ROUTINES

Buttocks Crunches

Place your hands and knees on your mat in a four-legged animal position, and look forward. Evenly distribute your weight on all four points, then transfer your weight to three points— your hands and left knee (you may need to move that knee a little). Extend and raise your right leg up to buttocks height. Bend your right knee to form a 90-degree angle. This is your starting position. Lift your thigh about 3 inches, keeping your leg bent and your foot parallel to the ceiling (imagine that your foot is balancing a tray of glasses), then return to starting position. When finished working both legs, lower your body into a fetal position, with your knees and forehead on the floor (this is called "child's pose" in yoga), and rest. **Repeat 15 times on each leg for 1 to 3 sets with a 10-second rest between sets.**

Where should I feel it? Buttocks.

Remember: Keep your head in line with your back and look forward. Breathe naturally.

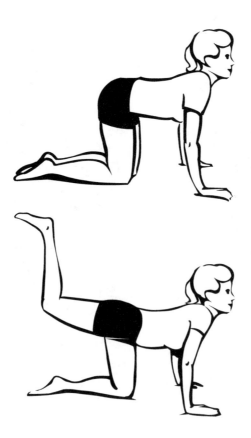

Fire Hydrant Leg Lifts

Place your hands and knees on your mat in a four-legged animal position, and look forward. Evenly distribute your weight on all four points, then transfer your weight to three points—your hands and left knee (you may need to move that knee a little). This will be your starting position. Raise your right leg to buttocks height (like a male dog at a fire hydrant), hold for a second, then return it slowly to starting position. When finished working both legs, lower your body into child's pose and rest. **Repeat 10 to 15 times on each leg for 1 to 3 sets with a 10-second rest between sets.**

Where should I feel it? Buttocks and thighs.

Remember: Keep your head in line with your back and look forward. Breathe naturally.

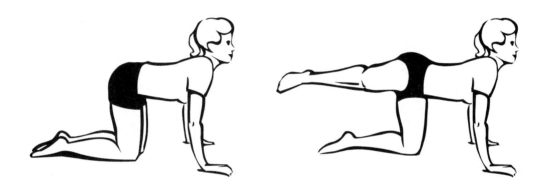

COOL DOWN STRETCHES

STAND WITH BOTH feet firmly on the ground. These after-exercise stretches will work all of your muscle groups, from your head to your toes.

Full Body: Standing with your feet together, raise your hands above your head as high as possible. Keep your stomach muscles engaged and your buttocks tight. Stretch up toward the sky, hold for 5 seconds, then lower your arms to your sides and take 2 deep breaths.

Neck: Hold your head up straight. This will be your starting position. Lower your chin to your chest gradually, then return to starting position. Slowly tilt your head back, then return to starting position. Keeping your chest facing forward, turn your head to the left and hold for 5 seconds, return to starting position, then turn to the right. Repeat 2 or 3 times.

Shoulders: Engage your stomach muscles. Roll your shoulders in circles backward 10 times, then forward 10 times.

Arms 1: Lift your right arm straight above your head. Bend it at the elbow and let your hand drop down behind your head to your shoulder. Gently pull your right elbow down with your left hand until you can feel the stretch. Repeat with the left arm.

Arms 2: Move your right arm across your chest and hug your left shoulder blade. Place your left hand on your upper right arm and gently pull it until you feel the stretch. Repeat with the left arm.

Back: Standing with your feet hip-width apart, place your hands on your hips. Keeping your back straight, slowly bend your torso forward from your hips. When you've gone down as far as you can, gently release your upper body and let it hang for 5 seconds. Return your hands to your hips and pivot up from your hips to raise your upper body. Repeat twice with a 10-second rest in between.

Thighs: If you need help balancing, brace yourself on a wall or chair. Standing straight, with your stomach muscles engaged, bend your right knee and grab your right foot with your right hand. Feel the stretch in your right thigh. Hold for 5 seconds. Repeat with your left leg.

Hamstrings: Place your hands on a wall and move your left foot back about 2 feet and your right foot back about 3 or 4 feet. Bend both knees. Lean forward until you feel the stretch in your right calf. Hold for 5 seconds. Repeat with your left leg.

Calves: Standing with your feet together and arms by your sides, engage your stomach muscles and raise your body so you are standing on the balls of both of your feet. Repeat 10 times.

▨ **CONVERSION CHARTS** ▨

VOLUME CONVERSIONS

AMERICAN	**METRIC (MILLILITERS)**	**FLUID OUNCES**
¼ teaspoon	1.25	
½ teaspoon	2.5	
1 teaspoon	5	
½ tablespoon (1½ teaspoons)	7.5	
1 tablespoon (3 teaspoons)	15	
2 tablespoons	30	1
¼ cup (4 tablespoons)	60	2
⅓ cup (5⅓ tablespoons)	75	2⅔
½ cup (8 tablespoons)	125	4
⅔ cup (10 tablespoons)	150	5
¾ cup (12 tablespoons)	175	6
1 cup (16 tablespoons; ½ pint)	250	8
1¼ cups	300	10
1½ cups	350	12
2 cups (1 pint)	500	16
3 cups	750	24
4 cups (1 quart, 2 pints)	1000 (1 liter)	32
5 cups	1250	40
16 cups (4 quarts, 1 gallon)	4000	128

AMERICAN	METRIC (GRAMS AND KILOGRAMS)
¼ ounce	7 grams
½ ounce	15 grams
1 ounce	30 grams
2 ounces	60 grams
3 ounces	90 grams
4 ounces	115 grams
5 ounces	150 grams
6 ounces	175 grams
7 ounces	200 grams
8 ounces	225 grams
9 ounces	250 grams
10 ounces	300 grams
11 ounces	325 grams
12 ounces	350 grams
13 ounces	375 grams
14 ounces	400 grams
15 ounces	425 grams
16 ounces (1 pound)	450 grams
1 pound 2 ounces	500 grams
1 pound 8 ounces	750 grams
2 pounds	900 grams
2 pounds 2 ounces	1000 grams (1 kilogram)
3 pounds	1.4 kilograms
4 pounds	1.8 kilograms
4 pounds 8 ounces	2 kilograms
5 pounds	2.4 kilograms

TEMPERATURE CONVERSIONS

To convert Fahrenheit into Centigrade, subtract 32, multiply by 5, and divide by 9.

To convert Centigrade into Fahrenheit, multiply by 9, divide by 5, and add 32.

EXAMPLE

$$100°C \times 9 = 900$$
$$900 \div 5 = 180$$
$$180 + 32 = 212°F$$

OVEN TEMPERATURES AT A GLANCE

DESCRIPTION	DEGREES FAHRENHEIT	DEGREES CENTIGRADE
Very Low	250–275	121–133
Low	300–325	149–163
Moderate	350–375	177–190
Hot	400–425	204–218
Very Hot	450–475	232–246
Extremely Hot	500–525	260–274

COMMON BAKING MEASUREMENTS

Butter: 1 stick = 4 ounces = 115 grams; 1 tablespoon = ½ ounce = 15 grams

All-purpose flour: 1 cup = 5 ounces = 160 grams

Granulated sugar: 1 cup = 7 ounces = 200 grams

Packed brown sugar: 1 cup = 6 ounces = 175 grams

Confectioners' sugar: 1 cup = 4½ ounces = 130 grams

▨ APPENDIX ▨

PREGNANCY-RELATED WEB SITES WORTH A BROWSE

www.MyPyramid.gov/

www.nlm.nih.gov/medlineplus/pregnancy.html#cat11

www.win.niddk.nih.gov/publications/two.htm

www.clevelandclinic.org/health/health-info/docs/1600/1674.asp?index=4724

www.teamnutrition.usda.gov/library.html

www.marchofdimes.com/pnhec/159_153.asp

www.vrg.org/nutrition/protein.htm

RECOMMENDED WEIGHT GAIN FOR PREGNANT WOMEN USING THE BODY MASS INDEX[1]

PREPREGNANCY WEIGHT CLASSIFICATION	OPTIMAL WEIGHT GAIN (LBS)	
	BMI (KG/M²)	POUNDS
Underweight	< 19.8	28–40
Normal	19.8–26	25–35
Overweight	26.1–29	15–25
Obese	> 29	< or equal to 15

CALORIE AND PROTEIN REQUIREMENTS
FOR PREGNANT WOMEN WITH A NORMAL BODY MASS INDEX

HEIGHT	PREGNANCY WEIGHT (LBS)	AVERAGE PREGNANCY WEIGHT (LBS)	CALORIE REQUIREMENT	AVERAGE CALORIE REQUIREMENT	MINIMUM PROTEIN (G) REQUIREMENT
5'0"	102–128	112	1,800–2,000	1,900	60
5'1"	106–132	116	1,800–2,300	2,000	60
5'2"	109–136	120	1,800–2,300	2,100	60
5'3"	113–141	124	1,900–2,400	2,100	60–65
5'4"	116–145	128	2,000–2,400	2,200	60–65
5'5"	120–150	132	2,000–2,500	2,300	60–65
5'6"	124–155	137	2,100–2,600	2,300	60–65
5'7"	127–159	140	2,100–2,700	2,400	60–70
5'8"	131–164	145	2,200–2,700	2,500	60–70
5'9"	135–169	149	2,200–2,700	2,500	60–70
5'10"	139–174	153	2,300–3,000	2,600	60–75
5'11"	143–179	158	2,300–3,000	2,600	65–75
6'0"	147–184	162	2,400–3,000	2,700	65–80

Body Mass Index Table

BMI	19	20	21	22	23	24	25	26	27	28	29	30	31	32	33	34	35	36	37	38	39	40	41	42	43	44	45	46	47	48	49	50	51	52	53	54
Category	Normal						Overweight					Obese										Extreme Obesity														
Height (inches)												Body Weight (pounds)																								
58	91	96	100	105	110	115	119	124	129	134	138	143	148	153	158	162	167	172	177	181	186	191	196	201	205	210	215	220	224	229	234	239	244	248	253	258
59	94	99	104	109	114	119	124	128	133	138	143	148	153	158	163	168	173	178	183	188	193	198	203	208	212	217	222	227	232	237	242	247	252	257	262	267
60	97	102	107	112	118	123	128	133	138	143	148	153	158	163	168	174	179	184	189	194	199	204	209	215	220	225	230	235	240	245	250	255	261	266	271	276
61	100	106	111	116	122	127	132	137	143	148	153	158	164	169	174	180	185	190	195	201	206	211	217	222	227	232	238	243	248	254	259	264	269	275	280	285
62	104	109	115	120	126	131	136	142	147	153	158	164	169	175	180	186	191	196	202	207	213	218	224	229	235	240	246	251	256	262	267	273	278	284	289	295
63	107	113	118	124	130	135	141	146	152	158	163	169	175	180	186	191	197	203	208	214	220	225	231	237	242	248	254	259	265	270	278	282	287	293	299	304
64	110	116	122	128	134	140	145	151	157	163	169	174	180	186	192	197	204	209	215	221	227	232	238	244	250	256	262	267	273	279	285	291	296	302	308	314
65	114	120	126	132	138	144	150	156	162	168	174	180	186	192	198	204	210	216	222	228	234	240	246	252	258	264	270	276	282	288	294	300	306	312	318	324
66	118	124	130	136	142	148	155	161	167	173	179	186	192	198	204	210	216	223	229	235	241	247	253	260	266	272	278	284	291	297	303	309	315	322	328	334
67	121	127	134	140	146	153	159	166	172	178	185	191	198	204	211	217	223	230	236	242	249	255	261	268	274	280	287	293	299	306	312	319	325	331	338	344
68	125	131	138	144	151	158	164	171	177	184	190	197	203	210	216	223	230	236	243	249	256	262	269	276	282	289	295	302	308	315	322	328	335	341	348	354
69	128	135	142	149	155	162	169	176	182	189	196	203	209	216	223	230	236	243	250	257	263	270	277	284	291	297	304	311	318	324	331	338	345	351	358	365
70	132	139	146	153	160	167	174	181	188	195	202	209	216	222	229	236	243	250	257	264	271	278	285	292	299	306	313	320	327	334	341	348	355	362	369	376
71	136	143	150	157	165	172	179	186	193	200	208	215	222	229	236	243	250	257	265	272	279	286	293	301	308	315	322	329	338	343	351	358	365	372	379	386
72	140	147	154	162	169	177	184	191	199	206	213	221	228	235	242	250	258	265	272	279	287	294	302	309	316	324	331	338	346	353	361	368	375	383	390	397
73	144	151	159	166	174	182	189	197	204	212	219	227	235	242	250	257	265	272	280	288	295	302	310	318	325	333	340	348	355	363	371	378	386	393	401	408
74	148	155	163	171	179	186	194	202	210	218	225	233	241	249	256	264	272	280	287	295	303	311	319	326	334	342	350	358	365	373	381	389	396	404	412	420
75	152	160	168	176	184	192	200	208	216	224	232	240	248	256	264	272	279	287	295	303	311	319	327	335	343	351	359	367	375	383	391	399	407	415	423	431
76	156	164	172	180	189	197	205	213	221	230	238	246	254	263	271	279	287	295	304	312	320	328	336	344	353	361	369	377	385	394	402	410	418	426	435	443

Source: Adapted from *Clinical Guidelines on the Identification, Evaluation, and Treatment of Overweight and Obesity in Adults: The Evidence Report.*

FORMULA FOR DETERMINING YOUR CURRENT BODY WEIGHT AND IDEAL BODY WEIGHT IN KILOGRAMS

TO DETERMINE YOUR IDEAL BODY WEIGHT (IBW):

The first 5 feet of your total height = 100 pounds

For every inch over the first 5 feet add 5 pounds

Your IBW should be within a plus/minus 10-pound range

For example: A woman who is 5'4":

5 feet = 100 pounds

4" x 5 pounds per inch = 20 pounds

100 + 20 = 120 pounds

Plus or minus 10-pound range: 110 to 130 pounds (Average = 120 pounds)

TO CONVERT POUNDS TO KILOGRAMS, DIVIDE BY 2.2:

For example: 120 pounds ÷ 2.2 = 55 kilograms

Plus or minus 10-pound range: 50 to 59 kilograms

FOOD SAFETY TIPS
ON MEAT, POULTRY, AND SEAFOOD[2]

Buying, Storing, and Thawing Meat, Poultry, and Seafood

- Read expiration dates on all meat, poultry, and seafood and give food a visual and smell test before purchasing. For meats and poultry, an inspection sticker from the U.S. Department of Agriculture (USDA) and grade mark should be displayed. Avoid any foods that look old, dehydrated, or freezer burnt and any that have an offensive odor.
- Judge the freshness of seafood by its appearance and odor. (See How to Buy and Cook Fish and Shellfish, page 316.)
- Store live shellfish (such as mussels, oysters, and clams) in a shallow dish covered with a damp dish towel. Never store them in water or in an airtight container or plastic bag—they need air to breathe. Live shellfish should have closed shells; if they do not, discard them. Other shellfish, such as shrimp, lobster, and scallops, should be stored in their original packaging in the coldest part of the refrigerator. Eat all types of fresh shellfish as soon as possible.
- After shopping, get fresh or frozen meat, poultry, or seafood into the freezer or refrigerator as soon as possible. (If you are not going home immediately, ask the fishmonger to store your seafood on ice in a plastic bag.) Do not leave these perishable foods out of the refrigerator for more than two hours. Ideally, the temperature of your refrigerator should be below 40°F and your freezer should be 0°F. Use a thermometer to check these temperatures if you have any doubts.
- Make sure that the packing is not leaking, then store fresh meat, poultry, or seafood in the coldest part of your refrigerator (your meat bin or the back of the bottom shelf).
- Regardless of the expiration or "sell by" date, freeze any fresh meat, poultry, or seafood if you are not going to use it within two days. The "sell by" date indicates the last day the item can be sold, not the last date it can be stored in your refrigerator. Almost all meats and poultry are "chill packed" and kept in the meat department's refrigerator at 28° to 32°F, versus the 40°F temperature of the home refrigerator. This increase in temperature in your own refrigerator creates the need to consume or freeze the product within two days.
- Before freezing, break down large quantities of meat, poultry, or seafood into appropriate serving sizes and place them in freezer bags. This will avoid having to defrost an entire 5-pound package of chicken parts to broil two breasts for dinner.
- Label and date all items in the freezer.
- Don't thaw frozen meat, poultry, or seafood on a kitchen counter at room temperature. Room temperature will promote the growth of bacteria on the outer

surface of the product even while the product remains frozen inside. Allow extra time to thaw foods on a plate (to catch the juices) in your refrigerator. If you are short on time, use the defrost setting of your microwave (use the manufacturer's guidelines); or thaw the unopened meat, poultry, or fish in a sink or large container filled with cold (not warm) water. Change the water about every 30 minutes to keep it cold.

- If it has been frozen and partially thawed, do not refreeze any meat, poultry, or seafood unless there are still ice crystals in the meat.
- Do not thaw pre-stuffed or precooked poultry, meat, or seafood dishes before cooking or reheating. Follow the manufacturer's instructions.

WELL-DONE TEMPERATURE GUIDE[3]

Beef	160°F
Pork (fresh)	160°F
Chicken and Turkey (whole)	165°F
Breast	165°F
Thigh	165°F
Ground	165°F
Stuffing (cooked alone or in the bird)	165°F
Ground Meat and Poultry	160°F
Casseroles	165°F

poultry freezer storage chart

PRODUCT		MAXIMUM STORAGE AT 0°F (MONTHS)
Uncooked Poultry		
Chicken	cut up	9
	giblets	3–4
	whole	12
	ground	3–4
Turkey	cut up	9
	whole	12
Cooked Poultry		
Poultry pieces, plain		4
Poultry pieces, in broth or gravy		4
Cooked poultry casseroles		4–6
Fried chicken		4
Chicken nuggets, patties		1–3
Stuffing, cooked		1
Processed Meat Products		
Chicken hot dogs		1–2
Luncheon meat		1–2
Turkey ham (cured turkey thigh meat)		Do not freeze

meat storage chart

PRODUCT	STORAGE PERIOD	
	Refrigerator *35–40°F (days)*	*Freezer* *0°F (months)*
Fresh Meat		
Chops: Beef/veal/lamb/pork	3–5	4–6
Roasts: Beef/veal/lamb/pork	3–5	4–12
Steaks: Beef/veal/lamb/pork	3–5	6–12
Stew meats	1–2	3–4
Ground meats	1–2	3–4
Variety meats	1–2	3–4
Sausage (raw)	1–2	1–2
Cooked Meats		
Cooked meat and meat casseroles	3–4	2–3
Gravy and meat broth	1–2	2–3
Pre-stuffed uncooked pork chops, lamb chops, or chicken breasts stuffed with dressing	1	Does not freeze well

seafood storage chart[4]

PRODUCT	STORAGE PERIOD	
	Refrigerator 34–40°F (hours)	*Freezer 0°F (months)*
Lean Fish		
Cod, flounder, haddock, halibut	36	6–8
Pollock, ocean perch, sea trout, rockfish	36	4
Fat Fish		
Rainbow trout, salmon, shad, smelt	36	4

HANDLING AND PREPARING
MEAT, POULTRY, AND SEAFOOD

- Wash your hands thoroughly with hot, soapy water before and after handling any raw meat, seafood, or poultry.
- Do not use a dish towel or sponge to clean up meat, poultry, or seafood juices—use a disposable paper towel. Sponges and damp dish towels are bacteria heaven, so replace them frequently. If you cannot afford to replace your sponges as often as you would like, boil them for 10 minutes to sterilize them.
- After handling raw meat, poultry, or seafood, wash all surfaces (countertops, sink surface, and cutting boards) and utensils (knives, dishes, etc.) with hot, soapy water or place them in the dishwasher. (Be sure your plastic cutting boards are dishwasher safe.) Nonporous, plastic cutting boards are recommended over wooden ones, which absorb juices from raw products.
- Do not use the plate that held raw products for cooked products. Raw juices can contaminate the cooked foods. For example, when grilling outdoors, use two separate plates—one for the raw foods and another for the cooked foods. Also, discard any marinades or sauces (such as barbecue sauce) that came in contact with the raw product. Do not serve them as a sauce and do not recycle them.
- Keep all marinating meat, poultry, or seafood covered and refrigerated. Do not marinate at room temperature.

COOKING AND STORING LEFTOVERS

- Poultry can go straight from the freezer to the oven if you allow one and a half times the normal cooking period. Frozen pre-stuffed poultry and frozen poultry dishes should never be thawed before cooking.

- Rinse (with cold water) and dry all meat, poultry, and seafood before cooking. Trim any excess fat from meat and poultry.

- Cook all meat, poultry, and seafood thoroughly, or to the well-done stage—this is especially important when you are pregnant. When pierced, juices from cooked meat and poultry should run clear and slightly yellow with no traces of pink. You can test fish and other seafood by cutting into it to make sure that the flesh is cooked through. Whether baking, broiling, or microwaving, use an instant-read thermometer to judge doneness of meat and poultry.

- Do not interrupt the cooking time (unless specified in a recipe). Partial cooking may promote bacterial growth.

- After cooking, transfer foods to shallow containers and refrigerate or freeze immediately. You do not have to let the food cool before refrigerating or freezing.

- Reheat leftovers thoroughly, to at least 165°F. Bring gravies and soups to a boil for 1 minute before serving.

- Stuffed poultry needs special attention because bacteria from raw poultry can grow in the stuffing. Ideally, the stuffing should be cooked in a separate dish, but that takes the fun out of it. To prevent bacterial growth, stuff the bird just before cooking. Stuff loosely (most stuffings will expand during cooking) to ensure uniform heating, and remove all of the stuffing from the cavity immediately after cooking.

SLOW COOKER SAFETY TIPS

COOKING IN A slow cooker is a convenient way to prepare meals, especially if you are at work or on the go all day. The temperatures of slow cookers usually range from 170° to 280°F, which is high enough to avoid bacteria growth. Here are a few basic points to keep in mind when using a slow cooker.[5]

- Always begin with a clean cooker, clean utensils, and a clean work area.
- Do not use the slow cooker for thawing, storing, or reheating food.
- Keep all food refrigerated until it is ready to be placed in the slow cooker. This reduces the chance of bacteria developing during the first few hours of cooking.
- Always completely defrost meat and poultry before placing it in the slow cooker.
- Cut foods into small pieces to ensure thorough cooking. Do not use the slow cooker for large pieces of meat or poultry, such as roasts or whole chickens, because the food will cook so slowly it could remain in the bacterial "danger zone" (temperatures between 40° and 140°F) for too long.
- Fill your cooker no less than half-full and no more than two-thirds full. Vegetables cook more slowly than meat and poultry in a slow cooker, so, if using them, put the vegetables in first, on the bottom and around the sides of the pot, then add the remaining ingredients.
- Keep the lid in place. Remove it only to check doneness or to stir.
- Ideally, turn the cooker on the highest setting for the first hour of cooking time, and then turn it to low, or to the setting called for in your recipe. It is perfectly safe to cook foods on the low setting the entire time.
- In case of power outage, throw away the food, even if it looks done. Or, if you are at home during the outage, immediately cook the food by some other nonelectrical means.
- Always use hot pads when removing the stoneware from the slow cooker.

SAFE COOKING IN THE MICROWAVE OVEN

MOST OF US could not live without our microwave ovens, and for good reason. However, microwave ovens can cook unevenly, leaving cold spots where harmful bacteria can survive. Here are a few tips to keep in mind.[6]

- Arrange foods evenly in a microwave-safe container, preferably not plastic. Add a little liquid if needed, then loosely cover with a lid or microwave-safe plastic wrap.
- Do not cook large cuts of meat on high power (100 percent). They should be cooked on medium power (50 percent) for longer periods. This allows the heat to reach the center without overcooking the outer areas.
- Stir or rotate food midway through the microwaving process to eliminate cold spots.
- After defrosting or partially cooking food in a microwave oven, immediately transfer it to the next heat source to finish the cooking process.
- Because the temperatures of microwave ovens can vary, always use an instant-read thermometer to check doneness. Refer to the Well-Done Temperature Guide on page 435.
- Cooking whole stuffed poultry in a microwave oven is not recommended.
- Heat ready-to-eat foods, such as hot dogs, luncheon meats, fully cooked ham, and leftovers, until steaming hot. An instant-read thermometer should read 165°F.
- Never use plastic wrap, brown paper, newspaper, or aluminum foil in the microwave oven.

TIPS FOR CLEANING FRESH PRODUCE

ARE THE FRUITS and vegetables you eat really clean? Probably not. Depending on the surface of the fruit or vegetable, washing with plain water is an effective means of removing particles of dust and dirt, and possibly some bacteria. Following are a few tips to help get your produce a bit cleaner.

- Wash produce under cool running water. Soaking can lead to cross-contamination, or bacteria floating from one item to another. The exception is leafy greens (such as spinach, Swiss chard, lettuce, and fresh herbs), which are best washed by plunging them into a sink or tub of water. Be sure to lift the greens out of the water, leaving the dirt behind—do not pour them into a colander to drain, which would throw the dirt right back on them. Repeat the procedure until no dirt or sand remains in the sink or tub. Dry with a salad spinner.
- Scrub produce with a vegetable brush if possible, as it causes friction and gets into hard-to-reach nooks and crannies.
- Always wash or scrub fruits and vegetables before they are peeled or sliced, as the blade of the knife or peeler can move bacteria from the skin to the interior. Large fruits such as melons or pineapples and vegetables such as winter squash should always be scrubbed before slicing.
- Produce-washing liquid solutions can be effective in removing more bacteria than plain water, but exactly how much more is unknown.
- Disinfecting fruits and vegetables with chlorine or iodine is not necessary unless the drinking water has been deemed unsafe, as in developing countries or after natural disasters.

TIPS FOR WASHING AND STORING GREENS

HAVING PREPARED SALADS on hand can save time and energy. A handful of greens can jazz up a sandwich and is perfect for throwing together a quick salad any time of day. It is important to wash all greens as thoroughly as possible to remove all dirt and any harmful bacteria. Wash greens under running water while rubbing gently with your fingertips to remove any particles. If you prefer to use a tub or sink filled with water, rub the leaves while washing them, then lift them out of the water and rinse them under running water. The following instructions should help to maximize the shelf-life of salad greens and fresh herbs.

- Large-leaf lettuce (romaine, red and green leaf, Boston, curly escarole, collard greens, kale, and mustard greens): Wash the leaves, discarding any badly bruised ones. Tear the leafy part of the lettuce into bite-size pieces, discarding the thick stems. Spin-dry the lettuce and, if not using immediately, place it in a zip-lock bag and store it in the vegetable bin of the refrigerator. Greens washed and stored this way will keep for three to five days.
- Small-leaf lettuce (watercress, Belgian endive, arugula, chicory, and radicchio): Wash the lettuce leaves, discarding any badly bruised ones, then spin-dry. Discard the thick stems of the watercress and break the leafy tops into bite-size pieces. Stack the endive or radicchio leaves and slice them just before adding them to the salad, or tear them into bite-size pieces. Store lettuce in a zip-lock bag in the vegetable bin of the refrigerator.
- Prepackaged baby greens and boxed lettuce (including mesclun or mixed baby greens): Wash and thoroughly spin-dry. These delicate greens tend to deteriorate quickly if a lot of moisture is left on them. Store in a zip-lock bag in the vegetable bin of the refrigerator.
- Prepackaged lettuce labeled "prewashed": Wash it anyway if you have the time.
- Prepackaged spinach: Always wash spinach, even if the package says that the spinach has already been washed three times (it can still be sandy).
- Fresh leafy herbs (such as parsley, cilantro, dill, basil, and chervil): Wash according to directions for prepackaged baby greens or boxed lettuce. Once washed, remove the leaves from the stems and store them in a zip-lock bag in the vegetable bin of the refrigerator.
- Woody-stemmed herbs (such as rosemary and thyme): These do not require immediate washing. Keep woody-stemmed herbs refrigerated in their containers and rinse them just before using.

TIPS TO HELP KEEP YOUR
KITCHEN WORKSPACE CLEAN

- Place a piece of plastic wrap over the top of your food processor or blender before you put the lid on.
- When grating slightly moist soft cheese, such as cheddar or mozzarella, lightly spray the grater with canola oil cooking spray to prevent sticking. Do the same for the grater attachment of a food processor.
- Spray canola oil cooking spray on measuring spoons and cups before measuring sticky substances such as molasses or honey.
- When grating lemon zest or Parmesan cheese, place a piece of plastic wrap or parchment paper under the grater to catch the zest.
- Use parchment paper to line baking sheets.
- Use foil to line baking sheets and baking dishes.
- Use a splatter lid when sautéing things that tend to splatter.
- Rinse a strainer or colander immediately after using it. This will prevent the starch from pasta or potatoes from drying on it.
- Keep a separate scrub brush for fruits and vegetables.
- Keep a separate plastic (not wood) chopping board for preparing raw poultry and meats.
- Line the container of your kitchen scale with plastic wrap, a paper towel, or parchment paper (depending on what you are weighing) to reduce cleanup.
- Choose one day a week to clean out your refrigerator—the day before you go grocery shopping or the day of trash pickup usually works well. This will help you keep track of your shopping needs and eliminate expired items.
- Store all opened packages and boxes of dry goods in zip-lock bags to avoid spills.
- Store all opened packages (especially hot dogs and luncheon meats) in zip-lock bags to avoid spills.

■ ENDNOTES ■

▶ *Introduction*

[1] Xiaoping Weng, Ph.D., Roxana Odouli, M.S.P.H., De-Kun Li, Ph.D., "Maternal Caffeine Consumption During Pregnancy and the Risk of Miscarriage: A Prospective Cohort Study," *American Journal of Obstetrics and Gynecology* 198, no. 3 (March 2008): 279.e1–299.e8. Web site requires a subscription.

[2] American College of Obstetricians and Gynecologists, "Food, Pregnancy, and Health," pamphlet (September 1986). Send a self-addressed, stamped, business-size envelope to the college, Resource Center, 409 12th Street SW, Washington, D.C. 20024.

[3] Mayo Clinic, Pregnancy Week by Week, "Pregnancy Nutrition: Healthy eating for you and your baby," February 19, 2008, http://www.mayoclinic.com/health/pregnancy-nutrition/PR00108.

[4] Carol J. Lammi-Keefe, Ph.D., R.D., Sarah C. Couch, Ph.D., R.D., and Elliot H. Philipson, M.D., editors, *Handbook of Nutrition and Pregnancy* (Totowa, NJ: Humana Press, 2008), 8.

[5] "Position of the American Dietetic Association: Nutrition and Lifestyle for a Healthy Pregnancy Outcome," *Journal of the American Dietetic Association* (2008): 554. The data for the chart, Daily Requirements for Pregnancy and Lactation, is from the Institute of Medicine, Dietary Reference Intakes: *The Essential Guide to Nutrient Requirements* (Washington, D.C.: National Academies Press, 2006). The values are Recommended Dietary Allowances except for energy (Estimated Energy Requirement) and total fiber, linoleic acid, alpha-linoleic acid, vitamin D, vitamin K, pantothenic acid, biotin, choline, calcium, manganese, chromium, sodium and potassium (adequate Intakes). The vitamin A value reflects RAE, retinol activity equivalents. The niacin value reflects NE, niacin equivalents.

[6] Gerard Hornstra, "Essential Fatty Acids in Mothers and Their Neonates," *American Journal of Clinical Nutrition* 71 (supplement; 2000): 1,262S-9S.

[7] Sheila M. Innis, "Dietary (n-3) Fatty Acids and Brain Development," *Journal of Nutrition* 37 (April 2007): 885–859, http://jn.nutrition.org/cgi/content/full/137/4/855.

[8] Martha Neuringer, Gregory J. Anderson, and William E. Connor, "The Essentiality of N-3 Fatty Acids for the Development and Function of the Retina and Brain," *Annual Review of Nutrition* 8 (July 1988): 517–541, cited in British Associate Parliamentary Food and Health Forum, *The Links Between Diet and Behavior: The Influence of Nutrition on Mental Health*, January 2008, 9, http://www.feingold.org/Research/PDFstudies/Health-Forum2008.pdf.

[9] Sjurour F. Olsen et al., "Gestational Age in Relation to Marine N-3 Fatty Acids in Maternal Erthrocytes: A Study of Women in the Faroe Islands and Denmark," *American Journal of Obstetrics and Gynecology* 164, no. 5 (May 1991): 1,203–1,209, cited in British Associate Parliamentary Food and Health Forum, *The Links Between Diet and Behavior: The Influence of Nutrition on Mental Health*, January 2008, 14, http://www.feingold.org/Research/PDFstudies/Health-Forum2008.pdf.; Sjurour F. Olsen et al., "Randomized Clinical Trials of Fish Oil Supplementation in High Risk Pregnancies: Fish Oil Trials in Pregnancy (FOTIP) Team," *BJOG: An International*

Journal of Obstetrics and Gynaecology 107, no. 3 (March 2000): 382–395, cited in British Associate Parliamentary Food and Health Forum, *The Links Between Diet and Behavior: The Influence of Nutrition on Mental Health*, January 2008, 14, http://www.feingold.org/Research/PDFstudies/Health-Forum2008.pdf.; C. M. Smuts et al., "A Randomized Trial of Docsahexaenoic Acid Supplementation During the Third Trimester Of Pregnancy," *Obstetrics and Gynecology* 101 (2003): 469–479. Study cited in *The Links Between Diet and Behavior: The Influence of Nutrition on Mental Health*, Report of an inquiry held by the Associate Parliamentary Food and Health Forum, January 2008, page 14.

[10] Lammi-Keefe, Couch, and Philipson, *Handbook of Nutrition and Pregnancy*, 96.

[11] Lammi-Keefe, Couch, and Philipson, *Handbook of Nutrition and Pregnancy*, 96.

[12] M. P. Freeman et al., "Evidence Basis for Treatment and Future Research in Psychiatry," *Journal of Clinical Psychiatry* 67 (2006): 1,954–1,967, cited in British Associate Parliamentary Food and Health Forum, *The Links Between Diet and Behavior: The Influence of Nutrition on Mental Health*, January 2008, 26, http://www.feingold.org/Research/PDFstudies/Health-Forum2008.pdf.

[13] "The long-chain omega-3 PUFAs, Eicosapentaenoic acid (EPA) and Docosahexaenoic acid (DHA) are mostly found pre-formed in appreciable quantities in fish and other seafood." British Associate Parliamentary Food and Health Forum, *The Links Between Diet and Behavior: The Influence of Nutrition on Mental Health*, January 2008, 12, http://www.feingold.org/Research/PDFstudies/Health-Forum2008.pdf.

[14] U.S. Food and Drug Administration, "FDA Announces Qualified Health Claims for Omega-3 Fatty Acids," *FDA News*, September 8, 2004, www.fda.gov/bbs/topics/news/2004/NEW0115.html.

[15] British Associate Parliamentary Food and Health Forum, *The Links Between Diet and Behavior: The Influence of Nutrition on Mental Health*, January 2008, 11, http://www.feingold.org/Research/PDFstudies/Health-Forum2008.pdf.

[16] "Omega-6 Fatty Acids," University of Maryland Medical Center, 2008, http://www.umm.edu/altmed/articles/omega-6-000317.htm.

[17] "Magnesium," Office of Dietary Supplements, National Institutes of Health, 2009, http://ods.od.nih.gov/factsheets/magnesium.asp; Lammi-Keefe, *Handbook of Nutrition and Pregnancy*, 213.

[18] Evira, "Consumption of liver and liver-based food during pregnancy—new information and new recommendations," August 15, 2007, http://www.evira.fi/portal/en/food/current_issues/?id=661.

[19] March of Dimes website at: March of Dimes, Pregnancy and Newborn Health Education Center, "Folic Acid," 2008 http://www.marchofdimes.com/pnhec/173_769.asp.

[20] American Dietetic Association, "Position of the American Dietetic Association: Nutrition and Lifestyle for a Healthy Pregnancy Outcome," *Journal of the American Dietetic Association* (2008): 555.

[21] Lammi-Keefe, *Handbook of Nutrition and Pregnancy*, 13.

[22] Lammi-Keefe, *Handbook of Nutrition and Pregnancy*, 67.

[23] National Heart, Lung, and Blood Institute, National Institutes of Health, "High Blood Pressure in Pregnancy," February 2009, http://www.nhlbi.nih.gov/health/public/heart/hbp/hbp_preg.htm.

[24] Lammi-Keefe, *Handbook of Nutrition and Pregnancy*, 13, 158.

[25] March of Dimes, Professionals and Researchers, "Diabetes in Pregnancy," December 2007, http://www.marchofdimes.com/14332_1197.asp.

▶ Chapter 1

1   Center for the Evaluation of Risks to Human Reproduction, National Institutes of Health,"Caffeine: Caffeine Levels in Foods and Drinks," April 23, 2008, http://cerhr.niehs.nih.gov/common/caffeine.html.

2   *The American Dietetic Association Manual*, Fifth Edition, "Nutrition Management During Pregnancy," Chicago, 1996, page 77.

3   Food Safety and Inspection Service. U.S. Department of Agriculture, "Shell Eggs from Farm to Table," August 2008, http://www.fsis.usda.gov/PDF/Shell_Eggs_from_Farm_to_Table.pdf.

4   Centers for Disease Control and Prevention, Division of Bacterial and Mycotic Diseases, "Salmonelosis," http://www.cdc.gov/nczved/dfbmd/disease_listing/salmonellosis_gi.html.

5   Center for Food Safety and Applied Nutrition, U.S. Food and Drug Administration, "Assuring the Safety of Eggs and Menu and Deli Items Made from Raw, Shell Eggs," April 2002, http://www.cfsan.fda.gov/~acrobat/fs-eggs2.pdf.

▶ Chapter 2

1   FDA CFSAN, U.S. Food and Drug Administration, Center for Food Safety and Applied Nutrition. *FDA Consumer*: "All About Eating for Two," By Judith Levine Willis, March 1984, www.cfsan.fda.gov/~dms/wh-preg1.html; Medline Plus Health Information, A Service of the U.S. National Library of Medicine. Medical Encyclopedia, "Pica," June 6, 2001, www.nim.nih.gov/medlineplus/ency/article/001538.htm.

2   Food Safety and Inspection Service, U.S. Department of Agriculture, "Keeping 'Bag' Lunches Safe," September 27, 2006, http://www.fsis.usda.gov/Fact_Sheets/Keeping_Bag_Lunches_Safe/index.asp.

3   Veni Gurd, "Which Plastic Bottles Don't Leach Chemicals?" Trusted.MD, March 29, 2007, http://trusted.md/blog/vreni_gurd/2007/03/29/plastic_water_bottles.

4   Center for the Evaluation of Risks to Human Reproduction, National Institutes of Health, "*Listeria* and Food Poisoning," April 23, 2008, http://cerhr.niehs.nih.gov/common/listeria.html.

5   Centers for Disease Control and Prevention, Division of Bacterial and Mycotic Diseases, "Listeriosis," March 27, 2008, http://www.cdc/gov/nczved/dfbmd/disease_listing/listerios_gi.html.

▶ Chapter 3

1   "US: High Pesticide Level Marks 'Dirty Dozen' Fruits and Vegetables," October 18, 2006, http//www.ewg.org/node/18866. For more information on the Environmental Working Group (EWG) contact 1436 U Street, N.W., Suite 100, Washington, D.C. 20009, 202-667-6982.

2   The American College of Obstetricians and Gynecologists, Education Pamphlet AP055, "Travel During Pregnancy," 2009, http://www.acog.org/publications/patient_education/bp055.cfm.

▶ Chapter 4

1   Carol J. Lammi-Keefe, Ph.D., R.D., Sarah C. Couch, Ph.D., R.D., and Elliot H. Philipson, M.D., editors, *Handbook of Nutrition and Pregnancy* (Totowa, NJ: Humana Press, 2008), 218.

2   Lammi-Keefe, Couch, and Philipson, *Handbook of Nutrition and Pregnancy*, 219.

3   Cleveland Clinic, "Nutrition During Pregnancy for Vegetarians," 2009, http://my.clevelandclinic.org/healthy_living/pregnancy/hic_nutrition_during_pregnancy_for_vegetarians.aspx.

4   The calcium availability from some fruits and vegetables depends upon the oxalic acid they contain. Oxalic acid combines in the digestive tract with calcium to form an insoluble compound, calcium oxalate. This calcium is not absorbed. Rhubarb, spinach, chard, and beet greens contain oxalic acid in appreciable amounts. Phytic acid, a phosphorus-containing compound found

principally in the outer husks of cereal grains (especially oatmeal), combines with calcium to form calcium phytate, which is insoluble and is not absorbed by the intestines. Marie V. Krasue, B.S., M.S., R.D., and L. Kathleen Mahan, M.S., R.D., *Food, Nutrition and Diet Therapy*, 6th edition (Philadelphia: W. B. Saunders, 1979).

5   British Associate Parliamentary Food and Health Forum, *The Links Between Diet and Behavior: The Influence of Nutrition on Mental Health*, January 2008, 12, http://www.feingold.org/Research/PDFstudies/Health-Forum2008.pdf.

6   Kannan Srimathi, Ph.D., "Factors in Vegetarian Diets Influencing Iron and Zinc Bioavailability," 2009, http://www.vegetariannutrition.net/articles/Iron-and-Zinc-Bioavailability-in-Vegetarian-Nutrition.php.

7   Srimathi, "Factors in Vegetarian Diets Influencing Iron and Zinc Bioavailability."

▶ *Chapter 5*

1   Centers for Disease Control and Prevention, Division of Foodborne, Bacterial and Mycotic Diseases, "*Escherichia coli*," March 27, 2008, http://www.cdc.gov/nczved/dfbmd/disease_listing/stec_gi.html.

2   March of Dimes, "Toxoplasmosis," October 2008, http://www.marchofdimes.com/professionals/14332_1228.asp.

3   Food Safety and Inspection Service, U.S. Department of Agriculture, "Parasites and Food-Borne Illness," May 2001, http://www.fsis.usda.gov/Fact_Sheets/Parasites_and_Foodborne_Illness/index.asp.

4   March of Dimes, "Toxoplasmosis," October 2008, http://www.marchofdimes.com/professionals/14332_1228.asp.

5   Evie Hansen and Cindy W. Snyder, *Seafood Twice a Week* (Richmond Beach, WA: National Seafood Educators, 1997), pp. 35–38.

6   EPA, U.S. Environmental Protection Agency [Internet]. Fish Advisories, Consumption Advice, Joint Federal Advisory for Mercury in Fish, "What You Need to Know about Mercury in Fish and Shellfish, 2004 EPA and FDA Advice for Women Who Might Become Pregnant, Women Who Are Pregnant, Nursing Mothers, and Young Children." August 14, 2008, www.epa.gov/waterscience/fishadvice/html.

7   Sierra Club, "When It Comes to Salmon, Buy Wild,." The essay leads readers to "Aquaculture's Troubled Harvest," an article by Bruce Barcott that appeared in the November/December 2001 issue of *Mother Jones*, http://www.motherjones.com/politics/2001/11/aquacultures-troubled-harvest, and *Salmon Nation: People, Fish, and Our Common Home*, an Ecotrust Book (Elizabeth Wooy et al., 2003), for further reading on the fate of wild salmon.

8   *Circulation*, "Fish consumption, Fish Oil, Omega-3 Fatty Acids, and Cardiovascular Disease," Penny M. Kris-Etherton, William S. Harris, and Lawrence J. Appel for the Nutrition Committee, November 2002; 106, 2747–2757. Available on the internet at http://circ.ahajournals.org/cgi/search?journalcode=circulationaha&fulltext=Fish=Consumption.

9   *eMedine Journal* [Internet]. "Salmonella Infection," Article by Robert Barrali, M.D., Volume 2, Number 10, October 4, 2001 [cited July 11, 2002]. Available from: www.emedicine.com/EMERG/topic515.htm.

► **Chapter 6**

1 *Diabetes and Pregnancy: What to Expect,* 4th edition (Alexandria, VA: American Diabetes Association, 2000), 30–31.

2 March of Dimes, "Fitness for Two," March 2008, http://www.marchofdimes.com/professionals/14332_1150.asp.

► **Chapter 7**

1 Lawrence M. Gartner, M.D., and Frank R. Greer, M.D., "Prevention of Rickets and Vitamin D Deficiency: New Guidelines for Vitamin D Intake," *Pediatrics* 111, no. 4 (April 2003): 908–910, http://aappolicy.aappublications.org/cgi/content/full/pediatrics;111/4/908.

2 Emily Oken et al., "Associations of Maternal Fish Intake During Pregnancy and Breastfeeding Duration with Attainment of Developmental Milestones in Early Childhood: A Study from the Danish National Birth Cohort" *American Journal of Clinical Nutrition* 88 (September 2008): 789–796.

3 Kathleen M. Rasmussen, Cs.M., Sc.D., R.D., and Chris L. Kjolhede, M.D. M.P.H., "Prepregnant Overweight and Obesity Diminish the Prolactin Response to Suckling in the First Week Postpartum," *Pediatrics* 111, no. 5 (May 2004): e465–e471, http://pediatrics.aappublications.org/cgi/content/full/113/5/e465; Christopher G. Owen, Ph.D., et al., "Effect of Infant Feeding on the Risk of Obesity Across the Life Course: A Quantitative Review of Published Evidence," *Pediatrics* 115, no. 5 (May 2005): 1,367–1,377, http://pediatrics.aappublications.org/cgi/content/full/115/5/1367.

4 Mayo Clinic.com Postpartum Depression, "Symptoms," June 7, 2008, http://www.mayoclinic.com/health/postpartum-depression/DSECTION=symptoms.

5 Jack F. Hollis, Ph.D., et al., "Weight Loss During the Intensive Intervention Phase of the Weight-Loss Maintenance Trial," *American Journal of Preventative Medicine* 35, no. 2 (2008): 118–126. For a more exact reading of your calorie needs, go to http://www.caloriecontrol.org/calcalcs.html and plug in your height, weight, age, and activity level, and you will get your estimated daily maintenance calorie needs.

► **Appendix**

1 Elizabeth Reifsnider, R.N., C., Ph.D., WHNP, and Sara L. Gill, R.N., Ph.D., IBCLC, "Nutrition for the Childbearing Years," *Journal of Obstetric, Gynecologic, and Neonatal Nursing* 29, no. 1 (January/February 2000): 46.

2 Food Safety and Inspection Service, U.S. Department of Agriculture "Doneness Versus Safety," April 3, 2006, http://www.fsis.usda.gov/Fact_Sheets/Doneness_Versus_Safety/index.asp.

3 Food Safety and Inspection Service, U.S. Department of Agriculture "Basics for Handling Food Safely," February 26, 2009, http://www.fsis.usda.gov/fact_sheets/Basics_for_Handling_Food_Safely/index.asp.

4 National Fisheries Institute, "Handling and Storage," AboutSeafood.com, 2009, http://www.aboutseafood.com/cooking/handling-storage.

5 Food Safety and Inspection Service, U.S. Department of Agriculture "Slow Cookers and Food Safety," February 13, 2009, http://www.fsis.usda.gov/Fact_Sheets/Focus_On_Slow_Cooker_Safety/index.asp.

6 Food Safety and Inspection Service, U.S. Department of Agriculture, "Cooking Safely in the Microwave Oven," April 3, 2006, http://www.fsis.usda.gov/Fact_Sheets/Cooking_Safely_in_the_Microwave/index.asp.

thanks!

THE SIMPLE WORDS "thank you" do not begin to describe the gratitude I feel toward so many people who have poured their expertise, time, energy, and creative ideas into this book. Matthew Lore, my gifted editor for six years, shared my vision and brought the first edition to life. But even more than that, he helped cultivate my writing career, for which I am forever grateful. Wendy Francis, my editor for the second edition, and her team brilliantly packaged a fully updated version for today's mothers-to-be. Lisa Ekus has been a superb agent for twelve years and a friend for even more.

My co-author, Rose Ann Hudson, combined her knowledge with decades of experience, and always kept things simple to understand. Shoshana Bennett, Ph.D.; Elaine Trujillo, R.D., L.D.; Linda Wade, Ph.D.; and Victor Palo contributed to the Nine Months Later chapter, making it a truly stellar and practical addition. Neal Rohrer illustrated the exercises. Their commitment to the wellness of women is overwhelming and truly admirable. I owe a special thanks to Elaine Trujillo for her insightful edits throughout the manuscript.

I am deeply indebted to all of my recipe contributors, from Chris Prouty, my website design guy who shared his blueberry muffin recipe, to my mother, Mary Abernethy, an extraordinary cook, who taught me the basics at a tender age. The recipes all work and taste great thanks to the enthusiasm and valuable comments from my team of recipe testers: Martha and Paul Grove, Nan Wood Mosher, Mary Mulard, Mary Fortino, Laura Wright, Melissa Alshab, Patricia Terry, Peggy Terry, Lynn Rudolf, Lisa Natanson, Annie Mozer, Margaret Jones, Carol Scheangold, Mari Webel, Jan Greenburg, Tina Wong, Thelma Javier, and Teresa Bacalla. Insightful editorial comments came from Shari Bistransky, Kathleen Luft, Judith Sutton (the best cookbook copyeditor in the business), Sue McCloskey, Peter Jacoby, and Bonnie Swart.

The profound importance of family is not fully understood until you start your own. You realize just how much your parents loved and nurtured you, how they sacrificed for you, and how in return you filled them with immeasurable love, pride, and happiness (and a bit of anguish from time to time). To my extended family, I say thank you for all of the support and encouragement you've given me over the years: my mother and step-father, Mary and Robert Abernethy; Brandon Grove, my father, and his late wife, Mariana; Evelyn Jones, my mother-in-law; Elizabeth; Jack and Hannah; Paul and Martha; Mark and Troy; Michele and David; and my beloved husband, Paul. My children, Aleksandra and Hale, give meaning to my world and bring me more joy than they will ever know.

—Catherine Jones

would like to thank my parents, Thomas and Lilian Angotti, who have always given me the love, guidance, and support I needed to achieve my goals. They have my deepest gratitude. Other members of my family have given a part of themselves to this project and I thank them: my wonderful husband, Mark, and beautiful daughters, Emily and Rachel, who gave me love and encouragement throughout; my sisters, Angela Angotti Morris and Antoinette Angotti, who have always been there for me; and my sister, Alma Angotti, who helped me organize my thoughts for this book on paper.

I thank my good friend Julian Safran, M.D., for sharing his expertise, and always offering words of encouragement; my colleagues, Mary Ellen Sabatella, R.D., and Martha Betts, R.D., for their careful review of the material. My gratitude also goes to my close friend, Laura Wright, for her unwavering enthusiasm for this project since its conception. Finally, I would like to thank Catherine Jones for her hard work and tremendous dedication, and for giving me the opportunity to be a part of this special book, which I hope will help pregnant women everywhere for years to come.

—Rose Ann Hudson

a mother's love
is the greatest love
there is.

Page references in **bold**
indicate boxed text.

Guacamole, Homemade
Guacamole, 173

vitamin D, 181
See also Recipes for
vegetarians/vegans;
Vegetarians/vegans
Vegemite, **52**
Vegetable oils, 14–15, **15**
Vegetables
healthiest choices, **138**
with most pesticides, **140**
safety issues, **129**, **140**
vitamin A/C and, **350**
See also *specific recipes*;
specific vegetables
Vegetables with Lemon, Olive
Oil, and Fresh Herbs, 153–
154
Vegetarian Curry, 206–207
Vegetarian Omelet for One,
229
Vegetarian Pad Thai, 220–221
Vegetarians
eggs and, **62**
food groups, **181**
Marmite, **52**
prenatal vitamins/
supplements, 180
See also Recipes for
vegetarians/vegans
Vegetarians/vegans
2000-calorie menus, **191–
198**
calcium, 181–182, **230**
diet classification, **213**
dips, 135
iodine, 183
iron, 180, 182, **230**
nutritional adjustments,
180
protein, 181, **184**
salads, 135
soups, 83
vitamin B$_{12}$ and, 21, 41, **72**,
182
vitamin D, 181
zinc, 180, 182, **230**, **231**
See also Recipes for
vegetarians/vegans
Veggie Burgers, 261–262
Veggie Cheese Wrap, 125
Very Simple Fried Rice with

Vegetables, 263–264
Vitamin A, 19, **20**, **350**
Vitamin B
B$_1$ (thiamine), 21–22
B$_2$ (riboflavin), 22
B$_3$ (niacin), 22, 183
B$_5$ (pantothenic acid), 23
B$_6$, 21, 183, 389
B$_7$ (biotin), 22
Vitamin B$_9$. *See* Folic acid
Vitamin B$_{12}$
cereals containing 100DV,
43
PPD and, 388
sources/overview, 21
vegetarians/vegans, 21, 41,
72, 182
Vitamin C
iron and, **66**
omega-3 fatty acids and,
183
overview, 19–20
sources, 19–20, **350**
Vitamin D
breastfed babies, 384
calcium and, 15, **15**
sources/overview, 19
sunlight and, 16, 20, 181,
389
toxic doses, 20, **20**
vegetarians/vegans, 181
Vitamin E, 20
Vitamin K, 20
Vitamins
fat-soluble vitamins, **20**, 42
functions overview, 19–23,
22
prenatal vitamins, 1, 8, 16,
44, 180, 381
sources overview, 19–23
toxic doses, 19, 20, **20**
water-soluble vitamins, **20**
See also *specific vitamins*
Volume conversions, **429**

▶ W

Wade, Linda, 390, 395, 399
Waffles

about, 53, 54, **54**
Whole Wheat Pecan
Waffles, 53–54
Walnuts
Banana Muffins with
Walnuts and Wheat
Germ, 69–70
Bran Muffins with Dried
Cranberries, Walnuts,
and Candied Ginger,
71–72
Roasted Beets with Goat
Cheese, Walnuts, and
Baby Greens, 158
Walnut Spice Coffee Cake,
375–376
Water
bottled water, **114**
importance of, **113**, **176**,
382, 389
plastic bottles, **114**
traveling and, **161**, **162**
Water-soluble vitamins, **20**
Web site resources, **432**
Weight
before conception, 2
conversion to kilograms,
435
determining ideal weight,
435
maintenance/weight loss
calories, **395**
obesity statistics, 23
See also Obese women
Weight gain with pregnancy
factors affecting, 5, 6–7, **7**
multiples, 5, 6–7, **7**
overview, 5–7, **5**, **6**, **7**, **432**
source of, **6**
teenage mothers, 5, 6–7, **7**
vegetarians/vegans, 181
Weight loss postpartum
1500-calorie menus, 399,
400–406
journaling, 393–394, 395–
397
maintenance/weight loss
calories, **395**
questions and answers/IFS
model, 390–394